Joint Education & Training Library

Hemangiomas and Vascular Malformations

R. Mattassi • D.A. Loose • M. Vaghi (Eds.)

Hemangiomas and Vascular Malformations

An Atlas of Diagnosis and Treatment

Foreword by
J. Leonel Villavicencio

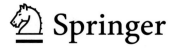
Springer

Editors

Prof. RAUL MATTASSI
Department of Vascular Surgery
Center for Vascular Malformations
"Stefan Belov"
"G. Salvini" Hospital
Garbagnate Milanese (Milan), Italy
rmattassi@yahoo.it

Dr. MASSIMO VAGHI
Department of Vascular Surgery
Center for Vascular Malformations
"Stefan Belov"
"G. Salvini" Hospital
Garbagnate Milanese (Milan), Italy
vaghim@yahoo.it

Prof. DIRK A. LOOSE
Center for Circulatory Disturbances
and Vascular Defects
Department for Angiology
and Vascular Surgery
Facharztklinik Hamburg
Hamburg, Germany
prof.loose@gmx.de

This is a revised, enlarged and completely updated version of the Italian Edition published under the title
"*Malformazioni vascolari ed emangiomi. Testo-atlante di diagnostica e terapia*" edited by
R. Mattassi, S. Belov, D.A. Loose, M. Vaghi
© Springer-Verlag Italia 2003
All rights reserved

Library of Congress Control Number: 2008938921

ISBN 978-88-470-0568-6 Springer Milan Berlin Heidelberg New York
e-ISBN 978-88-470-0569-3

Springer is a part of Springer Science+Business Media
springer.com
© Springer-Verlag Italia 2009

Cover design: Simona Colombo, Milan, Italy
Typesetting: C & G di Cerri e Galassi, Cremona, Italy
Printing and binding: Printer Trento Srl, Trento, Italy

Printed in Italy
Springer-Verlag Italia S.r.l., Via Decembrio 28, I-20137 Milan, Italy

Dedicated to our beloved teacher, Stefan Belov.
We grieve his untimely passing.
To him we dedicate the English edition of this atlas.
He showed us how to manage
the most difficult tasks in the field of angiology.
He taught us how to overcome loneliness
and how to defeat obscurantism with love, faith, and perseverance.
He led us to realize the critical difference between
simply getting good results and founding a new school of thought.
We hope that this atlas will contribute to the realization of his dream:
to systematize vascular malformations, to offer effective treatments,
and, finally, to expel angiodysplasias from the niche
of rare diseases for which no therapy is available.

Foreword

The field of congenital vascular malformations and the unfortunate patients that suffer from them will welcome this truly multidisciplinary international contribution to the study and treatment of a group of diseases that is gradually becoming better known, but not better liked, by the majority of our colleagues. Without question, the power of the internet with its access to world-wide medical literature, and the publication of complete issues of medical journals devoted to the subject of vascular malformations, have contributed to expanding knowledge and eliciting curiosity amongst physicians who some decades ago would not have wanted to deal with unusual, poorly understood and challenging diseases.

A group of authors from ten different countries, experts in their respective medical and surgical specialties, who have felt the pain of the many patients afflicted with vascular malformations, have made a combined effort to increase and update the growing knowledge of these diseases. The tremendous technological advances in non invasive as well as invasive diagnostic techniques, imaging, genetics, and therapeutic surgical and endovascular procedures, have given us new weapons with which to treat and improve the lives of many desperate patients afflicted by diseases that some years ago produced only sorrow, compassion and despair in their families and in the rare physicians who dared to tackle their problems.

Congenital vascular malformations exert a powerful and fascinating attraction in a small group of dedicated and compassionate physicians who see in these problems a challenge that is difficult to overcome. Often, the magnitude of the problem incites us to seek new avenues to solve it or, at least, to improve our patients' suffering.

A great deal of progress has been made in the understanding and management of congenital vascular anomalies. These new advances are shared with other physicians so that they can find, through the pages of this book, new ideas on how to treat their patients and hopefully, the solution to their patients' problems.

J. Leonel Villavicencio MD, FACS
Distinguished Professor of Surgery
Uniformed Services University School of Medicine
Bethesda, MD, USA

Preface

When a curious tourist travels through an unknown country following a guidebook, at the end of his trip he may have a number of different feelings. If the land he visited was interesting and the guidebook brought him to the remarkable places and clearly explained the meaning of what he was seeing and how to move through the country, he may remain interested in his trip, love the new country and want to return in order to explore it more in detail. If the guidebook was unclear, did not give him the correct explanations or guide him to the best places, he will leave without an interest in the land, will lay down his guidebook and will not come back.

The goal of this atlas is to guide the reader through the difficult field of hemangiomas and vascular malformations, help him to understand them and give him answers to questions, mainly about practical approaches to these diseases. All the authors have made an effort to explain their topics in the simplest way with text and pictures.

If we succeed in our effort and this small atlas is appreciated by readers, we will be happy that we have accomplished the goal given to us by our teacher and friend, Professor Stefan Belov, who dedicated his life to the study of these diseases and strongly desired to publish an atlas to help colleagues understand hemangiomas and vascular malformations in order to propagate knowledge and possibilities for treatment. He passed away before he could see his idea become reality, but we hope that our efforts fulfil his wishes.

We thank all the authors who spent their time making this book a reality. Special thanks to all our friends at Springer-Verlag in Milan, and particularly Antonella Cerri and Alessandra Born.

R. Mattassi
D.A. Loose
M. Vaghi

Contents

Part I   INTRODUCTION

1   Angiogenesis   3
A. Agliano

2   Historical Background   9
R. Mattassi

Part II   HEMANGIOMAS

3   Hemangiomas of Infancy: Epidemiology   17
M.R. Cordisco

**4   Classification of Infantile Hemangiomas and Other Congenital
Vascular Tumors**   23
H.P. Berlien

5   Diagnosis of Hemangiomas   35
J.C. López Gutiérrez

6   Visceral Hemangiomas   39
J.C. López Gutiérrez

**7   Principles of Therapy of Infantile Hemangiomas and Other
Congenital Vascular Tumors of the Newborns and Infants**   49
H.P. Berlien

8   Medical Treatment of Hemangiomas   57
J. Rössler, C.M. Niemeyer

9   Laser Therapy of Infantile Hemangiomas and Other Congenital Vascular Tumors of Newborns and Infants 65
H.P. Berlien

10   Surgery of Hemangiomas 79
G. Vercellio, V. Baraldini

11   Facial Hemangiomas 85
P. Rieu

12   Anogenital Hemangiomas 93
R. Grantzow, K. Schäffer

Part III VASCULAR MALFORMATIONS

13   Genetic Aspects of Vascular Malformations 99
N. Limaye, M. Vikkula

14   Epidemiology of Vascular Malformations 109
G. Tasnádi

15   Classification of Vascular Malformations 111
R. Mattassi, D.A. Loose, M. Vaghi

16   Non Invasive Diagnostics of Congenital Vascular Malformations ... 115
M. Vaghi

17   Nuclear Medicine in Diagnostics of Vascular Malformations 121
R. Dentici

18   Invasive Diagnostics of Congenital Vascular Malformations 135
J.H. Weber

19   Principles of Treatment of Vascular Malformations 145
R. Mattassi, D.A. Loose, M. Vaghi

20   Interventional Therapy in Arteriovenous Congenital Malformations 153
J.H. Weber

21   Diagnosis and Management of Soft Tissue Vascular Malformations with Ethanol 163
W.F. Yakes

22   Sclerotherapy in Vascular Malformations 171
J.C. Cabrera, D.A. Loose

23 Laser Therapy of Vascular Malformations 181
H.P. Berlien

24 The Combined Treatment of Arteriovenous Malformations 195
D.A. Loose

25 Multidisciplinary Surgical Treatment of Vascular Malformations ... 205
R. Mattassi

26 Treatment of Arterial Malformations 209
R. Mattassi, D.A. Loose

27 Treatment of Arteriovenous Malformations 215
D.A. Loose

28 Treatment of Venous Malformations 223
R. Mattassi

29 Treatment of Lymphatic Malformations 231
B.-B. Lee, J. Laredo, J.-M. Seo, R.F. Neville

30 Treatment of Vascular Malformations in Newborns and Infants ... 251
G. Tasnádi

Part IV TREATMENT PROBLEMS ACCORDING TO SPECIFIC LOCALIZATIONS

31 Introductory Remarks 275
R. Mattassi

**32 Management of Head and Neck Vascular Malformations:
an Overview** 277
J.A. Perkins

33 Surgical Treatment of Vascular Malformations in the Hand 287
P. Di Giuseppe

34 Management of Vascular Malformations in the Thorax Wall 293
F. Stillo, G. Bianchini

**35 Joint Involvement in Patients with Vascular Malformations.
Destructive Angiodysplastic Arthritis** 299
J. Hauert, D.A. Loose, F.M. Westphal

**36 Surgical Approach to Congenital Vascular Malformations
in the Foot** 305
G. Pisani, D.A. Loose

37 Diagnosis and Management of Vascular Malformations of Bone   319
W.F. Yakes

38 The Role of Syndromes   325
M. Vaghi

Conclusions   329

Subject Index   331

Contributors

ALICE AGLIANO
Hematology-Oncology Laboratory
European Institute of Oncology
Milan, Italy

VITTORIA BARALDINI
Center for Angiomas and Vascular
Malformations of Children
Vascular Surgery Unit
Children's Hospital "V. Buzzi"
Milan, Italy

HANS PETER BERLIEN
Department of Lasermedicine
Elisabeth Klinik
Berlin, Germany

GIOVANNI BIANCHINI
Department of Vascular Surgery
Multidisciplinary Center for Vascular
Malformations
IDI, Istituto Dermopatico dell'Immacolata
Rome, Italy

JUAN CARLOS CABRERA
Clinicas "Dr. Juan Cabrera"
Granada, Spain

MARIA ROSA CORDISCO
Pediatric Dermatology Service
Pediatric Hospital "Prof. Dr. G.P. Garran"
Buenos Aires, Argentina

ROBERTO DENTICI
Nuclear Medicine Service
"G. Salvini" Hospital
Garbagnate Milanese (Milan)
and Hospital "Caduti Bollatesi"
Bollate (Milan), Italy

PIERO DI GIUSEPPE
Plastic and Hand Surgery Unit
Hospital "Fornaroli"
Magenta (Milan), Italy

RAINER GRANTZOW
Department of Plastic Surgery
Haunerschen Pediatric Clinic
Ludwig-Maximilians-University Munich
Munich, Germany

JÜRGEN HAUERT
Department of Ortopedics and
Emergency Surgery
Clinic "Dr. Guth"
Hamburg, Germany

JAMES LAREDO
Department of Surgery
Division of Vascular Surgery
Georgetown University Hospital
Washington, DC, USA

BYUNG-BOONG LEE
Center for Vein, Lymphatics and Vascular
Malformation
Division of Vascular Surgery
Georgetown University School of Medicine
Washington, DC, USA

NISHA LIMAYE
Laboratory of Human Molecular Genetics
de Duve Institute, Université Catholique
de Louvain
Brussels, Belgium

DIRK A. LOOSE
Center for Circulatory Disturbances and
Vascular Defects
Department for Angiology and Vascular Surgery
Facharztklinik Hamburg
Hamburg, Germany

JUAN CARLOS LÓPEZ GUTIÉRREZ
Department of Pediatric Surgery
La Paz Children's Hospital
Autonomous University of Madrid
Madrid, Spain

RAUL MATTASSI
Department of Vascular Surgery
Center for Vascular Malformations
"Stefan Belov"
"G. Salvini" Hospital
Garbagnate Milanese (Milan), Italy

RICHARD F. NEVILLE
Department of Surgery
Division of Vascular Surgery
Georgetown University Hospital
Washington, DC, USA

CHARLOTTE NIEMEYER
Clinic IV of Pediatric Hematology and
Oncology
Centre for Pediatrics
University of Freiburg
Freiburg, Germany

JONATHAN PERKINS
Otolaryngology/Head and Neck Surgery
Children's Hospital and Regional
Medical Center
University of Washington
Seattle, WA, USA

GIACOMO PISANI
Center for Foot Surgery
Hospital "Fornaca di Sessant"
Turin, Italy

PAUL RIEU
Department of Surgery
Radboud University Medical Center Nijmegen
Nijmegen, The Netherlands

JOCHEN RÖSSLER
Division of Pediatric Hematology and Oncology
Department of Pediatrics and Adolescent
Medicine
University Hospital of Freiburg
Freiburg, Germany

KATHRIN SCHÄFFER
Hospital for Pediatric Surgery
Ludwig-Maximilians-University Munich
Munich, Germany

JEONG-MEEN SEO
Division of Pediatric Surgery
SamSung Medical Center &
Sungkyunkwan University
Kangnam-Ku, Seoul, Korea

FRANCESCO STILLO
Department of Vascular Surgery
Multidisciplinary Center for Vascular
Malformations
IDI, Istituto Dermopatico dell'Immacolata
Rome, Italy

GÉZA TASNÁDI
Professor of Pediatric Surgery
Budapest, Hungary

MASSIMO VAGHI
Department of Vascular Surgery and
Center for Vascular Malformations
"Stefan Belov"
"G. Salvini" Hospital
Garbagnate Milanese (Milan), Italy

GIANNI VERCELLIO
Plastic Surgery Unit II
Istituto Clinico Humanitas
Milan, Italy

MIIKKA VIKKULA
Laboratory of Human Molecular Genetics
de Duve Institute
Université Catholique de Louvain
Brussels, Belgium

JÜRGEN H. WEBER
Professor of Interventional Radiology
and Phlebology
Hamburg, Germany

FLORIAN MORITZ WESTPHAL
Department of Trauma
and Reconstructive Surgery
Berufsgenossenschaftliches
Unfallkrankenhaus Hamburg
Hamburg, Germany

WAYNE F. YAKES
Vascular Malformation Center
Swedish Medical Center
Englewood, CO, USA

Part I
INTRODUCTION

Angiogenesis

1

Alice Agliano

Abstract

The vascular system is a complex network of vessels that carries oxygenated blood and nutrients throughout our bodies. It comes as no surprise that angiogenesis, the process of growing new blood vessels, occurs not only in health, but also in serious disease, where it may be either up- or down-regulated. While the growth of the vascular system is one of the earlier events of embryogenesis, angiogenesis also occurs in adulthood, during wound healing and restoration of blood flow to injured tissues. The healthy body controls angiogenesis through a perfect balance of modulators, regulated by a strong interaction between growth factors and inhibitors, the imbalance of which can lead to disease. Angiogenesis is a "common denominator" shared by diseases affecting more than one billion people worldwide; these diseases are caused by both excessive angiogenesis (cancer, diabetic eye disease, rheumatoid arthritis), and insufficient angiogenesis (coronary heart disease, stroke, delayed wound healing) [1].

Introduction

This chapter describes processes involved in angiogenesis from positive and negative regulators, through endothelial cell (EC) and pericyte recruitment, to the importance of the therapeutic anti-angiogenic applications that have recently been made available.

Vascular endothelial cells (EC) cover the entire inner surface of blood vessels in the body, and the growth of the vascular system is primarily a development process occurring during embryogenesis and postnatal life.

Early during embryogenesis, blood islands composed of progenitors of blood cells (hematopoietic cells), and endothelial progenitor cells (EPCs or angioblasts) differentiate from the mesoderm. The formation of the earliest blood vessels and their organization into a primordial vascular structure through induction, differentiation and assembly of EPCs is called vasculogenesis [2]; it may initially be a random process that subsequently becomes refined by selective branch regression and expansion.

During development and in the postnatal life the process responsible for the formation of new blood vessels is called angiogenesis. It involves the formation of vascular sprouts from pre-existing vessels, resulting in a highly branched vascular plexus; this is remodeled several times until a mature vascular system is formed. EPCs released from the bone marrow are present in peripheral blood and differentiate into ECs in the setting of both physiological and pathological neovascularization. This discovery, in the 1990s, revealed that vasculogenesis occurs also during adult life (Fig. 1.1) [3]. Angiogenesis is a fundamental process in reproduction, development and wound healing, and under these conditions is highly regulated. The ability of an organism to spontaneously develop collateral vessels represents an important response to vascular occlusive diseases which determine the severity of residual tissue ischemia. Neovascularization of ischemic cardiac or skeletal muscle may be sufficient to preserve tissue integrity and function, and in response to tissue ischemia, constitutes a natural host defense intended to maintain tissue perfusion required for physiologic organ function. In adult organisms, both hypoxia and inflammation are usually considered to be the major stimuli for ischemia-induced neovascularization [5]. Aberrant, retarded or overshooting vascularization may severely impair organ function and is often associated with diseases [6]: in arthritis, new capillaries invade the joint and destroy cartilage; while ocular neovascularization, which is often associated

R. Mattassi, D.A. Loose, M. Vaghi (eds.), *Hemangiomas and Vascular Malformations*.
© Springer-Verlag Italia 2009

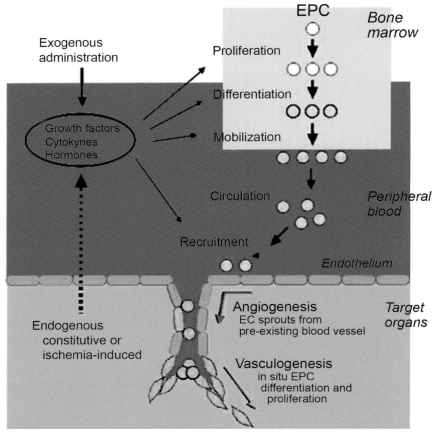

Fig. 1.1. Angiogenesis represents the classic paradigm for new vessel growth, as mature, differentiated endothelial cells (ECs) break free from their basement membrane (BM) and migrate and proliferate to form sprouts from parenteral vessels. Vasculogenesis involves participation of BM-derived endothelial progenitor cells (EPCs), which circulate to sites of neovascularization where they differentiate in situ into mature ECs. Growth factors, cytokines, or hormones released endogenously for therapeutic neovascularization act to promote EPC proliferation, differentiation, and mobilization from BM (via the peripheral circulation) to neovascular foci. Reproduced from [4], with permission

with diabetes, is the most common cause of blindness. Furthermore, uncontrolled angiogenesis may lead to psoriasis and juvenile hemangiomas, strongly vascularized lesions in which the number of newly formed vessels greatly exceeds the metabolic demand of the tissue concerned. Finally, tumor growth and metastasis are angiogenesis-dependent. A growing tumor needs an extensive network of capillaries to provide nutrients and oxygen. In addition, the new intratumoral blood vessels provide a way for tumor cells to enter the circulation and to metastasize to distant organs.

The Angiogenic Process

Angiogenesis is a complex process involving extensive interplay between cells, soluble factors and extracellular matrix components. The construction of a vascular network requires different steps, includ-

ing the release of proteases from "activated" ECs, the degradation of the basement membrane surrounding the existing vessel, the migration of the ECs into the interstitial space, their proliferation, and lumen formation. The next steps involve the generation of a new basement membrane with the recruitment of pericytes, the fusion of the newly formed vessels and finally the initiation of blood flow.

In theory, organ-specific vascular patterns may result from guided sprouting. A newly formed sprout that extends into the surrounding tissue may follow tracks and gradients that provide attractive and repulsive signals. Alternatively, an initial random sprouting and vascular plexus assembly may be followed by organ-specific vessel remodeling and pruning. As of today, evidence indicates the existence of both of these mechanisms [7].

Tubular morphogenesis relies on functional specialization of individual cells, and guidance of a tubular sprout is mediated through directed migration of tip cells that utilize filopodia to sense guidance clues. ECs situated at the tip of the growing angiogenic sprout extend multiple long filopodia, and the following stalk cells proliferate and form a vascular lumen [8].

The tip cell guidance and migration depends on the shape of the gradient of vascular endothelial growth factor (VEGF) located on the filopodia. Apparently VEGF receptor-2 (VEGFR-2) activation leads to fundamentally different functional responses in the tip cell, where filopodia extension is promoted, compared to proliferation in the stalk cell, which in turn determines the initial vascular pattern [9]. An imbalance between the two processes may explain why abnormal vascular patterns develop in pathological angiogenesis.

Intussusceptive angiogenesis refers to the process by which new blood vessels grow and develop from pre-existing vasculature through insertion of tissue pillars into the capillary lumen and expansion of the latter to form new capillary networks. Four consecutive steps are described: a zone of contact is established between opposite capillary walls, then a reorganization of the inter-EC junction and central perforation occurs. An interstitial pillar core is formed and is invaded by pericytes and myofibroblasts [10].

Contrast sprouting angiogenesis is a prolonged process characterized by extensive proliferation of ECs, degradation of extracellular matrix and an increase in vascular permeability. Intussusception occurs in the virtual absence of EC proliferation, and is achieved at low vascular permeability levels.

In the studies conducted so far, it has been shown that the vascular system is initiated by vasculogenesis followed by an early sprouting phase, forming the primary capillary plexus. During the second intussusceptive phase, capillary sprouting is supervened by trans capillary pillar formation. The putative inducers of sprouting angiogenesis include angiopoietins and their Tie-receptors [11], platelet-derived growth factor (PDGF-B) [12] and ephrins and their Eph-B receptors [13] probably also influence vascular remodelling. VEGF appears to be an early promoter of angiogenesis while the angiopoietins and Tie-2 as well as the ephrins and their receptors appear to act a somewhat later stage [14] and are probably associated with the regulation of intussusception.

VEGF promotes formation of new capillary segment and vascular maturation through pericytes and smooth muscle recruitment. Such periendothelial cells are important for vascular integrity and maturation. Three major functional roles have been ascribed to pericytes: contractility, regulation of EC activity, and macrophage activity [15]. We now know

that Tie-2/Angiopoietin-1 interactions maintain cell-cell contacts between ECs, stabilizing the vessel wall and promoting vessel maturation.

For angiogenesis to occur, profound changes in vessel architecture have to take place. Quiescent vessels are built up by a luminal lining in ECs, a basement membrane consisting of members of the collagen family, laminin and fibronectin, and an abluminal layer of perivascular cells, pericytes in capillaries and smooth muscle cells in larger veins and arteries. During angiogenesis, this structure needs to be temporarily destabilized. This is accomplished by secretion by ECs of matrix metalloproteinases (MMPs) which degrade the basal lamina, digest the extracellular matrix (ECM) and create additional space for the growing collateral vessel [16], and by secretion of angiopoietin-2 resulting in detachment of pericytes [17]. Another system plays a crucial role in the migration and invasion of ECs in fibrinous matrix – tissue-plasminogen activator (t-PA) and urokinase-plasminogen activator (u-PA) – where an interaction between integrins and u-PA receptor occurs. Perivascular fibrin serves as a substrate on which newly formed ECs can adhere and migrate to form new sprouts that develop into mature vessels. A considerable number of angiogenesis inhibitors have now been recognized that represent degradation products derived from extracellular matrix proteins or from proteases of the hemostatic system. The earliest recognized were angiostatin and endostatin; angiostatin exerts its anti-angiogenic activity by inducing endothelial apoptosis, while endostatin inhibits VEGF-induced migration and apoptosis [18].

During maturation, a new basement membrane is formed by the endothelium, and perivascular cells are recruited by secretion of angiopoietin-1. A number of functions have been proposed for pericytes: sensing of hemodynamic forces, the regulation of capillary blood flow and blood vessel morphogenesis. The recruitment of pericytes is mediated by PDGF-B signalling, expressed by ECs situated at the sprout tip, via PDGFRβ, expressed by the mural cells [19]. Also monocytes and macrophages contribute mechanistically and structurally to the formation of capillaries; the communication between them and ECs is bi-directional: the capillary advancement may be facilitated by monocyte presence, but their mobility can also be stimulated by ECs. Each process is mediated by VEGFR-1 which is highly expressed by monocytes. In order to form new capillaries ECs need to migrate. Since the tissue opposes mechanical resistance, the cells must create a "path" by degradation of the ECM. This process may be accomplished by monocytes and macrophages, which, because they are well equipped for tissue penetration, also provide soluble pro-angiogenic factors favouring capillary penetration and the engraftment of EPCs derived from bone marrow [20, 21]. The adhesion of circulating blood monocytes with the activated endothelium of a collateral arteriole is a pivotal step during the process of arteriogenesis. Important mediators of such cell-to-cell binding processes are selectins and intercellular adhesion molecules (ICAM-1 and ICAM-2) on ECs and integrins (Mac-1 and LFA-1) on monocytes. Factors like VEGF being potentially released by ECs have the ability to stimulate integrin expression on monocytes and increase cell adhesion. The monocyte interaction with the collateral endothelium is a complex multistep process. After the initial monocyte interaction with the vascular endothelium, called "rolling", mediated by several selectins, the tight monocyte adhesion to the collateral endothelium is triggered by integrins. The integrins interact with their corresponding adhesion molecules on the EC surface, preferably ICAM-1, ICAM-2 and VCAM-1, clustered in focal adhesion complexes [22]. While monocyte invasion, maturation into macrophages and appearance of typical signs of inflammation characterize the first phase of arteriogenesis, the subsequent growth phase is dominated by the proliferation of cells, mainly of smooth muscle and adventitial fibroblasts but also of ECs on the one hand, and extensive tissue remodelling on the other hand [23].

The angiogenic process is tightly controlled by a number of positive and negative regulators. Many negative regulators consist of proteolytic fragments of larger proteins. Well known examples are angiostatin and endostatin [24, 25]. Among the positive regulators, members of the VEGF family and the angiopoietins play prominent roles. One of the most potent and important angiogenic factors is VEGF-A. In a wide number of tumors VEGF-A correlates with vascular density and poor prognosis. VEGF-A induces migration and proliferation of ECs, expression of tissue factors and MMPs, tube formation, and regulates vascular permeability [26].

VEGFR-2 seems to mediate most of these activities: proliferation and migration, tyrosine phosphorylation of downstream targets, Ca2+ mobilization, prostacyclin (PGI2) production and ERK activation, nitric oxide (NO) production, and survival and phosphatidylinositol 3-kinase (PI3K)/Akt activity. The other VEGFR-1 has been proposed to be involved in migration, not only of ECs, but also of cells of hematopoietic origin like monocytes. Hypoxia, inducing expression of hypoxia-inducible factor-1 and 2 (HIF-1 and HIF-2), upregulates the transcription factors for VEGF. Thus, in hypoxic conditions, VEGF is secreted and binds to its receptors located on the surface of vascular ECs. Hypoxic upregulation of VEGF thus provide a compensatory mechanism by which tissues can increase their oxygenation through induction of blood vessel growth. In contrast, normoxia downregulates VEGF production and causes regression of some newly formed blood vessels. By these opposing processes, the vasculature exactly meets the metabolic demands of the tissue. Although hemodynamic forces such as shear stress are fundamental for remodelling, tissue hypoxia seems to play a crucial role in the coordinated expression of these factors; once oxygenation has reached normal levels, they are rapidly downregulated and HIF levels decrease [27]. It appears that VEGF, the angiopoietins, PDGF, the ephrins, erythropoietin and additional growth factors must act together in coordinated manner.

Despite the abundance of angiogenic factors present in different tissues, EC turnover in a healthy adult organism is remarkably low, in the order of thousands of days. The maintenance of endothelial quiescence is thought to be due to the presence of endogenous negative regulators. Moreover, positive and negative regulators often co-exist in tissues with extensive angiogenesis. These observations have led to the hypothesis that activation of the endothelium depends on a balance between these opposing regulators [28]. If positive angiogenic factors dominate, the endothelium will be activated, whereas quiescence is induced by negative regulators. Thus, the angiogenic process can be divided in an activation phase (initiation and progression of the angiogenic process) and a phase of resolution (termination and stabilization of the vessels). It is not yet clear whether the resolution phase is due to upregulation of endogenous inhibitors or exhaustion of positive regulators. A number of endogenous angiogenesis inhibitors have been described that act on ECs to block their migration, proliferation and/or their ability to form functional capillaries. These include proteins such as angiostatin or endostatin, platelet factor-4 (PF-4), thrombospondin-1 (TSP-1), interferon-α (IFN-α), tissue inhibitor of metalloproteinases (TIMPs), plasminogen activator inhibitors (PAIs) and others. Because the endothelium is the primary structure that maintains fluid and macromolecules in the bloodstream, it is a key regulator of the plasma leakage that is one of the hallmarks of inflammation. Since ECs upregulate adhesion proteins, which participate in leukocyte adhesion and extravasation during inflammation, pharmacologic agents that specifically limit the EC responses in inflammation might be useful for treating inflammatory diseases such as acute lung injury, rheumatoid arthritis, and psoriasis.

Angiogenesis Anomalies

Vascular anomalies comprise two main categories: malformations and tumors. Vascular malformations are believed to result from the aberrant development of vascular elements during embryogenesis and foetal maturation. These may be single vessel forms (capillary, arterial, lymphatic or venous), or combined. The progression of angiogenesis-dependent disorders depends on the remodelling of ECM. Excessive degradation of ECM by MMPs can lead to structural instability of vessels, causing disorders associated with the central nervous system. Human brain arteriovenous malformations (BAVMs), for example, are associated with abnormal expression of MMPs and TIMPs; a net balance between MMPs and TIMPs may determine a clinical course of unstable vascular lesions. Degradation of the ECM by MMP-9 seems to be a critical step for angiogenesis, and vascular remodelling; high levels of MMP-9 are detected in aneurysms and atherosclerotic arteries. Increased levels and altered expression of VEGF and VEGF receptors were also detected in BAVMs, so taken together, VEGF and MMPs may contribute to the development or maintenance of the disease vascular phenotype. There is an increase in the urinary level of MMPs, bFGF and VEGF in patients with vascular malformations; this could be taken in consideration when assessing a therapy that uses antiangiogenic drugs to suppress the clinical progression of these diseases [29–31].

Human tumors can remain "dormant" for years owing to a balance between cell proliferation and apoptosis which is maintained by a lack of angiogenesis or by the presence of angiogenesis inhibitors. When this balance is disrupted, an "angiogenic switch" may occur, followed by tumor outgrowth [32]. Because normal ECs are genetically stable, anti-angiogenic therapy was initially touted to be a treatment "resistant to tolerance" [33]. Initial xenograft studies supported the theoretical predictions of widespread activity, limited toxicity and no resistance [34]. As chemotherapy induces tumor cell death, the production of pro-angiogenic peptides decreases, leading to regression of the tumor-associated vasculature with increasing tumor hypoxia, stimulating an increase in VEGF production; however, the increased VEGF production in areas of tumors hypoxia may stimulate angiogenesis. Several studies have shown that combining anti-VEGF with chemotherapy results in greater anti-tumor effects that either treatment alone. Maximal anti-angiogenic therapy typically requires prolonged exposure to low drug concentrations (metronomic therapy), exactly counter to the maximum tolerated dose administered when optimal tumor cell kill is the goal. The combination of low, frequent dose chemotherapy plus an agent that specifically targets the EC compartment controls tumor growth much more effectively than the cytotoxic agent alone [35, 36]. The final tumor size is dependent only on the balance of positive and negative angiogenic factors and is independent of tumor size at the beginning of the treatment.

The preclinical and clinical studies of therapeutic angiogenesis performed to date have repeatedly shown that VEGF-induced angiogenesis is not indiscriminate or widespread but is instead restricted to sites of ischemia. The findings suggest that the fundamental mechanism by which therapeutic neovascularisation augments collateral development is by providing cytokine supplements to individuals who, because of their advanced age, diabetes, hypercholesterolemia, and/or other as yet undefined circumstances, are unable to appropriately upregulate cytokine expression in response to tissue ischemia. In this regard, ligand supplementation may be analogous to erythropoietin administration in patients with refractory anemia. Second, cytokine administration clearly represents only one aspect of the therapeutic intervention. Regardless of how much ligand is administered, the resident population of ECs competent to respond to an available level of angiogenic growth factors may also constitute a potentially limiting factor in strategies designed to promote neovascularization of ischemic tissues. A reasonable goal may therefore consist of developing a complementary strategy that would provide substrate together with ligand, a "supply side" version of therapeutic neovascularisation [4].

References

1. DeWitt N (2005) Angiogenesis. Nature 438(7070):931
2. Flamme I, Frolich T, Risau W (1997) Molecular mechanisms of vasculogenesis and embryonic angiogenesis. J Cell Physiol 173:206–210
3. Asahara T, Isner JM (2002) Endothelial progenitor cells for vascular regeneration. J Hematother Stem Cell Res 2:171–178
4. Isner JM, Asahara T (1999) Angiogenesis and vasculogenesis as therapeutic strategies for postnatal neovascularization. J Clin Invest 103:1231-1236
5. Carmeliet P (2000) Mechanisms of angiogenesis and arteriogenesis. Nat Med 6:389–395
6. Folkman J (1995) Angiogenesis in cancer, vascular, rheumatoid and other disease. Nat Med 1:27-31

7. Serini G, Ambrosi D, Giraudo E et al (2003) Modeling the early stages of vascular network assembly. EMBO J 22:1771–1779

8. Hacohen N, Kramer S, Sutherland D et al (1998) Sprouty encodes a novel antagonist of FGF signaling that patterns apical branching of the Drosophila airways. Cell 92:253–263

9. Gerhardt H, Golding M, Fruttiger M et al (2003) VEGF guides angiogenic sprouting utilizing endothelial tip cell filopodia. J Cell Biol 161:1163–1177

10. Djonov V, Schmid M, Tschanz SA, Burri PH (2000) Intussusceptive angiogenesis: its role in embryonic vascular network formation. Circ Res 86:286–292

11. Folkman J, D'Amore PA (1996) Blood vessel formation: what is its molecular basis? Cell 87:1153–1155

12. Hellstrom M, Kalen M, Lindahl P et al (1999) Role of PDGFR-beta in recruitment of vascular smooth muscle cells and pericytes during embryonic blood vessel formation in the mouse. Development 126:3047–3055

13. Gale NW, Baluk P, Pan L et al (2001) Ephrin-B2 selectively marks arterial vessels and neovascularization sites in the adult, with expression in both endothelial and smooth-muscle cells. Dev Biol 230:151–160

14. Augustin HG (2001) Tubes, branches, and pillars: the many ways of forming a new vasculature. Circ Res 89:645–647

15. Rucker HK, Wynder HJ, Thomas WE (2000) Cellular mechanisms of CNS pericytes. Brain Res Bull 15 51(5):363–369

16. Pepper MS (2001) Role of the matrix metalloproteinase and plasminogen activator-plasmin systems in angiogenesis. Arterioscler Thromb Vasc Biol 21:1104–1117

17. Holash J, Maisonpierre PC, Compton D et al (1999) Vessel cooption, regression, and growth in tumors mediated by angiopoietins and VEGF. Science 284:1994–1998

18. Eriksson K, Magnusson P, Dixelius J et al (2003) Angiostatin and endostatin inhibit endothelial cell migration in response to FGF and VEGF without interfering with specific intracellular signal transduction pathways. FEBS Lett 536:19–24

19. Gerhardt H, Golding M, Fruttiger M et al (2003) VEGF guides angiogenic sprouting utilizing endothelial tip-cell filopodia. J Cell Biol 161:1163–1177

20. Gunsilius E, Duba HC, Petzer AL et al (2000) Evidence from a leukaemia model for maintenance of vascular endothelium by bone-marrow-derived endothelial cells. Lancet 355:1688–1691

21. Anghelina M, Schmeisser A, Krishnan P et al (2002) Migration of monocytes/macrophages in vitro and in vivo is accompanied by MMP12-dependent tunnels formation and by neo-vascularization. Cold Spring Harb Symp Quant Biol LXVII:209–215

22. Hogg N, Henderson R, Leitinger B et al (2002) Mechanisms contributing to the activity of integrins on leukocytes. Immunol Rev 186:164–171

23. Moldovan NI (2002) Role of monocytes and macrophages in adult angiogenesis: a light at the tunnel's end. J Hematother Stem Cell Res 11(2):179–194

24. O'Reilly MS, Holmgren L, Shing Y et al (1994) Angiostatin: A novel angiogenesis inhibitor that mediates the suppression of metastases by a Lewis lung carcinoma. Cell 79:315–328

25. O'Reilly MS, Boehm T, Shing Y et al (1997) Endostatin: An endogenous inhibitor of angiogenesis and tumor growth. Cell 88:277–285

26. Dvorak HF, Brown LF, Detmar M, Dvorak AM (1995) Vascular permeability factor/vascular endothelial growth factor, microvascular hyperpermeability, and angiogenesis. Am J Pathol 146:1029–1039

27. Iruela-Arispe ML, Dvorak HF (1997) Angiogenesis: a dynamic balance of stimulators and inhibitors. Thromb Haemost 78:672–677

28. Jain RK (2003) Molecular regulation of vessel maturation. Nat Med 9:685–693

29. Hashimoto T, Wen G, Lawton MT et al (2003) Abnormal expression of matrix metalloproteinases and tissue inhibitors of metalloproteinases in brain arteriovenus malformations. Stroke 34:925–931

30. Lee CZ, Xu B, Hashimoto T et al (2004) Doxycycline suppress cerebral matrix metalloproteinase-9 and angiogenesis induced by focal hyperstimulation of vascular endothelial growth factor in a mouse model. Stroke 35:1715–1719

31. Marler JJ, Fishman SJ, Kilroy SM et al (2005) Increased expression of urinary matrix metalloproteinases parallels the extent of activity of vascular anomalies. Pediatrics 116:38–45

32. Folkman J, Merler E, Abernathy C, Williams G (1978) Isolation of a tumor factor responsible or angiogenesis. J Exp Med 133:275–288

33. Kerbel RS (1997) A cancer therapy resistant to resistance [news; comment] [see comments] Nature 390:335–336

34. Boehm T, Folkman J, Browder T, O'Reilly MS (1997) Antiangiogenic therapy of experimental cancer does not induce acquired drug resistance [see comments]. Nature 390:404–407

35. Kerbel RS, Kamen BA (2004) The anti-angiogenic basis of metronomic chemotherapy. Nat Rev Cancer 4(6):423–436

36. Klement G, Baruchel S, Rak J et al (2000) Continuous low-dose therapy with vinblastine and VEGF receptor-2 antibody induces sustained tumor regression without overt toxicity. J Clin Invest 105:R15–R24

Historical Background

Raul Mattassi

2

Visible abnormal vascular masses were the first congenital vascular malformations (CVM) reported in the literature. Probably the first report was that of Guido Guidi, personal physician of King Francis I of France in the XVI century. He described a young Florentine man with extremely dilated vessels of the scalp, which looked like enormous varices. He sent this patient to the famous surgeon Gabriele Falloppio who refused to operate on such a difficult case [1]. This case and several others were considered to represent abnormal dilated vessels because the concept of hemodynamics was not understood.

In 1628 William Harvey published his famous book "Excercitatio anatomica de motu cordis et sanguinis in animalibus" in Frankfurt, Germany, in which he explained blood circulation [2]. This discovery provided the basis upon which to understand abnormal circulation, such as arteriovenous (AV) connections. The first description of an AV fistula was by Lealis Lealis in 1707, in an uncommon site: between the spermatic artery and vein [3]. Between 1719 and 1721 Winslow described AV fistulas between the esophageal artery and left pulmonary vein; between the left bronchial artery and vein; and between the bronchial artery and azygos vein. In 1739 he also described a case of transposition of pulmonary veins [4]. Stenzel (1723) and Morgagni (1761) first described congenital stenosis of the aortic istmus [5, 6].

In 1757 William Hunter described typical signs of AV communications, such as the bruit that disappears by compression of the feeding artery or at the site of communication [7]. In 1827 George Bushe reported a congenital temporal AV fistula treated by ligation of the external carotid artery because of hemorrhage [8]. Sir Prescott Hewitt (1867) clearly described a congenital AV malformation of a lower limb with "heating" in the leg, vibratory thrill and super-

ficial dilated veins [9]. In the same year an Italian doctor, Gerini, reported at the French Society of Surgery at Paris on a case of a congenital pulsating tumor of the hand treated successfully by ligation of the radial and later of the ulnar artery [10].

In 1843 Norris performed a successful surgical treatment of an acquired AV fistula by double ligature of the artery [11], but later Breschet (1883) described two cases of ligature of the proximal artery in an AV fistula, followed by gangrene [12]. Nicoladoni in 1875 [13] and Branham in 1890 [14] described the pulse frequency reduction by compression of the fistula or the feeding artery, giving their name to this sign. A review of 447 published cases of AV fistulas was presented by Halsted to the American Surgical Association in 1889. This concluded that the great majority of AV fistulas were acquired [15]; but Rienhoff in another review found mainly congenital cases [16]. Other main reviews were carried out at the Mayo Clinic by Ward and Horton (1940) [17].

In the nineteenth century, many descriptions of cases of visible diffuse venous anomalies appeared. Von Pitha (1869) [18] described dilated superficial veins in the upper limb which Bockenheimer later called "diffuse phlebectasia" (1907) [19]. In 1869 Weber reported "diffuse phlebarteriectasia" [20].

The first descriptions of segmentary somatic hypertrophy coupled with vascular anomalies were published by Geoffroy-Saint-Hilaire in 1832 in his great teratological work "Histoire generale et particuliere des anomalies de l'organisation chez l'homme et les animaux" [21]. Later, other cases were described, such as the case of Foucher (1850), Broca (1859) [22], Krause (1862) [23], Friedberg (1867) [24] and others (Figs. 2.1, 2.2). In 1869 Trélat and Monod described a patient with hypertrophy of leg bones, nevus and varicose veins and reviewed different pub-

R. Mattassi, D.A. Loose, M. Vaghi (eds.), *Hemangiomas and Vascular Malformations*.
© Springer-Verlag Italia 2009

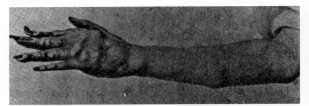

Fig. 2.1. Case described by Krause in 1862. Elongated left arm with visible pulsating "angiomata", present since the age of 7. At the age of 45, the arm was amputated after appearance of ulcers on the fingers [23]

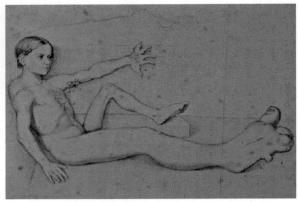

Fig. 2.2. Case described by Friedberg in 1867. A girl aged 10 with a hypertrophy of the right leg with a limb length discrepancy of 18 cm. This patient had also lymphangiomas on the left arm and hand with repeated episodes of phlebitis and lymphangitis, treated by wet packs and digitalis. She died of tuberculosis few years later [24]

lished cases. They expressed the opinion that this pathology was congenital and that the cause of the hypertrophy is the venous stasis [25]. The same concepts were presented 31 years later in the best known paper of the French neurologists Klippel and Trenaunay (1900). These authors noticed that the vascular defect involved only veins and capillaries, but not arteries. They also described "incomplete and subclinical forms" without the three signs: including only bone hypertrophy without nevus and varices; nevus without bone hyperthrophy and varices; and bone hypertrophy with nevus and no varices. They considered an infection of the embryo during pregnancy the cause of the defect [26].

Between 1907 and 1918 F. Parkes-Weber published different cases of limb hypertrophy and described signs of AV fistulas, as "…a definite thrill or pulsation… is transmitted to the veins". He put together different vascular dysplasias, ranging from lymphangioma, nevus, cirsoid aneurysm to diffuse AV fistulas and labelled all these cases as "haemangiectatic hypertrophy of limbs" [27–29].

The efforts of all these authors were limited by the lack of diagnostic technology and were therefore only based on clinical data.

The year 1923 marked a new step in diagnostics after the introduction of arteriography by Sicard and Forestier [30] using Lipiodol in France and by Berberich and Hirsch in Germany, injecting strontium bromide [31]. Arteriography made it possible to better study the hemodynamic of vascular malformations.

Dysplasias of the deep veins of the lower limbs were studied by Servelle with phlebographies. In 1962 he described stenosis of the popliteal vein due to compression of fibrous bands [32], but this data was not confirmed by others. Pathogenesis of limb overgrowth was considered to be due to the venous stasis. Soltesz demonstrated experimentally that AV shunts open by performing ligature of popliteal veins in young animals and arteriography; he concluded that limb hypertrophy is always due to AV fistulas [33].

A significant contribution towards comprehension of the different types of CVM was the paper of De Takats (1932) [34]; he made a clear distinction between AV malformations and other vascular defects, such as pure venous malformations and venous "angioma". Differentiation between hemangioma and vascular malformation was difficult. Even though Ewing in 1940 defined the hemangioma as a vascular tumor, different from a vascular malformation [35], only the publication of Mulliken and Young in 1988 was able to definitively clarify the difference [36].

Reports of cases with CVM of the limbs and limb shortening instead of hypertrophy were described later. In 1948 Servelle and Trinquecoste described two cases of venous hamartoma of the limbs with phleboliths and bone hypotrophy [37]. Martorell described a similar case in 1949 with "angiocavernomas" and severe bone destruction; he called this syndrome "angiomatosis braquial osteolitica" [38]. In 1957 Olivier distinguished two different types of "varicose angiomatosis", one superficial and one with deep-sited "angiomas" [39]. The opinion that even these venous-appearing malformations had AV communications was expressed by Pratt (1949) and Piulachs and Vidal Barraquer (1953) [40, 41].

Lymphatic dysplasia was described clearly in the nineteenth century. Cystic hygroma was first described by Wernher in 1843 [42]. Wegener (1877) divided lymphatic dysplasias or lymphangiomas into simplex, cavernosum and cysticum types, a classification which is accepted even today [43]. Extensive studies on diagnosis and treatment of lymphatic malformations were carried out by Kinmonth [44] and Servelle [45]. The rare condition of chylus reflux was first reported clearly by Servelle in 1949 [46]. Reports of combination of peripheral vascular malformations and lymphatic dysplasia were still included in some historical papers, like those of Klippel and Trenaunay and Parkes-Weber, but clear recognition of the lymphatic component was not achieved. Better data appeared only recently due to Pierer (1965) [47], Lindemayr (1967) [48], Partsch (1968) and also in the cited work of Kinmonth, among others.

In 1965 Malan published two papers in which he extensively analyzed all types of CVM, trying to clear problems of classification, diagnostics and treatment [49, 50].

The first monograph, "Abnormal Arteriovenous Communications", was published by Holman in 1968 [51] and was followed by the books of Belov in 1971 [52] and those of Giampalmo in 1972 [53]; the latter two had little diffusion because of their languages (Bulgarian and Italian). In 1974 Malan published his monograph in English with a report of 451 cases [56], followed by those of Schobinger (1977) [55]. Other remarkable works were due to Dean and O'Neal (1983) [17], Belov et al. (1985) [57] and Mulliken and Young (1988) [36].

Surgical treatment of CVM had been attempted for many years. Sometimes results were disappointing, as reported by Szilagyi in 1976 [58]; however, other authors, like Vollmar [59], Malan [54] and Belov [60] had better results. Belov was the first person to put surgery into a systematic level. Endovascular treatment was attempted first by Brooks in 1930: the author embolized a traumatic carotido-cavernous fistula with muscle fragments attached to a silver clip [61]. In 1960 Lussenhop and Spence embolized an intracranial AV malformation with spheres of methyl methacrylate through a surgically exposed common carotid artery [62]. Development of catheter technology and embolizing materials after 1970 increased the interest in these techniques. Zanetti and Sherman reported embolization with isobutyl 2-cyanoacrylate [63], Carey and Grace with gelfoam particles [64] while Gianturco created the coil in 1975 [65]. Yakes proposed the occlusion of CVM by alcohol injection through a direct puncture [66].

In 1976, Anthony Young (London) and John Mulliken (Boston) organized a small meeting with other colleagues interested in these problems, in order to exchange experiences and discuss difficult cases. Meetings were held every two years as interest in them increased. During the congress held in 1990 in Amsterdam, organized by Jan Kromhout, a group of experts agreed to found a scientific society to convene all the physicians interested in vascular malformations and hemangiomas, in order to obtain international acceptance. During the meeting held in Denver in 1992, organized by Wayne Yakes, the new society was founded. The first assembly agreed on the name International Society for the Study of Vascular Anomalies (ISSVA). The first President was Robert Schobinger (Switzerland). Today, ISSVA meets every two years. It brings together a multidisciplinary group of experts from all over the world dedicated to approaching these difficult topics. Interest in these diseases is growing and progress is on its way.

References

1. Guido Guidi, cited by Vichow R (1876) Pathologie des Tumeurs. Germer-Balliére, Paris
2. Whitterige G (1966) The anatomical lectures of William Harvey. Oxford
3. Lealis Lealis, cited by Malan E, Puglionisi A (1965) Congenital angiodysplasias of the extremities (Note II: Arterial, arterial and venous and hemolymphatic dysplasias). J Cardiovasc Surg 6:255–345 (reference 50)
4. Winslow, cited by Malan E, Puglionisi A (1965) Congenital angiodysplasias of the extremities (Note II: Arterial, arterial and venous and hemolymphatic dysplasias). J Cardiovasc Surg 6:255–345 (reference 50)
5. Stenzel ZG (1723) Dissertatio anatomico-pathologica de steatomatibus in principio aortae repertis. Vittembergae, 4
6. Morgagni GB (1761) De sedibus et causis morborum. Typografia Remondiniana, Venezia
7. Hunter W, cited by Fairbairn JF, Bernatz PE (1972) Arteriovenous fistulas. In: Fairbairn GF, Juergens JL, Spittel JA (eds) Peripheral vascular diseases. Saunders, Philadelphia
8. Bushe G (1827–1928) Temporal aneurysm: a case where, after an excision of an anastomoting aneurysm from the right temple, ligature of the external carotid became necessary to restrain hemorrhage. Lancet 2:413
9. Hewitt P (1867) A case of congenital aneurismal varix. Lancet 1:146
10. Gerini (1867) Societé Imperial de Chirurgie. Séance du Juin 1867. Gas d. Hosp de Paris, p 303
11. Norris cited by Fairbairn JF, Bernatz PE (1972) Arteriovenous fistulas. In: Fairbairn GF, Juergens JL, Spittel JA (eds) Peripheral vascular diseases. Saunders, Philadelphia

12. Breschet cited by Malan E, Puglionisi A (1965) Congenital angiodysplasias of the extremities (Note II: Arterial, arterial and venous and hemolymphatic dysplasias). J Cardiovasc Surg 6:255–345 (reference 50)

13. Nicoladoni C (1875) Phlebarteriectasie der rechten oberen Extremität. Arch Klin Chir 18:252– 274

14. Branham HH (1890) Aneurismal varix of the femoral artery and vein following a gunshot wound. Int J Surg 3:250–251

15. Callander CL (1920) Study of arteriovenous fistula with analysis of 447 cases (relation about the report of Halsted in 1889). John Hopkins Hosp Rep 19:259

16. Rienhoff WF jr (1924) Congenital arterio-venous fistula. An embyological study with the report of a case. John Hopkins Hosp Bull 35:271

17. Ward CE, Horton BT (1940) Congenital arteriovenous fistula in children. J Pediat 16:763

18. von Pitha, cited by Malan E, Puglionisi A (1965) Congenital angiodysplasias of the extremities (Note II: Arterial, arterial and venous and hemolymphatic dysplasias). J Cardiovasc Surg 6:255–345 (reference 50)

19. Bockenheimer P (1970) Über der genuine diffuse Phlebektasie der oberen Extremität. Festschrift f. G.E. von Rindfleisch. Leipzig 38:311

20. Weber KO, cited by Malan E, Puglionisi A (1965) Congenital angiodysplasias of the extremities (Note II: Arterial, arterial and venous and hemolymphatic dysplasias). J Cardiovasc Surg 6:255–345

21. Geoffroy-Saint-Hilaire, cited by Labitzke R, Rauterberg W (1970) Die Medizinische Welt. 19:891–896

22. Broca (1856) Des aneurysmes et de leur traitement. Paris

23. Krause W (1862) Traumatische angiectasis des linken Armes. Arch Klin Chir 2:143. Published in: Deutsche Gesellschaft für Chirurgie (1947) Langenbecks Archiv für klinische Chirurgie ... vereinigt mit Deutsche Zeitschrift für Chirurgie. Springer-Verlag, Germany

24. Friedberg H (1867) Riesenwuchs des rechten Beines. Virchows Archiv 40(3–4):343–379

25. Trelat U, Monod A (1969) De l'hypertrophie unilatérale ou totale du corps. Arch Gen Med 536

26. Klippel M, Trenaunay I (1900) Du noevus variqueux et ostéohypertrophique. Arch Gen Med 3:641–672

27. Weber FP (1907) Angioma formation in connection with hypertrophy of limbs and hemihypertrophy. Brit J Derm Syph 19:231–235

28. Weber FP (1908) Haemangiectatic hypertrophies of the foot and lower extremity, congenital or acquired. Med Press, London 136:261

29. Weber FP (1918) Haemangiectatic hypertrophy of limbs – congenital phlebarteriectasis and so-called congenital varicose veins. Brit J Chil Dis 15:13–17

30. Sicard JA, Forestier G (1923) Injections intravasculaires d'huile iodeé sous control radiologique. C R Soc Biol 88:1200–1202

31. Berberich J, Hirsch S (1923) Die roenthgenographische Darstellung der Arterien und Venen am Lebenden. Munch Klin Wschr 49:2226

32. Servelle M (1962) Oedémes chroniques des members chez l'enfant et l'adulte. Masson, Paris

33. Soltez L (1965) Contribution of clinical and experimental studies of the hypertrophy of the extremities in congenital arteriovenous fistulae. J Cardiovasc Surg [Suppl] 260

34. de Takats G (1932) Vascular anomalies of the extremities. Report of five cases. Surg Gynecol Obst 55:227

35. Ewing J (1940) Neoplastic diseases: a treatise on tumors. Saunders, Philadelphia, p 1160

36. Mulliken JB, Young AE (1988) Vascular Birthmarks: Hemangiomas and malformations. Saunders, Philadelphia

37. Servelle M, Trinquecoste D (1948) Des angiomes veineux. Arch Mal Coeur 41:436

38. Martorell F (1949) Hemangiomatosis braquial osteolìtica. Angiologia 1(4):219–123

39. Olivier CL (1957) Maladies des veins. Masson, Paris

40. Pratt GH (1949) Arterial varices. A syndrome. Am J Surg 77(4):456–460

41. Piulachs P, Vidal Barraquer F (1953) Pathogenetic study of varicose veins. Angiology 4:59–99

42. Wernher A (1843) Die angeborenen Kysten-hygrome und die ihnen verwandten Genschwulste in anatomischer, diagnostischer und therapeutischer Beziehung. Giessen, Germany: GF Heyer, Vater

43. Wegener G (1877) Über Lymphangiome. Arch klin Chir 20:641–707

44. Kinmonth JB (1972) The lymphatics. Diseases, lymphography and surgery. Edward Arnold, London

45. Servelle M (1975) Pathologie vasculaire. 3. Pathologie lymphatique. Masson, Paris

46. Servelle M, Deysson H (1949) Reflux du chyle dans les lymphatiques jambieres. Arch Mal Coeur 12:1181

47. Pierer H (1965) Klippel-Trenaunay-Weber syndrome from the surgical viewpoint. Klin Med Osterr Z Wiss Prakt Med 20(6):265–272

48. Lindemayr W, Lofferer O, Mostbeck A, Partsch H (1967) Lymphatic system in Klippel-Trenaunay-Weber's phakomatosis. Z Haut Geschlechtskr 1;43(5):183–188

49. Malan E, Puglionisi A (1964) Congenital angiodysplasias of the extremities (Note I: generalities and classification; venous dysplasias). J Cardiovasc Surg 5:87–130

50. Malan E, Puglionisi A (1965) Congenital angiodysplasias of the extremities (Note II: Arterial, arterial and venous and hemolymphatic dysplasias). J Cardiovasc Surg 6:255–345

51. Holman E (1968) Abnormal arteriovenous communications. Charles C Thomas, Springfield

52. Belov S (1971) Congenital angiodysplasia and their surgical treatment. Medicina I Fizkultura, Sofia

53. Giampalmo A (1972) Patologia delle malformazioni vascolari. Società Editrice Universo, Roma

54. Malan E (1974) Vascular malformations (angiodysplasias). Carlo Erba Foundation, Milan

55. Schobinger RA (1977) Periphere Angiodysplasien. Hans Huber, Bern

56. Dean RH, O'Neill Jr (1983) Vascular disorders of childhood. Lea & Febiger, Philadelphia

57. Belov S, Loose DA, Müller E (1985) Angeborene Gefäßfehler. Einhorn Presse, Reinbek
58. Szilagyi DE, Smith RF, Elliott JP, Hageman JH (1976) Arch Surg 11(4):423–429
59. Vollmar J (1963) Arteriovenöse Fisteln. Ihre Pathophysiologie Klinik und Behandlung. Med Welt 20
60. Belov S (1990) Surgical treatment of congenital vascular defects. Int Angiol 9(3):173–182
61. Brooks B (1930) The treatment of traumatic arteriovenous fistula. South Med J 23:100–106
62. Lussenhop AJ, Spence WT (1960) Artificial embolization of cerebral arteries: report of use in a case of arteriovenous malformation. JAMA 172:1153–1155
63. Zanetti PH, Sherman FE (1972) Experimental evaluation of a tissue adhesive as an agent for the treatment of aneurysms and arteriovenous anomalies. J Neurosurg 36(1):72–79
64. Carey LS, Grace DM (1974) The brisk bleed: control by arterial catheterization and gelfoam plug. J Can Assoc Radiol 25(2):113–115
65. Gianturco C, Anderson JH, Wallace S (1975) Mechanical devices for arterial occlusion. Am J Roentgenol Radium Ther Nucl Med 124(3):428–435
66. Yakes, WF, Pervsner PH, Reed MD et al (1986) Serial embolizations of an extremity arteriovenous malformation with alcohol via direct percutaneous puncture. AJR 146:1038–1040

Part II
HEMANGIOMAS

Hemangiomas of Infancy: Epidemiology

3

Maria Rosa Cordisco

Abstract

Few reports about the epidemiology of infantile hemangiomas (IH) exist and prospective studies are
missing; it is difficult to provide some data. The incidence in the general newborn population is between
1.1 and 2.6%, but increases to up to 12% by one year
of age. About 30% of IH are noticed at birth and
70–90% appear during the first four weeks of life.
The majority of hemangiomas occur sporadically;
however, familial occurrence of IH has been reported.

Although IH can be seen in all races, they are more
common in Caucasian infants, and less common in
those of African or Asian descent. In a prospective
cohort study ongoing in the United States, data in
1058 patients revealed that 68.9% of patients were
Caucasian, 14.4% were Hispanic and 2.8% were
African-American. The female-to-male ratio was
2.4:1.0, which is similar to the previously published
ratio. Premature babies and those with a low birth
weight have a significantly higher incidence of IH.

According to the new clinical classification proposed by Chiller, distribution of IH according to the
different types are: localized 72%, segmental 18%,
indeterminate 9%, and multifocal 3%. Twenty-four
percent of patients experience complications related
to their hemangiomas. Ulceration is the most common complication (16%), followed by threat to vision (5.6%), airway obstruction (1.4%), auditory canal
obstruction (0.6%) and cardiac compromise (0.4%).

PHACE, a neurocutaneous syndrome that refers to
the association of large, plaque-like, "segmental" hemangiomas of the face, with one or more of other anomalies, represents about 2 to 3% of patients with IH overall, and at least 20% of patients with segmental IH of
the face. Cerebral and cerebrovascular anomalies of
PHACE are the greatest potential source of morbidity.

Concepts

Hemangiomas of infancy (HOI) are the most common benign tumors in children. The incidence in the
general newborn population is between 1.1% and
2.6%, but increases to up to 12% by one year of age
[1]. About 30% of HOI are noted at birth and 70–90%
will appear during the first four weeks of life [1].

Prior to 1980, the nomenclature used to describe
vascular birthmarks, including hemangiomas, was
confusing due to the lack of both a uniformly accepted classification and a clear understanding of the
natural history of these birthmarks [2]. No prospective
studies examining the incidence of hemangiomas have
been published for several decades. The nomenclature
used to describe lesions has not been uniform between
studies. In 1982, Mulliken and Glowacki [3] helped to
clarify this confusion and proposed a biological classification of vascular anomalies: as either hemangiomas
or malformations, based on clinical appearance, cellular features and natural history. A key feature of this
classification is rapid neonatal growth phase followed
by gradual involution. A modification of this classification was adopted by the International Society for the
Study of Vascular Anomalies in 1996 [4]. A clear distinction was drawn between vascular tumors, which are
characterized by endothelial proliferation, and malformations, which are true errors in vascular morphogenesis with little endothelial mitotic activity.

Kilcline and Frieden [5], in an interesting and systematic review of medical literature of HOI, explained the methodological limitations of the few relevant studies which make it impossible to determine
the true incidence of HOI. This is due to problems
in definition, study design and population selection.
The authors think the incidence of HOI is lower than
10% and likely closer to 4–5%.

R. Mattassi, D.A. Loose, M. Vaghi (eds.), *Hemangiomas and Vascular Malformations*.
© Springer-Verlag Italia 2009

Ideally, studies should include a careful skin examination at around 3 to 4 months of age, a time where nearly all HOI are apparent.

Although HOI can be seen in all races, they are more common in Caucasian infants, but are less common in those of African or Asian descent. It is the commonest childhood vascular tumor seen in Singapore [6].

HOI exhibit a female preponderance [7] and it is widely accepted that HOI are more frequent in premature infants, especially in those weighing less than 1500 g [7–9]. In a prospective cohort study ongoing in the United States, data from 1058 patients revealed that 68.9% of patients were Caucasian and non Hispanic and there was a low proportion of African-Americans (2.8%), while 14.4% were Hispanic patients. The female-to-male ratio was 2.4:1.0, which is similar to the previously published ratio. The cause of this is unknown, but may be related to hormonal differences.

Premature birth and low birth weight were significantly more common in children with HOI: 20% were preterm (defined as younger than 37 weeks gestational age); 5.7% were very preterm (defined as younger than 32 weeks gestational age); 5.3% had very low birth weight (defined as less 1500 g), 13.3% had low birth weight (defined as 1500–2499 g) and 81.5% had normal birth weight (defined as less or equal to 2500 g) [10].

Chorionic villus sampling (CVS) during pregnancy has also been suggested to result in a higher risk of hemangioma development [11, 12]. In this study only a small group of patients (3.5%) had this antecedent. On the other hand, amniocentesis and transabdominal CVS does not produce a significant difference in hemangioma incidence [13].

There is preliminary evidence to indicate that elevated maternal age, multiple gestations, placenta previa and pre-eclampsia might also be risk factors for the development of HOI [12].

The majority of hemangiomas occur sporadically, as evidenced by a review of the literature by Burns et al. [14]; a recent study showed that the incidence of HOI in monozygotic and dizygotic twin pairs does not differ statistically [15].

Nonetheless, familial occurrence of HOI has been reported. Blei et al. [16] documented the autosomal dominant transmission of HOI and vascular malformations in six kindred and the locus involved has been identified at 5q 31–33 [17].

During the last few years, HOI have been classified into three groups according to the level of the affected skin: superficial, deep, and mixed hemangiomas.

Chiller et al. [18] proposed a new clinical classification, in which HOI were divided into four groups: localized, segmental, indeterminate, and multifocal hemangiomas.

Segmental hemangiomas were those hemangiomas or clusters of hemangiomas with a configuration corresponding to a recognizable and/or significant portion of a developmental segment.

A segmental hemangioma was defined as a hemangioma with plaque-like morphology, showing linear and/or geographic patterning over a specific cutaneous territory.

Localized hemangiomas were defined as those hemangiomas that seem to grow from a single focal point or were localized to an area without any apparent linear or developmental configuration.

Indeterminate hemangiomas were those that were not readily classified as either localized or segmental.

Lastly, multifocal hemangiomas were defined as such when more than ten cutaneous hemangiomas were present.

Chiller et al. [18] did a prospective study reviewing 327 patients in an ambulatory referral center. The results of the 472 hemangiomas studied were as follows: 72% were localized, 18% were segmental, 9% indeterminate and 3% multifocal.

They found that segmental lesions had a higher frequency of complications and associated abnormalities. This type of hemangioma seems to be present with increased frequency in Hispanic infants.

The most frequent complication is ulceration, but hemangiomas may also affect ophthalmologic, auditory, or respiratory functions.

Haggstrom et al. [19], in a prospective cohort study in 1058 children with HOI, reported similar findings.

The majority of hemangiomas were classified as localized (66.8%), whereas 13.1% were segmental, 16.5% were indeterminate and 3.6% were multifocal.

Twenty-four percent of patients experienced complications related to their hemangioma(s) and 38% of our patients received some form of treatment during the study period.

Of the complications found during the study period, ulceration was the most common (16%); threat to vision was found in 5.6%; airway obstruction in 1.4%; auditory canal obstruction in 0.6%; and cardiac compromise in 0.4%. Hepatic hemangiomas were detected in 0.1% of the patients. Patients with segmental hemangiomas were 11 times more likely to experience complications and eight times more likely to receive treatment than those with localized hemangiomas, even when controlled for size.

The authors concluded that although both size and location were important predictors, morphologic subtype was the best single predictor for development of complications and need for treatment. Demographic and perinatal factors, including gender, ethnicity, prematurity, birth weight, family history, and maternal chronic illness did not predict higher rates of complications or need for treatment [20].

In a prospective study of 252 patients with hemangiomas we described demographic, prenatal and perinatal characteristics [21]. We found a female predominance (71.5%); males represented 28.5% of the patients; 39% were Caucasian and 61% were Latin American.

The study found a positive family history of vascular lesions in 16.6% of cases: 87.5% had hemangiomas, while 2.8% of cases were the product of multiple gestations. The median birth weight was 2875 g, and only 22.68% presented low birth weight (defined as 1500–2499 g). A very low birth weight (less than 1500g) was present in 7.5% of cases.

Of these patients, 3.9% were born prematurely (defined as younger than 37 weeks gestational age) and 0.78% were born very prematurely (defined as younger than 32 weeks gestational age). Obstetric antecedents were relevant in 37.6% of the cases and perinatal pathology was observed in 4.3%.

The head and neck were the most commonly affected locations (72.5%). Sacrococcygeal and trunk locations were found in 11% and limb involvement in 5.5%.

The number of lesions ranged between 1 and 47, but 75% of the patients had three hemangiomas or less. In 45% of the cases, the lesions were present at birth.

Most patients had localized lesions (94%). Seven percent were segmental, 7% multifocal and 3% indeterminate. We found, however, increased morbidity, associated anomalies, and less favorable outcomes with segmental hemangiomas than with the other lesion types.

Consultation was more frequent during the first year of life.

Ulceration was the most frequent complication (36.5%); and more observable in segmental lesions.

Other important features were bleeding, ophthalmologic impairment, auditory canal occlusion, airway compromise, and visceral involvement.

Treatment with oral antibiotics and corticosteroids was needed in 26.6% of the patients and in three cases local corticoid infiltration was necessary.

Seven patients had associated abnormalities. In three cases we arrived at a diagnosis of PHACE association. Hypergalactosemia was another important pathology associated with multifocal hemangiomas.

Five of our patients also had cutaneous vascular malformations (port wine stain). Evidence for this association had been previously described by Garzon

et al. [22]. The complication rates and associated anomalies in our study were high.

Segmental HOI are plaque-like and show linear or geographic "patterning" over the skin. The patterns observed in facial segmental HOI do not appear to correspond to facial dermatomes or lines of Blaschko, but they do correspond at least partially to developmental facial prominences [23]

PHACE (OMIM# 606519) is a neurocutaneous syndrome that refers to the association of large, plaque-like, "segmental" hemangiomas of the face, with one or more of the following anomalies: posterior fossa brain malformations, arterial cerebrovascular anomalies, cardiovascular anomalies, eye anomalies, and ventral developmental defects, specifically sternal defects and/or supraumbilical raphe [24]. The etiology and pathogenesis of PHACE is unknown, and potential risk factors for the syndrome have not been systematically studied.

Recent studies estimate that PHACE probably represents about 2% to 3% of patients with HOI overall, and at least 20% of patients with segmental HOI of the face [25, 26].

Although the true incidence of PHACE is unknown, this syndrome is uncommon, but not rare, and may be as common, or more so, than Sturge-Weber syndrome, a more well-known neurocutaneous syndrome.

Metry et al. [27] undertook a prospective cohort study of 1096 children with hemangiomas, 25 of whom met criteria for PHACE. Compared to previous reports, our PHACE patients had a higher incidence of cerebrovascular and cardiovascular anomalies.

PHACE patients represented 2.3% of children with hemangiomas in this study. In comparison, they were of slightly older gestational age and born to slightly older mothers, and were even more likely to be female. None of the patients was a product of a multiple gestation, our incidence of placenta previa was low and none of our mothers had a history of pre-eclampsia.

The underlying pathogenesis of PHACE syndrome is unknown. A strong female predominance exists, leading some to suggest that PHACE may represent an X-chromosome linked dominant condition, with potential lethality in male patients. However, no familial cases have been reported.

The 78% female incidence noted in this study is lower than prior reports, but still substantiates the known marked female predominance in PHACE.

Metry et al. [28] reported 17 male infants with PHACE syndrome and reviewed a database of 270 published PHACE reports. They compared the incidence of syndrome-associated anomalies between 59 reports of male patients with PHACE syndrome (17 new and 42 published) versus 213 published reports of female patients with PHACE. They found only a statistically significant difference for structural brain anomalies, which were more common in male patients.

The structural cerebral and cerebrovascular anomalies of PHACE are not only the most common findings of the syndrome, but also the greatest potential source of morbidity. They may result in acquired, progressive vessel stenosis and acute ischemic stroke.

In conclusion, methodological limitations of the few relevant studies which do exist make it impossible to determine the true incidence of HOI. In the future it will be necessary to do prospective epidemiologic studies on primary care settings in different countries using the currently accepted classification of vascular lesions.

Data on demographic and perinatal factors, including gender, ethnicity, prematurity, birth weight, family history, maternal chronic disease, size and location of hemangiomas should be included to determine the possible risk factor and the true incidence of this common vascular tumor of infancy.

References

1. Jacobs AH, Walton RG (1976) The incidence of birthmarks in the neonate. Pediatrics 58:218–222
2. Waner M, Suen JY (1999) The natural history of hemangiomas. In: Waner M, Suen JY (eds) Hemangiomas and vascular malformations of the head and neck. Wiley-Liss, New York, pp 13–46
3. Finn MC, Glowacki J, Mulliken JB (1983) Congenital vascular lesions: clinical application of a new classification. J Pediatr Surg 18:894–899
4. Enjolras O, Mulliken JB (1997) Vascular tumors and vascular malformations (new issues). Adv Dermatol 13:375–423
5. Kilcline C, Frieden IJ (2008) Infantile hemangiomas: how common are they? A systematic review of the medical literature. Pediatr Dermatol 25:168–173
6. Guidelines of care for cutaneous haemangiomas: Chan YC, Giam YC (2005) Ann Acad Med Singapore 34:117–123
7. Mulliken JB, Fishman SJ, Burrows PE (2000) Vascular anomalies. Curr Probl Surg 37:517–584
8. Powell TG, West CR, Pharoah PO, Cooke RW (1987) Epidemiology of strawberry haemangioma in low birth-weight infants. Br J Dermatol 116:635–641
9. Drolet BA, Haggstrom AN, Baselga E et al (2004) Risk factors for haemangioma of infancy – A cohort prospective study. 15th International Society for the Study of Vascular Anomalies, Wellington, New Zealand (abstract)
10. The hemangioma investigator group: Haggstrom AN, Drolet BA et al (2007) Prospective study of hemangiomas: demographic, prenatal, and perinatal characteristics. J Pediatr 150:291–294
11. Drolet BA, Haggstrom AN, Baselga E et al (2004) Risk factors for haemangioma of infancy – A cohort prospective study. 15th International Society for the Study of Vascular Anomalies, Wellington, New Zealand (abstract)
12. Burton BK, Schulz CJ, Angle B, Burd LI (1995) An increased incidence of haemangiomas in infants born following chorionic villus sampling (CVS). Prenat Diagn 15:209–214
13. Van der Vleuten C, Bauland CG, Bartelink LR et al (2004) The effect of amniocentesis and choriovillus sampling on the incidence of haemangiomas. 15th International Society for the Study of Vascular Anomalies, Wellington, New Zealand (abstract)
14. Burns AJ, Kaplan LC, Mulliken JB (1991) Is there an association between hemangioma and syndromes with dysmorphic features? Pediatrics 88(6):1257–1267
15. Cheung DS, Warman ML, Mulliken JB (1997) Hemangioma in twins. Ann Plast Surg 38(3):269–274
16. Blei F, Walter J, Orlow SJ, Marchuk DA (1998) Familial segregation of hemangiomas and vascular malformations as an autosomal dominant trait. Arch Dermatol 134:718–722
17. Walter JW, Blei F, Anderson JL et al (1999) Genetic mapping of a novel familial form of infantile hemangioma. Am J Med Genet 82:77–83
18. Chiller KG, Passaro D, Frieden IJ (2002) Hemangiomas of infancy: clinical characteristics morphologic subtypes and their relationship to race ethnicity and sex. Arch Dermatol 138:1567–1576
19. Haggstrom AN, Drolet BA, Baselga E et al (2006) Prospective study of infantile hemangiomas: clinical characteristics predicting complications and treatment. Pediatrics 118:882–887
20. Waner M, North PE, Scherer KA, Frieden IJ et al (2003) The nonrandom distribution of facial hemangiomas. Arch Dermatol 139:869–875
21. Cordisco MR, Castro C, Pierini (2008) Hemangioma of infancy: prospective study of 252 patients. 17th international Workshop on Vascular Anomalies, Boston (abstract)
22. Garzon MC, Enjorlas O, Frieden IJ (2000) Vascular tumors and vascular malformations: Evidence for an association. J Am Acad Dermatol 42:275–279
23. Haggstrom AN, Lammer EJ, Schneider RA et al (2006) Patterns of infantile hemangiomas: New clues to hemangioma pathogenesis and embryonic facial development. Pediatrics 117:698–703
24. Frieden IJ, Reese V, Cohen D (1996) PHACE syndrome: The association of posterior fossa brain malformations, hemangiomas, arterial anomalies, coarctation of the aorta and cardiac defects, and eye abnormalities. Arch Dermatol 132:307–311

25. Metry DW, Dowd CF, Barkovich AJ, Frieden IJ (2001) The many faces of PHACE syndrome [published correction appears in J Pediatr 139:117–123]
26. Phan TA, Adms S, Wargon O (2006) Segmental hemangiomas of infancy: a review of 14 cases. Autralas J Dermatol 47:242–247
27. Metry DW, Haggstrom BA, Baselga E et al (2006) A prospective study of PHACE syndrome in infantile hemangiomas: demographic features clinical findings and complications. Am J Med Gen 140A:975–986
28. Metry DW, Siegel DH, Cordisco MR et al (2008) A comparison of disease severity among affected male versus female patients with PHACE syndrome. J Am Acad Dermatol 58:81–87

Classification of Infantile Hemangiomas and Other Congenital Vascular Tumors

4

Hans Peter Berlien

Abstract

Congenital vascular tumors have a wide variety of origins. The most common congenital vascular tumor is the GLUT-1 positive infantile hemangioma. This has to be differentiated from the congenital hemangioendothelioma. While the majority of infantile hemangiomas have a high rate of spontaneous regression, severe complications are possible and it is important to identify the dangerous forms as early as possible and start early treatment to prevent secondary complications.

Introduction

The general term "strawberry hemangioma" covers a series of diverse hereditary vascular abnormalities. In order to determine the type of therapeutic procedure to employ – active or restrained – early differentiation is essential [1]. Infantile hemangiomas are proliferating embryonal tumors that possibly stem from placental tissue or resemble it (they are GLUT-1-positive). Congenital hemangioendotheliomas are not part of the infantile hemangiomas and are GLUT-1-negative. Both have to be differentiated from arterial, venous, lymphatic and combined vascular malformations, including glomangiomas and systemic congenital glomangiomatosis such as hamartomatous abnormalities. They show no spontaneous regression but rather steady growth, with the exception of the abortive forms of port-wine stains (PWS) such as Unna's nevi, certain forms of cutis marmorata telangiectatica and isolated monocytic lymphangiomas of the neck, such as hygroma colli.

Classification of Congenital Vascular Tumors

Infantile hemangiomas (IH) have to be classified according to stage, growth pattern, appearance and organ specificity. Congenital hemangioendotheliomas (HE) are classified according to their progression, growth pattern, appearance and organ specificity, while vascular malformations (VM) have to be classified according to their growth pattern, appearance and organ specificity, but also according to the embryological disorder and their predominant vascular origin [2]. This means that a common feature of all congenital vascular abnormalities is that they can appear in all organs and regions of the body. Another joint feature is that they can appear in singular, multiple or disseminated forms and may vary in their growth pattern, with well-demarcated to diffuse infiltrating shapes. Any classification therefore has to answer the three central questions: what, where and how (Table 4.1). The "Hamburg Classification" has become the standard procedure for classification of vascular malformations [1]. Because of the sometimes difficult differential diagnosis, a classification of congenital vascular tumors should be modeled accordingly.

Stage/Type ("What")

Infantile Hemangioma

Prodromal Phase

Clinical Symptoms

Infantile hemangiomas (IH) (Fig. 4.1) only appear days or weeks after birth, but about half of them show precursor lesions such as circumscribed telangiectasias, anemic, reddish-blue or blue maculae and

R. Mattassi, D.A. Loose, M. Vaghi (eds.), *Hemangiomas and Vascular Malformations*.
© Springer-Verlag Italia 2009

Table 4.1. Classification of congenital vascular anomalies. The three major questions of what, where and how are valid both for vascular malformations and for congenital vascular tumors. Therefore this classification follows the Hamburg Classification of vascular malformations

	Vascular Tumor		Vascular Malformation		
	Infantile hemangioma	**Hemangio-endothelioma**	**Origin**	**Embryological defect**	**Compartment**
What	Stage I Prodromal II Initial III Proliferation IV Maturation V Regression	Type Rapid involuting (RICH) Non involuting (NICH) "Tufted" angioma Kaposiform	Venous Lymphatic Arterial Arteriovenous Capillary Mixed	Aplasia Hypoplasia Dysplasia Hyperplasia Hamartoma	Truncular Extratruncular
Where	Intra/subcutaneous Intracranial	Intra/submucous Parenchymatous	*Organ* Intramuscular Intracavitar	Intraosseous/intra-articular Mesenterial	
Singular			*Number* Multiple		Disseminated
	Peri/intra-orbital Perimammary	Peri/intra-auricular Peri/enoral Anogenital/intra-anal/ intestinal	*Localization* Laryngo-tracheal Trunk (other)	Face (other) Acral/hand/feet	Head/neck Extremities (other)
How	Limited		*Growth* Moderate infiltrative		High infiltrative
	Exulceration Excess growth	Infection Bleeding Cardiac failure Vent. obstruction Feeding problems	*Complication* Intravasc. coagulopathy Intestinal obstruction	Assoc. defects Visual obstruction	

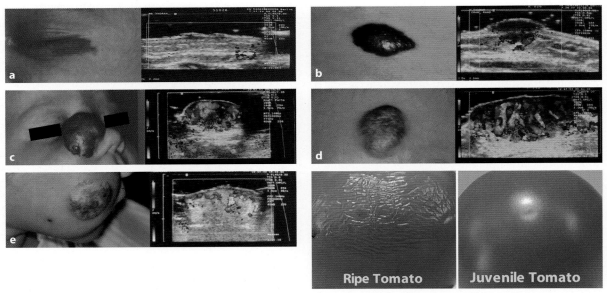

Fig. 4.1. The typical clinical and sonographic findings of the different stages of the infantile hemangioma. **a** I Prodromal Phase. Clinically no difference to PWS (*left*) but the ultrasound (*right*) shows a ballooning of the dermis which is never found in PWS. **b** II Initial phase: the early onset (*left*) looks like a fresh tomato with a shiny surface. Note that the dermal part and the subcutaneous part can have different stages (*right*). **c** III Proliferation phase: clinically the cutis shows regression (*left*), but subcutaneously the color-coded duplex sonography (CCDS) shows increasing microcirculation as a sign of aggressivity (*right*). **d** IV Maturation phase: the dermis shows shrinking like a ripe tomato (*left*), the CCDS shows development of larger drainage veins (*right*). **e** V Regression phase: clinically remaining teleangiectasias can occur (*left*), the CCDS shows hypersonic areas with enlarged veins (*right*)

port-wine stain lesions [3]. They sometimes cannot be detected, particularly in newborns with a high hematocrit or hyperbilirubinemia. Color-coded duplex sonography (CCDS) does not yet provide a typical result, but in case of intracutaneous manifestation, there is sometimes already a ballooning of the dermal double lamina structure (Table 4.2).

Differential Diagnoses

Pronounced lesions at birth should include the differential diagnosis "congenital hemangioendothelioma" or "vascular malformation". A port-wine stain is already evident at birth as a macular reddening of differing extents and on ultrasound reflects no disintegration of the normal double laminar structure. This is a decisive differential diagnostic criterion for the prodromal phase of infantile hemangioma. In addition, port-wine stains in newborns almost never progress, so that an increase in color intensity, size or a change in the typical skin texture is almost proof of the presence of the most aggressive form of infantile hemangioma (Fig. 4.2).

Initial Phase

Clinical Symptoms

In the early or initial phase, infantile hemangiomas may partially appear within a few days. Depending on the type of growth, limited or infiltrative (see below),

Table 4.2. Classification of infantile hemangioma. Correlation of clinic and CCDS

Stage	Clinic	CCDS
I. Prodromal phase	Red/white spot; teleangiectasia blurred swelling	Structureless; low echo space; no signs of pathological vessels
II. Initial phase	Loss of typical skin structure; increasing thickness and induration	Hyposonoric center; hypervascularization beginning at edges
III. Proliferation phase	Bright red cutaneous infiltration; flat spreading subcutaneous growth of thickness; infiltration of surroundings possibly even at organ borders	Increasing intratumoral hyperperfusion; center vessel density; nutrition tumor vessels; drainage veins with arterial flow profile
IV. Maturation phase	Pale and livid color; possible central exulceration; decreasing growth	Declining central vessel density; increasing ectatic drainage veins; declining arterialization of drainage veins; central increasing hypersonore
V. Regression phase	Hypopigmentation; wrinkled skin/teleangiectasis; surrounding subcutaneous drainage veins; subcutaneous palpable induration	Circumscribed hypersonoric area; loss of typical tissue structure; nearly no central tumor vessels; residuals supplying tumor arteries; residuals of ectatic drainage veins

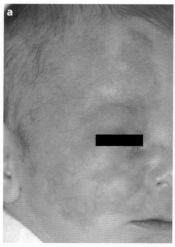 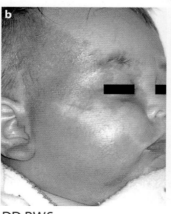 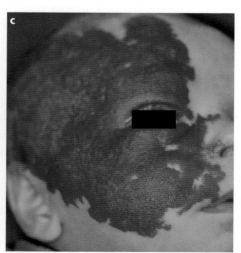

At birth   DD PWS   At the age of 1 month

Fig. 4.2. Infantile hemangioma. **a** Prodromal phase. **b** Clinical findings after 1 month. **c** The differential diagnosis of PWS and infantile hemangioma is that in PWS at birth there are never ectasic veins

they are diffuse, infiltrating the surrounding tissue or, in case of limited growth, are sharply demarcated. The latter frequently clearly protrude from the skin, are light reddish in color and shine brightly, causing parents to show these to a physician more readily than the infiltrative hemangiomas. By CCDS often only a diffuse hyposonic structure will be seen, similar to the image of a fresh hematoma without visible vessels or capillarization. In intracutaneous hemangiomas, the typical double lamina structure of the skin vanishes.

Differential Diagnoses

The venous malformation is also rarely very pronounced at birth with little tissue proliferation, so that in newborns a venous malformation is easily "squeezable", in contrast to an infantile hemangioma. Early forms of angiokeratomas and a lymphangioma circumscriptum can be easily differentiated from the initial phases of infantile hemangiomas simply by their rather livid color.

Proliferation Phase

Clinical Symptoms

During the proliferation phase, a cutaneously located hemangioma proliferates at a different pace while spreading in size, by exophytic or endophytic subcutaneous growth, sometimes also in combination. Hemangiomas of limited growth usually only expand minimally. Primary subcutaneous hemangiomas appear at a later stage and grow for a longer period of time. The co-existence of two forms is common, whereby a dissociated growth of the two parts is possible. With CCDS, hypercapillarizations can now be seen: the stronger they are, the more active the proliferation of the hemangioma. Thus, CCDS is the only method with which to dependably check the activity and aggressiveness of an infantile hemangioma. In addition to hypersonic parts which are already regressing, hyposonic, early proliferative parts may exist in the very same hemangioma (Fig. 4.3). In case of very excessive growth, secondary capillarization cannot keep up, so there may be trophic disturbances with exulcerations.

Differential Diagnosis

The hereditary glomangioma is already dark-bluish at birth, as infantile hemangiomas only appear in their late phases. Congenital glomangiomas are actin antibody positive and thus clearly differ from the late phases of infantile hemangiomas, which always, even after regression, remain GLUT-1-positive.

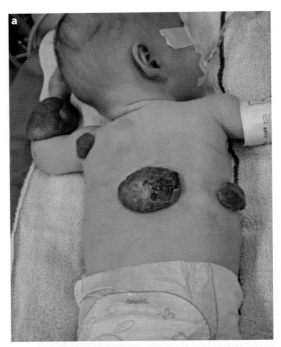

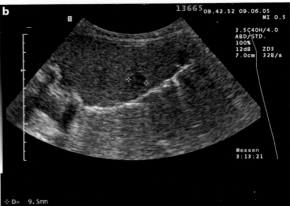

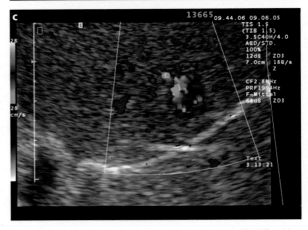

Fig. 4.3. "Benign" neonatal hemangiomatosis (BNH). **a** Not all infantile hemangiomas regress spontaneously, some grow rapidly with complications, such as ulcerations. **b** Even in BNH liver hemangiomas can occur. **c** The CCDS shows the typical hyperperfusion in the hemangioma

Maturation Phase

Clinical Symptoms

A maturation phase follows in which proliferation comes to a halt. In intracutaneous hemangiomas, this can be seen by a reduction of the bulk and accompanying wrinkles of the epidermis. In addition, gray regression areas form in the dark red hemangioma. The tissue is rather plastic: sonography reveals hypersonic areas as signs of maturation. Duplex sonography, on the one hand, shows that microcirculation decreases, on the other, drainage veins are formed, which usually run vertical to the surface. If a biopsy is performed at this point, the pathologist finds large veins with only a single-layered endothelium, which are responsible for the term "cavernous hemangioma". They can trigger ulceration by the steal effect. The smaller the distance from these drainage veins to the epidermis, the greater the risk.

Differential Diagnosis

The bluish color of pure subcutaneous infantile hemangiomas also may occur in venous vascular malformations, but this it not expressible and with CCDS shows ectatic caverns with little or no spontaneous flow.

Regression Phase

Clinical Symptoms

The regression phase is usually finished by the sixth birthday as a rule faster in cutaneous localized hemangiomas than in diffuse infiltrating cutaneous or subcutaneous hemangiomas. CCDS is now hypersonic as an expression of a fibrolipomatous transformation. Large, reticular veins remain in the vicinity for a number of years; these appear as a secondary change and show normal vessel walls. Small hemangiomas, which at the end of the proliferation phase and the beginning of regression had not yet caused secondary destruction of the surrounding tissue, can completely heal without residues. Larger hemangiomas often leave telangiectasias, areas of atrophic, multiple foldable skin, cutis laxa, hyper- or hypopigmentations or prune belly-like lumps of fibrolipomatous tissue. The larger the hemangioma prior to the entry into the quiescent and regressive phase, the more pronounced the residue.

Table 4.3. Differential diagnosis (DD) of congenital vascular tumors. In atypical clinical courses, other congenital malignant tumors should be considered

Hemangioma (esp. primary subcutaneous hemangioma)
DD: Congenital hemangioendothelioma (kapoisform, tufted angioma, RICH, NICH)
DD: Glomangioma/-atosis
DD: Eruptive angioma
DD: Skin metastasis of congenital neuroblastoma
DD: Hemangiosarcoma, teratoma

Vascular Malformation
DD: Secondary varicosis
DD: Kaposiform congenital hemangioendothelioma
DD: Rhabdomyosarcoma
DD: Angiolipoma
DD: Neurofibromatosis
DD: Proteus

Differential Diagnosis

An infantile hemangioma will not become active again after regression. There is no recurrence. A hemangioma which begins or develops during infancy is not an infantile hemangioma. The most probable differential diagnoses are vascular malformations, but also vasculitis, and cutaneous metastases of malignant tumors may have to be excluded by a biopsy. Plexiform neurofibromas may appear as part of a venous or lymphatic malformation (Table 4.3).

Congenital Hemangioendothelioma (HE)

The congenital hemangioendothelioma is a real vascular tumor [4], but has to be differentiated from the hemangioendothelioma of adults, as the acquired ("adult") hemangioendothelioma belongs to the "borderline" tumors with uncertain biological behavior, whereas a congenital hemangioendothelioma has never been reported to have turned malignant [5]. Unlike in the case of the infantile hemangioma, the primary intracutaneous form is less common, but in case of aggressive growth, a secondary involvement of the dermis is possible. The clinical appearance of the cutis marmorata may be similar to the dermal findings of a congenital hemangioendothelioma, but the cutis marmorata lacks subcutaneous proliferation. Depending on their proliferation pattern, entirely different forms must be differentiated before establishing the indication for any therapy. During healing, spontaneously or following therapy, they all show the same picture: atrophy of the subcutis to the fascia and cutis laxa (Table 4.4).

Table 4.4. Differential diagnostic algorithm of the appearance of first symptoms, color and consistency, but not the course of the treated or untreated disease. The algorithm gives a probability of a diagnosis

	Time														Color								Consistency									
	Prepartal	Partal	Postpartal	1M	3M	6M	9M	12M	2Y	4Y	8Y	16Y	25Y	35Y	Pale red	Dark red	Livid	Bluish	Petechial	Stained	Mappy	Grey	No changes	Chalasia	Atrophied	Bulging elastic	Tough	Pasty	Squeezeable	Buzzing	Hyperthermic	Hypothermic
Vascular tumors																																
Infantile hemangioma (IH)																																
Prodromal phase			━	━	━										X								X									
Initial phase			━	━	━	━									X											X			X		X	
Proliferation phase				━	━	━	━	━								X										X					X	
Maturation phase						━	━	━	━							X											X		X			
Regression phase						━	━	━	━	━	━											X		X			X					X
Cong. hemangioendothelioma (HE)																																
RICH	━	━	━															X		X		X	X	X		X						
NICH	━	━	━														X												X			
"Tufted angioma"						━	━	━	━												X								X			
Kaposiform KHE	━	━	━														X			X	X								X		X	
Vasc. malformation																																
Hamartoma																																
Glomangioma	━	━	━	━								━	━				X										X					X
Angioma racemosum											━	━	━			X				X							X		X	X	X	
Lymph-angiokeratoma	━	━	━	━	━	━	━	━	━	━	━				X		X		X								X	X				
Extratruncular																																
PWS	━	━	━	━											X					X	X		X									
Cutis marmorata	━	━	━	━	━	━	━	━									X				X					X						X
Truncular																																
Lymphangioma	━	━									━	━	━				X	X				X							X			
Venous malformation	━	━	━	━	━	━	━	━									X												X			X
AV malformation	━	━	━	━						━	━	━	━	━		X				X							X			X		X
	Time of appearance of first clinical signs, not the course of the treated or untreated anomaly																															

The Rapidly Involuting Congenital Hemangioendothelioma (RICH)

This tumor is totally matured prenatally ("prenatal mature hemangioma") and should be clearly differentiated from an infantile hemangioma because it is negative for GLUT-1. Because of its bluish hue which often shines through the skin, it is often mistaken for a venous vascular malformation. However, unlike this malformation, which at birth is always soft and "squeezable", the congenital hemangioendothelioma is tough. Ultrasound reveals the initial fibrosis as a hypersonic area. Intratumoral vessels are rare and frequently there are bowl-like veins. Unlike the pure venous vascular malformation, which is usually hypothermic due to blood pooling, thermography shows a normothermic image. The skin above may be shimmering and bulging, but there are never any inflammatory symptoms. Within a few days of birth, the spontaneous regression begins, noticeable by a decrease in turgor. Regression as a rule is completed within three months, but as a primary destructive tumor of the subcutis, it leaves a lesion in the subcutaneous tissue with chalasis of the dermis on top and occasionally muscle atrophy and an atrophy of the fascia below due to the pressure (Fig. 4.4). A teratoma must be excluded by differential diagnosis, especially in case of presacral localization.

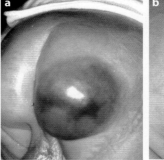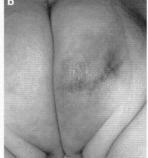

Fig. 4.4. Rapid involuting congenital hemangioendothelioma (RICH). **a** Clinical picture at birth. **b** Clinical picture at 6 months. Clinically difficult to discriminate from a teratoma, the CCDS shows typical signs. The result of spontaneous healing is, as in all other congenital hemangioendotheliomas, a chalasia of the skin and an atrophy of subcutis and fascia

The Non-involuting Congenital Hemangioendothelioma (NICH)

Contrary to RICH, NICH may be only sparsely developed at birth. The skin above is not directly infiltrated, but often shows a light bluish change in coloring along with a more pronounced telangiectasia. This sometimes makes it difficult to differentiate it from a hamartomatous extratruncular arteriovenous malformation known as angioma racemosum. Unlike the arteriovenous malformation, which by sonography always shows a massive hyperperfusion even without direct evidence of an arteriovenous shunt and in thermography shows a pronounced hyperthermia; sonography in NICH reveals – besides lobular hypersonic areas – arteries and veins running vertically to the surface, and thermography shows a clear but rather weak hyperthermia. In the first few years of the child's life there is progressive growth, increased by infections. In some cases, there is spontaneous regression, recognizable in the sonography by an increasing fibrosis and a decrease in vascularization, and similar to RICH, a remainder of a chalasia of the cutis and an atrophy of the subcutaneous fat. On the other hand, as long as NICH is still active, transition to a Kaposi-like hemangioendothelioma is possible at any time with the formation of a Kasabach-Merritt syndrome. Therefore, in all NICH patients, regular control of thrombocytes and, if necessary, clotting parameters is mandatory.

The "Tufted Angioma"

It is not yet clear if the "tufted angioma" is a separate entity to the congenital hemangioendothelioma or only a delayed occurrence of a NICH variation. Ultrasound reveals separate lobular structures with vessels along the edges. Multiple lesions are reported in the "tufted angioma" (Fig. 4.5).

The Kaposi-like Congenital Hemangioendothelioma (KHE)

At birth, a result similar to NICH may be seen. In most cases, however, the skin covering the tumor does not show any signs of infection, but a tough infiltration which, besides erysipelas, is differential-diagnostically reminiscent of a mixed intracutaneous-subcutaneous lymphangioma ("wasp sting symptom") (Fig. 4.6). Thermography shows significant hyperthermia, while ultrasound reveals almost structureless interstitial gaps sited between lobular hypersonic areas. Color-coded duplex sonography clearly shows an increased microcirculation which is not located in the center, as

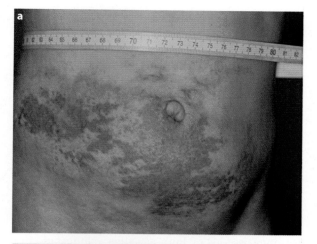
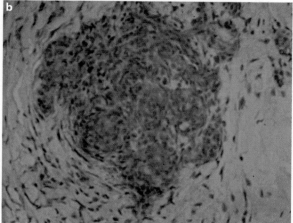

Fig. 4.5. Congenital hemangioendothelioma. **a** Disseminated late onset (before treatment). **b** Typical histological findings

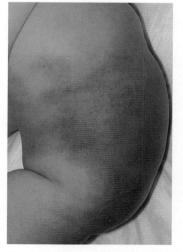

Fig. 4.6. Early transition of NICH into kaposiform hemangioendothelioma. In spite of massive swelling with local pain (wasp sting syndrome), there are no general symptoms of disease, but continuously decreasing thrombocytes and normal clotting parameters

in active infantile hemangiomas, but at the lobuli divided by septa. There are no symptoms at this point.

Clinical and sonographic signs are present before the beginning of a disseminated intravascular coagulopathy in Kasabach-Merritt symptoms, so that at this point thrombocytes and fibrinogen or rather fibrin degradation products may still be quite normal (Fig. 4.7).

Organ/Number/Localization ("Where")

Organs

An intra-osseous or intra-articular manifestation of hemangioma described in the literature is probably a faulty classification and has been ascribed to vascular malformations. Otherwise all soft tissue, solid organs or hollow viscera can be affected (Table 4.5). Most commonly affected are certainly the cutis and subcutis, but the mucous membranes and submucosa of the aerodigestive tract and the urogenital and anogenital region can be affected as well. Of the parenchymal organs, the liver is mainly affected, particularly in case of multiple hemangiomas [6]. The parotid gland and the mammary glands are seldom affected primarily by the infantile hemangioma, but excessively proliferating infantile hemangiomas can lead to secondary displacement or infiltration.

Hemangioendotheliomas affect soft tissue rather than the cutis. If body cavities (pleura and peritoneum) or the lungs are affected, or in case of an intracranial effect in the meninx, an infantile hemangioma is unlikely and a malignant neoplasm should be ruled out by biopsy. The most important differential diagnosis besides (a benign) congenital systemic glomangiomatosis (glomuvenous malformation) is a congenital neuroblastoma (stage IV).

Number

Even though a single site is the rule in most children, several infantile hemangiomas may also develop, possibly at different times. For this reason, if there are more than three infantile hemangiomas, a thorough check-up should be performed, clinically and with the aid of ultrasound, to identify occult hemangiomas, particularly in the liver, as early as possible.

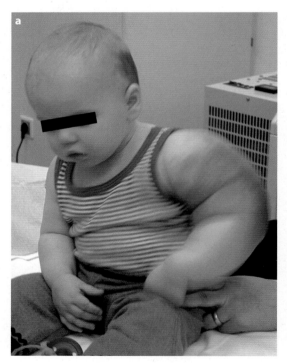

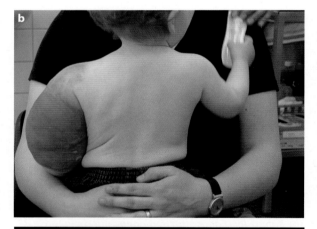

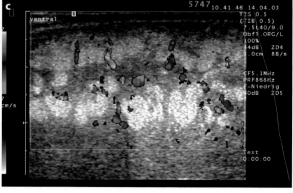

Fig. 4.7. Hemangioendothelioma. **a, b** Early onset of a kaposiform hemangioendothelioma. **c** CCDS shows interstitial hypersonoric areas with palisade like vessels which are pathognomonic for congenital hemangioendothelioma

Table 4.5. Evaluation of vascular tumors. These different criteria are not equally important, but as an indication for therapy they are counted for their risk of complication

What					Where				How		
IH Phase		HE Type		Organ		Number		Localization		Growth	Complication
Prodromal	2	RICH	1	Intracutan	1	Singular	1	**Life-threatening**		Limited 1	Exulceration 5
Initial	3	NICH	3	Intramucous	3	Multiple	2	Tracheal	7	Moderate Infiltrative 2	Infection 5
Proliferation	5	"Tufted angioma"	5	Subcutan	3	Disseminated	5	Pharyngeal	6	High infiltrative 3	Bleeding 10
Maturation	2	KHE	10	Submucous	4			Intestinal	5		Cardiac failure 10
Regression	1			Intramuscular	3						DIC 10
				Intraosseous	3			**High risk**			LIC 5
				Intraarticular	5			Parabulbar	4		Assoc. defects 3
				Intracranial	5			Enoral	4		Excess growth 5
				Parenchymatous	5			Intraanal	4		Vent. obstruction 10
								Columella	4		Feeding problems 5
				(mixed lesions add up)				Finger/toe	4		Intestinal obstruction 10
											Visual obstruction 10
								Medium risk			Ear obstruction 5
								Periorbital, -oral	3		
								Periauricular	3		
								Praeauricular	3		(combinations add up)
								Paranasal	3		
								Perineal	3		
								Breast	3		
								Vulva/urethra	3		
								Hand/foot	3		
								Low risk			
								Hairy head	2		
								Neck	2		
								Axilla	2		
								Perianal	2		
								Remaining face	2		
								No risk			
								Remaining Trunk	1		
								Arm/leg	1		

The systemic hemangiomatosis has a special status here. Two biologically completely different clinical courses should be noted [7]. The most common is the so-called "benign" neonatal hemangiomatosis (BNH), in which multiple tiny, pinhead size intracutaneous hemangiomas pop up within a few days and quickly stop growing. Except for tight monitoring, therapy is not required. It should be considered, however, that there also may be a few fast growing vast subcutaneous hemangiomas, which then are an indication for treatment. Rather rare is the aggressive diffuse hemangiomatosis ("disseminated neonatal hemangiomatosis" [DNH]), which may involve the organs, particularly the gastrointestinal tract and the liver (Fig. 4.8). This type more often forms primarily enlarged solitary lesions. Hemangioendotheliomas, especially RICH and NICH, tend to be solitary. Tufted hemangioendotheliomas may appear

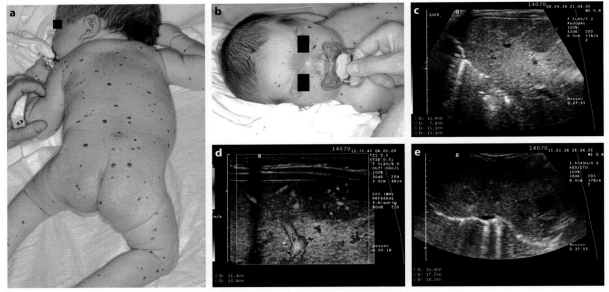

Fig. 4.8. Disseminated neonatal hemangiomatosis (DNH). **a, b** The skin involvement does not reveal the severity of the disease. **c–e** Extended clinical investigation of abdomen and cranium is mandatory (e.g., CCDS shows diffuse hemangiomatosis in the liver)

at multiple sites, the Kaposi-like hemangioendothelioma may be – besides its monstrous size – lobular, and thus seem to be multiple.

Localization

While the criteria listed so far are decisive for the diagnosis, the following determine the indication for therapy.

Besides the proliferation pattern, localization is the most important criterion for the occurrence of complications that require therapy. This is why it is of utmost importance in the score (Table 4.6).

Eyelid, peri- or intraorbital infantile hemangiomas may hamper the orbit and thus lead to irreversible amblyopy, and by compression of the eyeball lead to anisometropy and astigmatism and may be accompanied by primary cataract.

Strongly vascularized hemangiomas of the ears often cause hypertrophy of ear growth and cartilage destruction. A relocation of the ear canal may trigger infections due to fluid retention and secondary deafness. This is why all hemangiomas of the ear, peri- and preauricular, require otoscopy. Similar precautions have to be taken for the nose with the consequence of skeletal malformations or obstruction of nasal breathing. Perioral localization can hamper food intake, lead to permanent deformation of lips and, in extreme cases, to abnormalities of the lower jaw

and irregular dentition. In perioral localization and involvement of the mucous membranes of the oropharynx or the pretracheal skin, tracheal involvement must be excluded. In hemangiomas in the face, residues (ptosis, facial asymmetry) can be very irritating and lead to functional impairment depending on their size and extension. Here it is important, to initiate – by active treatment – the quiescent or regression phase as early as possible.

Hemangiomas localized in the anogenital area also have a high risk of ulceration and often cause complications such as bleeds, infections, pain and dermatitis.

Proliferation Pattern/Complications ("How")

Growth Pattern

In case of non-progressive infantile hemangiomas that are not very extensive, complications as a rule do not interfere, especially when localized on the trunk or upper and lower extremities. Hemangiomas that grow rapidly and infiltrate, on the other hand, can cause intertriginous ulcerations at all sites with the risk of secondary infections, bleeds and pain. In diffuse growing, infiltrating hemangiomas, proliferation can be very quick and there is a greater danger of remaining residues after regression. Dif-

Table 4.6. Example of therapy score from Table 4.5 for typical lesions. In cases with multiple hemangiomas, the most endangered hemangioma gives the indication. In cases with foreseeable progress the indication is broader; for example, in cases with high risk of complications there may even be an indication for adjuvant prednisolone therapy

		Phase/Type/Form	Organ	Number	Localization	Growth pattern	Complication	Score	No treatment, no control necessary	Preferably no treatment, but control necess	Close control, laser therapy in progress	Definite laser indication	Add. adjuvant systemic therapy
Grade									1	2a	2b	3	4
Ser. No	**Localization**	1-10	1-5	1-5	1-5	1-3	5-10	**Sum**	>5	6-8	9-11	<12	<15
1	Trachea	5	3	1	7	5		16					X
2	Tharynx	3	4	1	6	2		13				X	
3	Cheek	5	3	1	3	2		9	X				
4	Cheek	5	4	1	3	3	5	16					X
5	Back	2	1	1	1	1		4					
6	Breast	5	3	1	3	2	5	14				X	
7	Oral	2	4	1	4	1		10			X		
8	Leg	2	3	1	1	1		6		X			
9	Finger	3	4	1	4	2		11			X		
10	Neck	2	1	1	2	1		5	X				X
11	Neck	5	4	1	2	1		8		X			
12	Eye	5	4	1	4	3	10	22					X

fuse growing, infiltrating infantile hemangiomas of the face are described as "segmental" by some authors, although they follow neither dermatome nor nerve supply patterns. As a result, nearly a third of the diffuse infiltrating growing infantile hemangiomas of the face are classified as "not determinable" [8]. This view fails completely for the extremities, the body and the anogenital area, although proliferation in these regions does not differ from the face.

Complications

Hemangiomas of the face and head may be associated with malformations of the central nervous system (CNS) [9], the intra- and extracranial arteries, the heart, the eyes and sternal clefting (PHACES syndrome) [10]. The association with urogenital and anal malformations as well as spina bifida occulta has been described as PELVIS syndrome. The expression "syndromal hemangiomas" for these infantile hemangiomas is erroneous, and suggests that they form a separate entity of hemangiomas. In reality, these infantile hemangiomas do not differ in their phases or proliferation from other sites or in their relation to organs, but only in their biological activity. It is important that for these typical findings a careful, more extensive diagnosis is performed, to identify and avoid later complications. Kasabach-Merritt syndrome does not appear in infantile hemangiomas, even in extended complicated infantile hemangiomas, but only in Kaposi-like hemangioendotheliomas and rarely in tufted hemangioendotheliomas [11]. Very large and widely spread hemangiomas with or without ulcerations may lead to cardiac problems, complications of the systemic circulation, infections and hemorrhage.

References

1. Berlien H-P, Cremer H, Djawari D et al (1993/94) Leitlinien zur Behandlung angeborener Gefäßerkrankungen. Pädiatr Praxis 46:87–92
2. Enjolras O, Wassef M, Chapot R (2007) Color atlas of vascular tumors and vascular malformation. Cambridge University Press, Cambridge
3. Urban P, Algermissen B, Berlien HP (1999) Stadieneinteilung kindlicher Hämangiome nach FKDS-Kriterien. Ultrasschall in Med 20:36
4. Tsang WYW, Chan JKC, Fletcher CDM (1991) Kaposi-like infantile haemangioendothelioma: a distinctive vascular neoplasm of the retroperitoneum. Am J Surg Pathol 15:982–929
5. Stevens M (2005) Solide Tumore bei Kindern, Annales Nestle 63:127–139
6. Herman TE, McAllister PW, Dehner LP, Skinner M (1997) Beckwith-Wiedemann syndrome and splenic hemangioma: report of a case. Pediatr Radiol 27:350–352
7. Poetke M, Jamil B, Müller U, Berlien H-P (2002) Diffuse neonatal hemangiomatosis associated with Simpson-Golabi-Behmel syndrome: A case report. Eur J Pediatr Surg, in press
8. Waner M, North PE, Scherer KA et al (2003) The nonrandom distribution of facial hemangiomas. Arch Dermatology 139:869–875
9. Burns AJ, Kaplan LC, Mulliken JB (1991) Is there an association between hemangioma and syndromes with dysmorphic features? Pediatrics 88:1257–1267
10. Poetke M, Frommeld T, Berlien H-P (2002) PHACE Syndrome. New views on diagnostic criterias. Eur J Pediatr Surg 10:125–129
11. Zuckerberg LR, Nickoloff BJ, Weiss SW (1993) Kaposifom hemangioendothelioma of infancy and childhood: an aggressive neoplasm associated with Kasabach-Merritt syndrome and lymphangiomatosis. Am J Surg Pathol 17:321–328

Diagnosis of Hemangiomas

5

Juan Carlos López Gutiérrez

Abstract

Diagnosis of hemangiomas is based first on the medical history. The presence of a lesion at birth supports a diagnosis of a vascular malformation or congenital hemangioma. Infantile hemangiomas are characterized by an initial rapid proliferation phase in the first 6–9 months of life, followed by a slow involution phase and, in many cases, complete regression. Physical examination should allow a hemangioma to be classified as superficial, deep, or mixed type. On imaging, Doppler ultrasound (US) can assess the flow dynamics of a hemangioma, but the most important tool is contrast-enhanced magnetic resonance imaging (MRI), which demonstrates the extent of the lesion and can help to differentiate between a hemangioma and another disorder. The type of lesion can usually be determined based on the physical examination and Doppler US. MRI is mostly useful for confirming the clinical diagnosis, estimating the extent of the lesion, and determining the feasibility of surgical resection. If the diagnosis is in question after a thorough history, physical examination and radiological findings, a skin biopsy can be helpful in distinguishing unusual or atypical hemangiomas from other vascular lesions.

Introduction

Referral for treatment of hemangiomas is dependent on an accurate diagnosis of these lesions by the primary care physician. Because the management of vascular anomalies frequently crosses medical disciplines, specialists must agree on a uniform terminology in order to facilitate communication and develop treatment protocols.

The nomenclature of vascular lesions is confusing and one may find terms such as capillary hemangiomas, strawberry hemangiomas and cavernous hemangiomas in the recent medical literature [1].

Diagnosis of Hemangiomas is Based First on the Patient's Medical History

Two questions are of paramount importance when diagnosing a hemangioma: was the lesion present at birth? Did proportional or disproportional growth of the lesion occur after birth? The presence of the lesion at birth supports a diagnosis of a vascular malformation or congenital hemangioma. Infantile hemangiomas are characterized by an initial rapid proliferation phase in the first 6–9 months of life, followed by a slow involution phase and, in many cases, complete regression. Congenital hemangiomas are fully developed at birth, present as erythematous warm vascular plaques or nodules with a rim of pallor, and do not undergo postnatal growth. Congenital hemangiomas are divided into two categories: rapidly involuting congenital hemangiomas (RICH) and non-involuting congenital hemangiomas (NICH). As their name implies, RICH lesions begin to involute almost immediately after birth, and in many cases fully involute by 1 year of age (Fig. 5.1). A NICH may partially involute or soften, but full resolution does not occur. Despite the fact that normally RICH rapidly involute, usually much faster than common hemangiomas, some patients may develop significant health problems (e.g., cardiac failure or bleeding) due to arteriovenous shunting [2, 3].

R. Mattassi, D.A. Loose, M. Vaghi (eds.), *Hemangiomas and Vascular Malformations*.
© Springer-Verlag Italia 2009

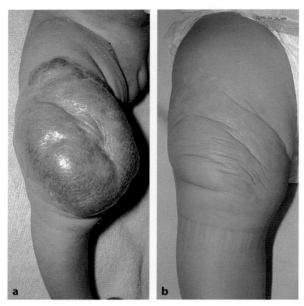

Fig. 5.1. Rapidly involuting congenital hemangioma (RICH) (**a**, **b**)

Physical Examination

After physical examination hemangiomas should be classified as superficial, deep, or mixed type, according to their location in the skin and subcutaneous tissue. Superficial infantile hemangiomas may be mistaken for capillary malformations (port-wine stains). Deep infantile hemangiomas may resemble lymphatic, venous, or mixed (venous and lymphatic) malformations (Fig. 5.2). Congenital hemangiomas may be confused with venous malformations or mixed malformations. Infantile hemangiomas can present as superficial (bright red plaques), deep (blue subcutaneous nodules), or mixed (both components) type. A RICH cannot be distinguished from a NICH at birth and only clinical observation allows differentiation. In the newborn, lesions may not be evi-

dent or may present as a red, white, telangiectatic or blue patch. A peripheral rim of pallor due to vasoconstriction may be seen at this stage. As the tumor proliferates, the lesion may take on the more classic appearance, which depends on the depth of the lesion and stage of evolution [4, 5].

Imaging

On imaging, Doppler ultrasound can assess the flow of a hemangioma, characterized by a shunt pattern with decreased arterial resistance and increased venous velocity, but the most important tool is contrast-enhanced magnetic resonance imaging (MRI), which demonstrates the extent of the lesion and can help to differentiate between a hemangioma and another disorder. Hemangiomas have a typical solid appearance with intermediate intensity on a T1-weighted spin-echo image, which is more intense compared with venous or lymphatic malformations. During the proliferative stage, hemangiomas show a relatively low intensity in a T2-weighted spin-echo image, while in the involution phase, they have a very low intensity. Contrast-enhanced T1-weighted MRI shows moderate intensity with prominent flow voids during the proliferative stage due to the high flow. In contrast, hemangiomas show low intensity during involution as a result of the low flow at that stage. The appropriate diagnostic tests for congenital hemangiomas are also ultrasonography with Doppler (the lesions are uniformly hypoechoic, mostly confined to the subcutaneous fat and diffusely vascular tissue traversed by multiple tubular vascular channels), and MRI (RICH has areas of inhomogeneity and larger flow voids) (Fig. 5.3). Angiography is only indicated if embolization has to be performed (large and irregular feeding arteries in disorganized patterns, arterial aneurysms, direct arteriovenous shunts, and intravascular thrombi are common features of RICH and

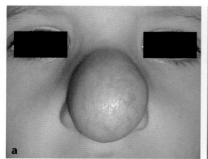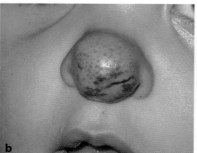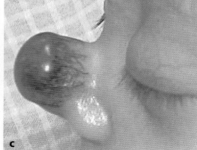

Fig. 5.2. Deep (**a**), mixed (**b**) and superficial nasal tip (**c**) hemangiomas

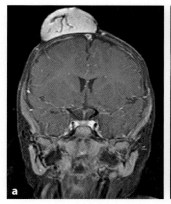
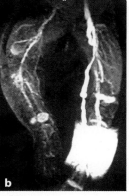

Fig. 5.3. MRI of scalp hemangioma (**a**) and lower limb RICH (**b**)

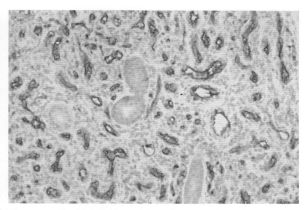

Fig. 5.4. Glut-1 positive stain in hemangiomas

are rarely seen in infantile hemangiomas) [6, 7].

The type of lesion can usually be determined based on Doppler US and MRI. MRI is mostly useful for confirming the clinical diagnosis, estimating the extent of the lesion, and determining the feasibility of surgical resection.

The differential diagnosis also includes angiosarcoma, glioma, infantile fibrosarcoma, infantile myofibromatosis, kaposiform hemangioendothelioma, pyogenic granuloma and teratoma, tufted angioma or rhabdomyosarcoma.

If the diagnosis is in question after a thorough history, physical examination and radiological findings, a skin biopsy can be helpful in distinguishing unusual or atypical hemangiomas from other vascular lesions. Specimens may be evaluated by routine histological examination and immunohistochemical analysis.

The histologic appearance of RICH differs from NICH and common infantile hemangioma, but some overlap is noted among the three lesions. RICH is composed of small-to-large lobules of capillaries with moderately plump endothelial cells and pericytes; the lobules are surrounded by abundant fibrous tissue. One-half of the specimens have a central involuting zone characterized by lobular loss, fibrous tissue, and draining channels that are often large and abnormal.

Additionally, hemangiomas have a unique vascular phenotype demonstrated by glucose transporter-1 (GLUT-1) staining (Fig. 5.4). Since its first description by North in 2000 [8], staining for GLUT-1 has become widespread by clinicians and researchers in the field of vascular anomalies. Endothelial cells in RICH and other vascular tumors or malformations do not express GLUT-1 protein [8].

References

1. Hand JL, Frieden IJ (2002) Vascular birthmarks of infancy: resolving nosologic confusion. Am J Med Genet 108:257–264
2. Chiller KG, Passaro D, Frieden IJ (2002) Hemangiomas of infancy: clinical characteristics, morphologic subtypes, and their relationship to race, ethnicity, and sex. Arch Dermatol 138:1567–1576
3. Boon LM, Enjolras O, Mulliken JB (1996) Congenital hemangioma: evidence of accelerated involution. J Pediatr 128:329–335
4. Haggstrom AN, Drolet BA, Baselga E et al (2006) Prospective study of infantile hemangiomas: clinical characteristics predicting complications and treatment. Pediatrics 118(3):882–887
5. Frieden IJ, Haggstrom AN, Drolet BA et al (2005) Infantile hemangiomas: current knowledge, future directions. Proceedings of a research workshop on infantile hemangiomas, April 7-9, 2005, Bethesda, Maryland, USA. Pediatr Dermatol 22(5):383–406
6. Frieden I, Enjolras O, Esterly N (2003) Vascular birthmarks and other abnormalities of blood vessels and lymphatics. In: Schacner LA, Hansen RC (eds) Pediatric dermatology, 3rd edn, Mosby Publishers, St Louis, pp 833–862
7. Burrows PE, Laor T, Paltiel H, Robertson RL (1998) Diagnostic imaging in the evaluation of vascular birthmarks. Dermatol Clin 16:455–488
8. North PE, Waner M, Mizeracki A, Mihm MC Jr (2000) GLUT1: a newly discovered immunohistochemical marker for juvenile hemangiomas. Hum Pathol 31:11–22

Visceral Hemangiomas

6

Juan Carlos López Gutiérrez

Abstract

A small but significant percentage of hemangiomas develop at an extracutaneous location. The location has important prognostic and therapeutic implications. These hemangiomas are difficult to detect on physical examination and imaging studies are required in order to assess both size and behavior. An extracutaneous hemangioma is more serious than a cutaneous one. When detected in an infant, immediate intervention is required. In this chapter we describe the unique characteristics of central nervous system hemangiomas (that occur on the surface of the brain and spinal cord), parotid gland hemangiomas (in which the high overall response rate to pharmacological treatment does not exclude surgical treatment), thoracic hemangiomas (emphasizing the difficult differential diagnosis of intramuscular and congenital heart hemangiomas), and abdominal hemangiomas (with special focus on the management of focal, multicentric and diffuse liver hemangiomas – formerly known as hemangioendotheliomas – as well as the less common group of intestinal or genito-urinary hemangiomas).

Introduction

Accurate diagnosis of visceral hemangiomas remains a challenge for physicians because of confusing terminology, lack of knowledge regarding lesion behavior, and poor understanding of diagnostic criteria on the part of physicians. Despite distinct clinical, radiological, and histological findings, visceral vascular anomalies are often misdiagnosed. This complicates both the care of the patient and interpretation of the medical literature. As for their cutaneous counterparts, the most common misdiagnosis

in visceral vascular anomalies is the use of the term hemangioma to refer to venous malformations. Visceral hemangioma exists only in young children. This misconception can easily lead to incorrect triaging and mistreatment [1].

Focal cutaneous hemangiomas of infancy are common in the general pediatric population, are usually easily diagnosed, and generally do not require treatment. However, a small but significant percentage of hemangiomas may develop at extracutaneous locations. This has important prognostic and therapeutic implications. Multiple hemangiomas of the skin have traditionally been recognized as an indicator of potential visceral hemangioma, and any infant with multiple cutaneous hemangiomas should be closely assessed for possible visceral involvement [2].

Additionally, segmental hemangiomas of the skin are commonly found in association with visceral hemangiomatosis. The most common site of internal organ involvement is the liver, followed by the gastrointestinal tract, the brain, the mediastinum and the lung.

Head and Neck Hemangiomas

Brain

Hemangiomas of the central nervous system are uncommon. These lesions have imaging characteristics similar to those of subcutaneous hemangiomas, such as diffuse contrast enhancement and vascular flow voids. Most of them are on the surface of the brain and spinal cord (associated with dysraphism). They always regress. Infants with large segmental hemangiomas of the face are at increased risk of arterial ischemic stroke caused by both structural arterial anomalies and development of intracranial hemangiomas.

R. Mattassi, D.A. Loose, M. Vaghi (eds.), *Hemangiomas and Vascular Malformations*.
© Springer-Verlag Italia 2009

Infants presenting with a large facial hemangioma should be evaluated for central nervous system (CNS), arterial, cardiac and ocular abnormalities in the first weeks of life. Head magnetic resonance imaging (MRI) and magnetic resonance angiogram (MRA), chest MRI, cardiac ultrasound and head sonogram should be considered for all such infants [3].

Thyroid

Thyroid nodules are more uncommon in children than in adults, but the risk of malignancy is much higher. As thyroid hemangioma is extremely uncommon, fine-needle aspiration biopsy of a suspected thyroid hemangioma is mandatory in order to confirm diagnosis.

Parotid

Hemangioma is by far the most common tumor of the parotid gland in children, and shows a high overall response rate to pharmacological treatment (propanolol steroids or interferon), as it does in other locations (Fig. 6.1). Current parotid hemangioma treatment regimens include propanolol systemic or intralesional steroids and surgery. Unfortunately, there are no controlled prospective studies comparing these

treatments. In 1975, Scheunemann [4] reviewed the indications for parotid hemangioma surgical treatment and only partially recommended it as the therapy of choice. Thirty years later there is still no consensus on indications for excision of proliferative parotid hemangiomas in early childhood. Although surgeons may dispute indications and timing, most would agree that facial hemangiomas causing functional disturbance or serious psychological distress should be surgically excised before the age of expected spontaneous regression and that the abstention rule should not be applied, as surgery can provide active treatment with excellent results and minimal morbidity [5].

For some of these significantly disfiguring tumors or those that impact upon physical function, the surgical scar may be preferable to the presence of the tumor. Nevertheless, permanent facial nerve dysfunction is a potential complication of parotid surgery and should be taken into consideration.

In a study of a series of conservative parotidectomies with facial nerve dissection to treat benign tumors, rates of facial weakness and Frey's syndrome ranged from 2 to 7%. Even though there is significant evidence that the superficial musculoaponeurotic system (SMAS) flap should be considered the standard of care for preventing Frey's syndrome in patients with parotid hemangioma, the type of lesion and its topography, the age of the patient and operative indications, postoperative complications and aesthetic and func-

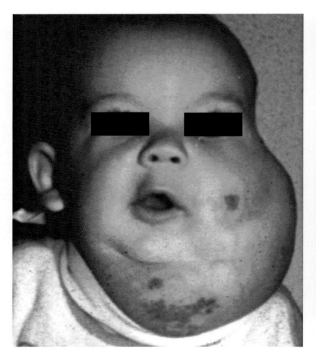
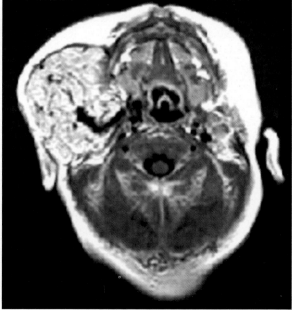

Fig. 6.1. Parotid hemangioma

tional results should be considered individually in each patient. An early multidisciplinary check-up to identify cases with a predictably long involution phase or large fibrofatty residuum after complete resolution of the angioma would help to select future cases where early surgical correction would be most beneficial.

Late secondary procedures such as preauricular excision of redundant skin or fibrofatty tissue and auricular revision are often necessary in order to improve facial contours.

Thoracic Hemangiomas

Mediastinum

Vascular anomalies, including hemangiomas and vascular malformations, comprise 3–6% of mediastinal masses in childhood. Correct diagnosis can almost always be established by history, bronchoscopy, and/or radiographic studies.

Lung

Focal pulmonary hemangiomas (Fig. 6.2) are exceptionally rare in childhood and even more so in infancy. They may involve the airways or parenchyma, and may be localized or multifocal. If asymptomatic, pharmacological and surgical treatments are not indicated.

Pulmonary capillary hemangiomatosis is a rare and distinct disease characterized by widespread capillary proliferation in the lung, infiltrating the interstitium and the alveolar walls. This causes severe pulmonary hypertension.

Pleura

In rare cases, hemangiomatosis involving the pleura may cause bloody pleural effusion in the neonate. When associated with congestive heart failure, the prognosis is particularly grave.

Heart

Vascular tumors of the heart are also rare in children, and include small subgroups of congenital hemangiomas in newborns and intramuscular hemangiomas in older children. Intramuscular hemangiomas do not respond to corticosteroids, while congenital hemangiomas exhibit spontaneous or

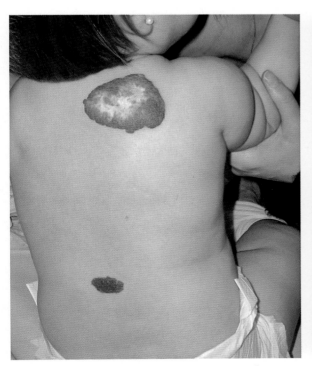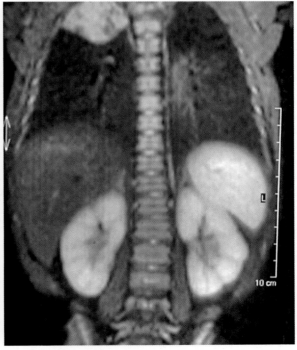

Fig. 6.2. Hemangioma of the lung in patient with cutaneous scapular hemangioma

pharmacotherapy-induced regression [6]. It is important that the physician understands the difference between these two groups in order to provide appropriate prognostic and therapeutic advice to the parents of affected children.

The presence of hemangioma in the heart valve is an exceptional finding. Normally, transesophageal echocardiography is used to establish a diagnosis of cardiac tumor, though careful interpretation is needed to avoid diagnostic errors, such as of prolapsing left atrial myxoma.

Esophagus

Despite the fact that there are a large number of reports of "esophageal hemangiomas" in the medical literature, the majority of these have been misdiagnosed and are, in fact, venous malformations.

Thymus

Thymic hemangiomas are usually identified as diffusely infiltrating tumors that extend into the pericardium and up the carotid sheath. They typically present with stridor at the proliferative phase.

Abdominal Hemangiomas

Stomach

As is the case in the esophagus, in the medical literature a wide variety of gastric vascular anomalies are incorrectly referred to as hemangiomas. Significant differences must be taken into consideration before any surgical approach towards hemangiomas and venous malformations of the stomach is chosen. Although bleeding is the most common symptom of both gastric hemangiomas and venous malformations, treatment of the two conditions differs. Pharmacological angiogenesis inhibition is the mainstay of hemangioma therapy. Endoscopic vascular obliteration is extremely useful in treating the much more common venous malformations. There is no indication for endoscopic sclerotherapy of gastric hemangiomas, but this treatment is clearly the first option to consider when treating gastric venous malformations. Gastrectomy should be seen as a life-saving procedure to be used only when bleeding is out of control and several attempts at sclerosis have failed.

Intestine

Hemangiomas of the small bowel are rare. Once again a proper use of nomenclature is crucial to prevent the institution of improper therapies [7]. Hemangiomas have a pathognomonic appearance on endoscopy. In case of doubt, glucose transporter-1 (GLUT-1) immunohistochemistry on a biopsy specimen will aid a correct diagnosis. Capsule endoscopy can be performed safely in pediatric patients after ingestion or endoscopic placement of the capsule in order to diagnose bleeding vascular tumors after negative results from gastroscopy and colonoscopy.

Although intussusception caused by a hemangioma of the small bowel is a rare condition (commonly found in blue rubber bleb nevus syndrome), it should be taken into consideration in the differential diagnosis of abdominal pain of doubtful origin.

Sigmoidoscopy reveals hemangiomas in only 1% of patients with minor rectal bleeding.

Hemangiomas of the greater or lesser omentum are not exceptional and are very often asymptomatic in the context of diffuse neonatal hemangiomatosis [8].

Liver

Hemangiomas are the most common benign liver tumors in children. They can be difficult to diagnose and complex to treat. Differential diagnosis must be accurate in any patient with atypical presentation of liver hemangioma. An important differentiating factor in the evaluation of pediatric hepatic masses is the age of the patient. Hepatoblastomas, mesenchymal hamartomas, and metastatic disease from Wilms' tumor or neuroblastoma are usually seen in the first 3 years of life, whereas hepatocellular carcinoma, focal nodular hyperplasia, hepatic adenoma, and metastases from lymphoma are more common in older children.

Several current studies are attempting to determine the frequency of liver hemangiomas in children with infantile hemangiomas by comparing liver ultrasound results in hemangioma patients (with one to four cutaneous hemangiomas, five or more cutaneous hemangiomas, or at least one large hemangioma), to ultrasound results in children without hemangiomas. These studies will also identify specific risk factors in patients who have liver hemangiomas.

Vascular anomaly specialists must be able to distinguish hemangiomas from various vascular malformations, as well as to appreciate their dynamic course over time. Several attempts have been made to classify pediatric liver vascular tumors, resulting in an unhelpful plethora of confusing terminology. Recently, immunohistochemistry has been used to study hemangiomas and this supports a new classification of these tumors based on GLUT-1 expression [9]:

1. GLUT-1 positive expression is usually demonstrated in multifocal and diffuse hepatic infantile hemangioma, which shares clinical and morphological features with cutaneous infantile hemangioma. Diffuse neonatal hemangiomatosis is a frequently fatal disorder characterized by multiple cutaneous and visceral hemangiomas. Complications include high-output cardiac failure, hemorrhage, hepatic failure, and consumption coagulopathy. Levels of type 3 iodothyronine deiodinase activity need to be determined in every patient with multifocal or diffuse lesions: a diagnosis of consumptive hypothyroidism can be made if increased activity is found. Myocardial depression secondary to hy-

pothyroidism in children with hepatic hemangioma has been reported. The child's hypothyroidism improves coincident with the involution of the hemangioma.

2. GLUT-1 negative vascular liver tumors with unique clinical, imaging and pathological features occur in neonates. They differ from diffuse hemangioma in terms of earlier presentation as a solitary mass with central necrosis, rapid involution and pathologic features showing a notable, often prolific, lymphatic compliment that immunoreacts positively with the monoclonal antibody D2-40.

Following the parallels with cutaneous anomalies, it has been suggested that the term hepatic congenital hemangioma be applied to these tumors, comparing their behavior with the rapid involuting congenital hemangiomas (RICH) described in skin and subcutaneous locations.

In summary, hepatic hemangiomas can fall into one of three different categories of lesions: focal (Fig. 6.3), multicentric (Fig. 6.4) or diffuse (Fig. 6.5).

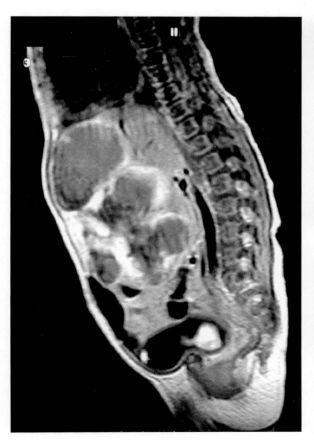

Fig. 6.3. Focal liver hemangioma

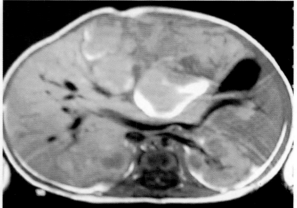

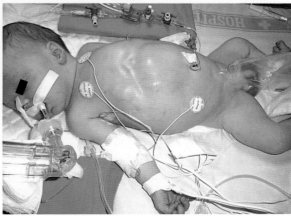

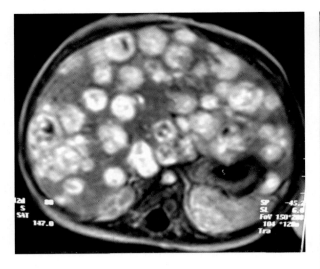

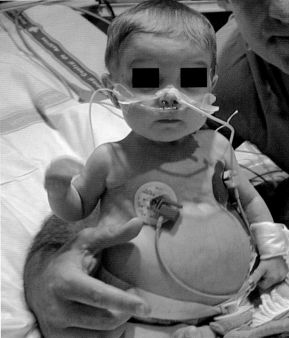

Fig. 6.4. Multifocal liver hemangioma

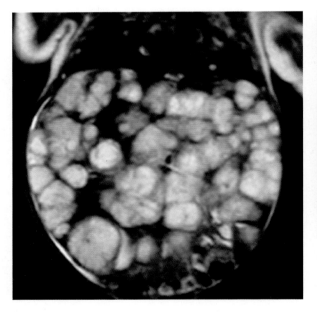

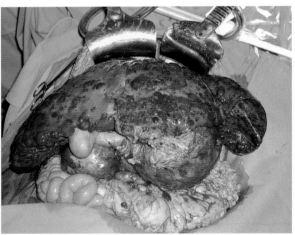

Fig. 6.5. Diffuse liver hemangioma. Liver transplantation

Treatment

The natural history of focal hemangiomas is spontaneous regression in the first year of life; however, shunt embolization or complete surgical excision is required in case of cardiac failure. Sometimes the lesions are detected antenatally, in which case maternal corticosteroid therapy should be considered if the fetal heart progressively enlarges.

For multifocal liver hemangiomas, high-dose steroids (3–5 mg/kg/d) are initially given for 3–5 weeks. Supportive care may include liberal use of diuretics and digitalis to improve cardiac function. This regimen is discontinued if no response is observed, in order to avoid steroid-induced complications. Daily subcutaneous administration of interferon-alpha (3×10^6 U/m^2/kg) may lead to hemangioma involution. Up to 50% regression has been reported [10]; however, the response time is slow, and lesions can rebound once the drug treatment is stopped. Very young children also have a risk of developing spastic diplegia. Selective hepatic artery embolization may not be as successful in multifocal lesions as in focal lesions. On occasion, liver transplantation may be indicated for diffuse disease that is unresponsive to steroid and interferon therapy. Currently, there is data available on the effect of propanolol on the clinical course of liver emangiomas.

In patients with severe acquired hypothyroidism resulting from both increased type 3 iodothyronine deiodinase activity and increased production of thyroid stimulating hormone (TSH)-like hormone from hepatic hemangiomas, L-thyroxin replacement should be considered if the patient is less than 3 years of age. Intravenous triiodothyronine can be used to preoperatively stabilize an infant with hypothyroidism undergoing liver hemangioma surgery.

Spleen

Hemangiomas involving the spleen are rare and seldom symptomatic. These are not to be confused with littoral cell angioma (LCA), a different benign vascular tumor of the spleen that most commonly presents in adults as an enlarged spleen containing multiple nodules with constitutional symptoms (low grade fever and fatigue) and signs of hypersplenism (anemia and thrombocytopenia). Hemangiomatosis of the spleen and omentum is also a finding in patients with diffuse neonatal hemangiomatosis.

Pancreas

The pancreas is an unusual site for hemangioma in an infant. Hemangioma should be considered as a possibility in a patient younger than 6 months who presents with a history of jaundice, pale stools and dark urine. Abdominal ultrasound scan and MRI will show an enhancing mass in the pancreas of the affected patients. Pancreatic resection should be avoided. Biliary diversion with a Roux-en-Y hepaticojejunostomy is the procedure of choice in case of obstructive jaundice.

Urinary Tract

Despite several cases in the medical literature of neonatal hematuria caused by a bleeding hemangioma of the kidney or bladder, clinical and radiological findings for hemangiomas of the urinary tract are typical of venous malformations. In the largest published series of patients with bladder "hemangioma" the mean patient age at the time of diagnosis was 58 years (range, 19–76 years)!

Penis

Hemangiomas of the glans penis (Fig 6.6) are a more common entity. Treatment with surgical excision, Nd:YAG laser or cryotherapy gives optimal cosmetic results.

Testicle

Hemangioma of the testis most commonly presents as a painless scrotal mass. It may be similar to a malignant testicular tumor in terms of clinical symptoms, as well as on ultrasonography and MRI, and therefore this should be included in the differential diagnosis.

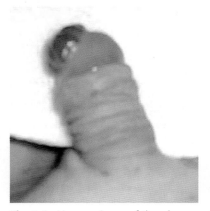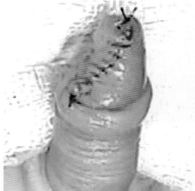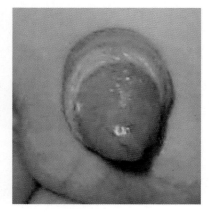

Fig. 6.6. Hemangioma of the glans penis

Female Genital Tract

Vascular tumors are rare in the female genital tract, considering its very rich vascular supply (vulvar and scrotal hemangiomas are common but they must be considered as cutaneous and not visceral tumors). They are often an incidental finding at surgery and are rarely associated with systemic manifestations. It is important to remember that adnexal torsion is common in cases of associated enlarged ovary mass. The presence or absence of flow by Doppler sonography is not helpful for diagnosis. Hemangiomas of the uterine cervix or vagina are uncommon. Irregular vaginal bleeding during the proliferative phase is the main symptom.

Breast

Hemangiomas of the breast are not uncommon. They usually involve the nipple-areola complex and cause significant contour deformity and sequelae in late childhood. In consequence, reconstructive breast surgery should be considered before puberty (Fig. 6.7).

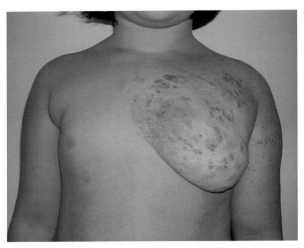

Fig. 6.7. Breast hemangioma

Conclusion

After diagnosis of a visceral vascular tumor, the physician should be able to recognize the typical clinical presentation of hemangioma, including common symptoms and physical examination findings. This will allow the physician to generate an appropriate differential diagnosis, to select the appropriate imaging and diagnostic studies to confirm the diagnosis and to recognize associated histological findings, leading to appropriate pharmacological or surgical care (Fig. 6.8). Only specially trained surgeons should perform surgical excision of visceral hemangiomas because of the risk of hemorrhage and the potential for damage to vital structures associated with the hemangioma [11].

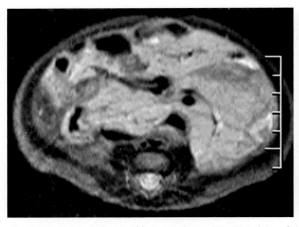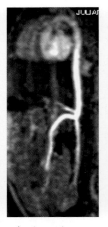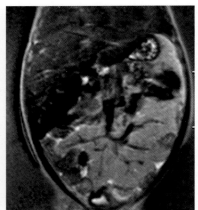

Fig. 6.8. Giant abdominal hemangioma (GLUT-1+) involving the intestine

References

1. Haggstrom AN, Drolet BA, Baselga E et al (2006) Prospective study of infantile hemangiomas: clinical characteristics predicting complications and treatment. Pediatrics 118(3):882–887
2. Frieden IJ, Haggstrom AN, Drolet BA et al (2005) Infantile hemangiomas: current knowledge, future directions. Proceedings of a research workshop on infantile hemangiomas. Pediatr Dermatol 22(5):383–406
3. Poindexter G, Metry DW, Barkovich AJ, Frieden IJ (2007) PHACE syndrome with intracerebral hemangiomas, heterotopia, and endocrine dysfunction. Pediatr Neurol 36(6):402–406
4. Scheunemann H (1975) Conservative parotidectomy in infancy and childhood. J Maxillofac Surg 3:37–40
5. Greene AK, Rogers GF, Mulliken JB (2005) Management of parotid hemangioma. Plast Reconstr Surg 116(2):676–677
6. Mackie AS, Kozakewich HP, Geva T et al (2005) Vascular tumors of the heart in infants and children: case series and review of the literature. Pediatr Cardiol 26(4):344–349
7. Fishman SJ, Fox VL (2001) Visceral vascular anomalies. Gastrointest Endosc Clin N Am 11(4):813–834
8. Fishman SJ, Burrows PE, Leichtner AM, Mulliken JB (1998) Gastrointestinal manifestations of vascular anomalies in childhood: varied etiologies require multiple therapeutic modalities. J Pediatr Surg 33(7):1163–1167
9. Christison-Lagay ER, Burrows PE, Alomari A et al (2007) Hepatic hemangiomas: subtype classification and development of a clinical practice algorithm and registry. J Pediatr Surg 42:62–67
10. Blei F, Orlow SJ, Geronemus R (1997) Multimodal management of diffuse neonatal hemangiomatosis. J Am Acad Dermatol 37(6):1019–1021
11. Enjolras O, Riche MC, Merland JJ, Escande JP (1990) Management of alarming hemangiomas in infancy: a review of 25 cases. Pediatrics 85(4):491–498

Principles of Therapy of Infantile Hemangiomas and Other Congenital Vascular Tumors of the Newborns and Infants

7

Hans Peter Berlien

Abstract

As hemangiomas frequently involute spontaneously, a wait-and-see principle is common. However, some cases need early treatment: these include "dangerous hemangiomas" of the face, anogenital region and rapidly growing hemangiomas. The goal of treatment should be to stop proliferation, speed up regression of large hemangiomas and prevent functional problems. The most common treatments are drug therapy, laser treatment, and surgical excision. Treatments such as X-ray and sclerotherapy are no longer indicated, and cryotherapy has been replaced by laser, while embolization is only indicated as a final treatment option.

Introduction

The two main kinds of congenital vascular tumors look so similar – in the past some authors used the term hemangioma to classify both – yet the approach to them is so different (Fig. 7.1). In general, congenital vascular tumors behave differently to acquired vascular tumors, as also seen in congenital malignancies where the congenital malignant neuroblastoma has the potential for spontaneous maturation [1]. This does not mean that the congenital vascular tumors have malignant potential, but there are several similarities: aggressive growth, high proliferation rate and potential for spontaneous regression.

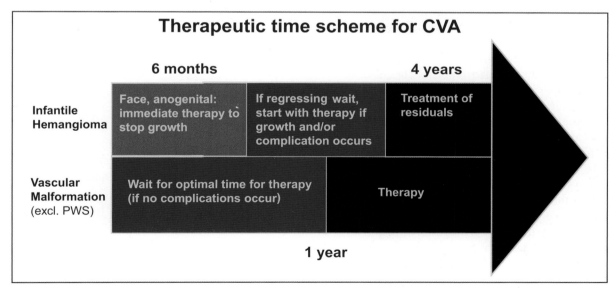

Fig. 7.1. In contrast to vascular malformations, where a spontaneous regression never occurs, in congenital vascular tumors such as infantile hemangiomas there is a great potential for spontaneous regression. However, the indication for active therapy is wider and earlier in endangered regions than it is in other regions. *PWS*, port-wine stain; *CVA*, congenital vascular anomalies

R. Mattassi, D.A. Loose, M. Vaghi (eds.), *Hemangiomas and Vascular Malformations*.
© Springer-Verlag Italia 2009

Indication for Treatment of Congenital Vascular Tumors

Due to their mesenchymal origin, vascular tumors do not primarily involve the epithelial layer either in the epidermis or in the mucous membrane. This means that any treatment has to avoid secondary effects from growth and additional damage caused to the epithelium by therapy.

Spontaneous Course

Because hemangiomas may involute spontaneously, waiting for spontaneous regression remains a viable therapeutic option. But the wait-and-see principle is always wrong. If it means that treatment arrives too late, then "see-and-wait" as a control is correct, because at the first sign of progression of complication an action can be taken. Therefore, in case of small, uncomplicated infantile hemangiomas in non-problematic areas (extremities, body) without any tendency to proliferate, especially in coetaneous hemangiomas, one can "see-and-wait". If delayed growth cannot be excluded, frequent controls are required. Clinical check-ups alone may not be sufficient, as subcutaneous infantile hemangiomas may remain unnoticed as they grow deeply and are then only recognized after complications result. This is why a periodic duplex scan control is mandatory. For hemangiomas in the quiescent or regression phase, a "see-and-wait" attitude should normally be recommended. However, if complications are expected from ulcerations, treatment is also required for these forms. As therapy may cause adverse systemic or cutaneous side-effects, particularly scarring, sometimes intervention has been reserved for patients with significant complications. Therefore, it is difficult to choose a therapy that eliminates hemangiomas before the development of complications and without systemic side effects [2].

For this reason, the following infantile hemangiomas must be considered as "problem hemangiomas", for which active treatment is mandatory (Table 7.1):

- Hemangiomas of the face, particularly periorbitally, periorally, in the areas of the ear, lips and nose.
- Hemangiomas at the mammary gland, in the anogenital area, particularly the vulva, the urethral orifice and the anal derma.
- Rapidly growing, diffuse infiltrating hemangiomas at any anatomic site.
- Hemangiomatosis, aggressive diffuse or involving an organ.

Hemangiomas in problem zones (face, anogenital region) should be treated in their early stages to prevent complications. This is the rule for hemangiomas near the eyes (threat to vision), lips (little regression tendency) and nose area (malformations of the nose – Cyrano nose). Approaches to these hemangiomas are discussed in detail in Chapter 9.

Treatment is also indicated when hemangiomas are located on the fingers (tactile problems), toes (shoe problems expected later on), breast, and cleavage area in women. Extended, highly proliferating hemangiomas or those already causing complications, as well as diffuse infiltrating hemangiomas, should be treated actively. Early treatment initiation can be decisive for the further course. In particular, as a rule, diffusely growing, infiltrating hemangiomas also require a systemic approach.

Of the hemangioendotheliomas, rapidly involuting congenital hemangioendothelioma (RICH) needs only frequent ultrasound controls. For non-involuting congenital hemangioendothelioma (NICH), provided there is tight color-coded duplex sonography (CCDS) and thrombocyte monitoring, one may wait for a possible spontaneous regression as in RICH. If transition to a Kaposi-like hemangioendothelioma is suspected, however, due to an increase in inflammatory infiltrates and a thickening of interstitial septae in the sonogram, therapy should be started prior to manifestation of a Kasabach-Merritt Syndrome (KMS). In addition to a local Nd:YAG laser therapy, high-dose prednisone treatment is required. A treatment with cytostatics can thus often be avoided (Fig. 7.2).

Induction of Regression

Treatments have included laser therapy, radiation therapy, electrosurgery, cryosurgery, surgical excision, sclerotherapy, embolization, and drug therapy (Table 7.2).

The aim of therapy in cases of infantile hemangiomas as a rule is not the immediate removal, but should:

- Stop proliferation of the hemangioma.
- Speed up regression of large hemangiomas.
- Avoid or remove functional problems (eye).
- The earlier the growth is stopped, the better the results achieved in regression.

An early halt to progression is the best basis for a good outcome. If the hemangioma does not spontaneously halt, early treatment is recommended.

Table 7.1. Exemplary grading of typical localizations of infantile hemangioma

Ser. No	Localization	Phase/Type/Form	Organ	Number	Localization	Growth pattern	Complication	Score	No treatment, no control necessary	Rather no treatment, but control necessary	Close control, laser therapy in progress	Definite laser indication	add. adjuvant systemic therapy
	Grade*								1	2a	2b	3	4
	Localization	1-10	1-5	1-5	1-5	1-3	5-10	Sum	>5	6-8	9-11	<12	<15
1	Trachea	5	3	1	7	5		16					X
2	Pharynx	3	4	1	6	2		13				X	
3	Cheek	5	3	1	3	2		9	X				
4	Cheek	5	4	1	3	3	5	16					X
5	Back	2	1	1	1	1		4					
6	Breast	5	3	1	3	2	5	14				X	
7	Oral	2	4	1	4	1		10			X		
8	Leg	2	3	1	1	1		6		X			
9	Finger	3	4	1	4	2		11			X		
10	Neck	2	1	1	2	1		5	X				X
11	Neck	5	4	1	2	1		8		X			
12	Eye	5	4	1	4	3	10	22					X

* Grade 1 means uncomplicated hemangioma with no risks; Grade 2a hemangiomas with low risk factors need controls; G2b with risk factors need close controls and laser therapy if any progress is observed; Grade 3 has a laser indication due to risks of complication and Grade 4 requires additional systemic therapy

Local Procedures

Physical Procedures

The application of physical energy can be divided into direct tissue removal or destruction and secondary apoptosis by primary inflammation.

Cryotherapy

Cryotherapy at −30° (electrical) or at −176° (liquid nitrogen) is used in the contact procedure for the therapy of small plane hemangiomas with a maximal diameter of 1 cm. Cryotherapy has no specific absorption in the tissue and causes a severe frostbite with a congelatio escharotica III [3]. Because of the physi-cal principle of thermal conductivity, treatment is only possible by destroying the overlying epithelial layer (Fig. 7.3). Complications include hypopigmentations (10–15%) and scars or atrophies. After application blisters and crusts occur. For infiltrated or disseminated and subcutaneous hemangiomas this method is not suitable. Furthermore, there is no place for cryotherapy in treating any type of hemangioendothelioma.

Scarification Techniques

Due to the observation that hemangiomas can start involution after trauma or infection, one principle used in the past for treatment was the scarifica-

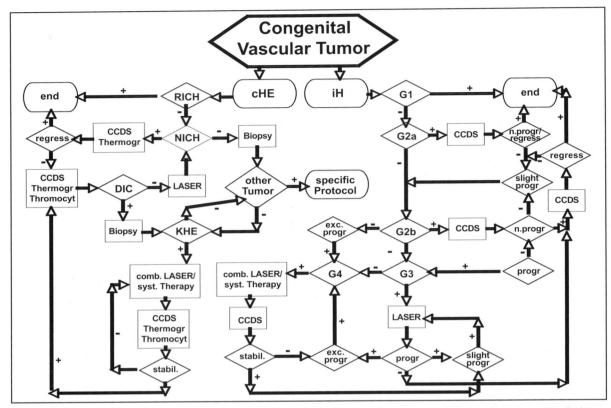

Fig. 7.2. Therapeutic algorithm for infantile hemangiomas and congenital hemangioendotheliomas. The symbols are according to ISO 9000. The grading for infantile hemangioma is given in Table 7.1. The therapeutic principle is a downgrading to an uncomplicated form either of infantile hemangioma or congenital hemangioendothelioma to allow the spontaneous regression. Abbreviations: *DIC*, disseminated intravasal coagulopathy; *CCDS*, color coded duplex sonography; *cHE*, congenital hemangioendothelioma; *iH*, infantile hemangioma; *RICH*, rapid involuting congenital hemangioendothelioma; *NICH*, non involuting congenital hemangioendothelioma; *KHE*, kaposiform congenital hemangioendothelioma; *Thermogr*, infrared thermography

Table 7.2. Overview of the therapeutic principles. Some are mentioned only for historical reasons

1. Spontaneous course
2. Induction of regression

Local procedures	Systemic therapy
Physical	Antiproliferating drugs
Cryosurgery	Cytostatic
Scarification	Interferon.
Laser	
X-ray	
Mechanical	Antiangiogenesis
Compression	Corticoids
Ligation	Vascular growth inhibitors
Embolization	
Chemical	
Sclerotherapy	
MG-seeds	
Interstitial corticoid crystals	
Topical Imiquimod	

3. Removal
   Early complications
   Residuals

tion technique with needle radiofrequency. However, this procedure, like cryotherapy, causes scars on the skin, so the reason for reporting it here is purely historical. Furthermore, there is a high risk of massive bleeding, especially in proliferation hemangiomas. At the beginning of the laser era some surgeons started using CO_2-laser scarification, but the results were similar to radiofrequency. While the prior techniques treat hemangiomas only by destruction, the following induces inflammation.

Laser Therapy

Due to the high specific absorption of the correct selected wavelength in the dermal or subcutaneous layer, laser therapy has been demonstrated as effective and safe for the treatment of congenital vascular tumors in children, while significantly minimizing any cutaneous adverse effects. Several clinical

Aim of treatment

Due to the mesenchymal origin of any congenital vascular anomalies
– primarily only the dermis and not the epidermis is affected

This means
– any therapeutic technique has to preserve the epithelial layer and not destroy it

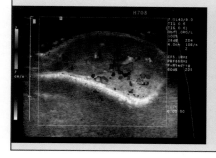 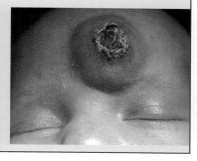

Fig. 7.3. Cryotherapy results in a congelatio with consequent epithelial damage. This means that cryotherapy will not fulfil the requirements for a safe therapy

trials have been reported positively. Through laser treatment an early and careful therapy of hemangiomas has also become possible, so that hemangiomas can be treated in early or prodromal phases to avoid enlargement [4].

However, laser treatment is required in rapidly growing hemangiomas of the head, when these lesions interfere with important functions (e.g., hands and feet), or when they endanger delicate structures because of their location (e.g., eye, anogential region). Treatment of large hemangiomas also may desirable (Fig. 7.4).

X-Ray Therapy

Comparable to the procedure in X-ray therapy of keloids or other inflammatory diseases, radiotherapy has also been used. The principle of tissue interaction is comparable to laser therapy: induction of inflammation followed by regression. Both techniques will not affect the unintended epithelial layer. However, in laser therapy the specific reaction causes selective absorption, in radio therapy the specific reaction of this radiation is more effective in highly proliferative tissue. So it appears to be an ideal tool for hemangioma treatment, except for the fact that in contrast to laser therapy, radio therapy is an ionizing radiation that carries a high risk of mutagenity and carcinogenity. Furthermore, a secondary cataract is a major complication near the eyes. Therefore, for infantile hemangiomas and kaposiform hemangioendothelioma X-ray therapy is discussed here only as a historical treatment and is no longer applicable today.

Mechanical Procedures

Compression

The idea of the compression technique of infantile hemangioma comes from burn scar therapy to prevent keloids. Due to the biological behaviour of the proliferating tumor this causes only ulcerations by pressure to the primarily unaffected epithelial layer. Therefore, this report is purely historical.

Ligation

Ligation and embolization [5] follow the experiences of acquired malignant tumors: occlusion of feeding arteries induces a necrosis of the tumors. But this is a misunderstanding of the biology of congenital vascular tumors such as infantile hemangioma. The ori-

Aim of laser treatment

Infantile hemangiomas & other benign vessel tumors
– Induction of regression through inflammatory processes after intravascular absorption and vessel occlusion

Vascular malformation
– Destruction of pathologic capillarization (extratruncular VM) and occlusion of cavernous vessel spaces and small AV-fistulas (truncular malformations)

Fig. 7.4. In contrast to vascular malformations in congenital vascular tumors, the aim of laser therapy is not to remove or completely destroy the hemangioma, but only to induce a halt of progression and initiation of regression

gin is a highly proliferative tissue which has secondary vessels. So any occlusion either by ligature or embolization will be compensated immediately by the formation of new nutritional arteries.

Embolization

Comparable to ligation due to the collaterals of congenital vascular tumors, embolization is nonsensical [6]. One exceptional indication for embolization is in infantile liver hemangiomas with massive cardiac failure or massive bleeding from ulcerated hemangiomas [7]. In special cases of kaposiform hemangioendothelioma such as KMS, which cannot be treated successfully by cytostatics and laser, an embolization may be considered, but only as the last option.

Chemical Procedures

The basis of chemical agents for the therapy of congenital vascular tumors is comparable to the indication of physical energy: induction of inflammation.

Sclerotherapy

Polidocanol is the main drug for sclerotherapy of varices, where it is a safe and successful procedure. However, in infantile hemangioma or in congenital hemangioendothelioma there is a diffuse microcirculation which does not allow a complete compression to avoid a systemic outflow. In newborns even low concentrations of this drug can cause myocarditis. So the indication for sclerosing drugs is replaced by laser therapy [8].

Interstitial Magnesium Seeds

Therapy with oxidizing metals such as copper and magnesium is outdated. The biological reaction is the production of free radicals in contact with the tissue. The application is not controllable; the technique is the seed technique known from radiotherapy which carries a high risk of puncture failure and complete necrosis. As with sclerotherapy, this procedure has been completely replaced by the different laser techniques.

Interstitial Corticoid Crystals

An interstitial direct corticoid crystal injection has been reported for localized infantile hemangiomas. In the eye there is a high risk of crystal embolization of the artery resulting in permanent blindness. Topical corticoid creams can cause skin atrophy and systemic side effects due to uncontrolled resorption [9].

Imiqiumod (Aldara®)

Imiquimod was introduced for the therapy of intraepithelial neoplasias induced by human papilloma viruses (HPV). The basis is a local production of cytokines and it has replaced the topical application of interferon. However, due to the mesenchymal origin of congenital vascular tumors, this principle works only by destruction and ulceration of the epithelial layer followed by a secondary inflammation in the hemangioma itself. So this treatment is comparable to the scarification techniques and has no effect on deep dermal or subcutaneous hemangiomas, which are the main indication for any therapy. In congenital hemangioendothelioma due to epidermal barrier this procedure has no effect.

Systemic Procedures

The basics and principles of systemic therapy are discussed in Chapter 8.

There is no specific systemic treatment for infantile hemangioma or congenital hemangioendothelioma. Two main principles are in use: antiproliferating drugs [10] and antiangiogenesis.

Antiproliferative Drugs

The higher the proliferation rate, the more effective the therapy with antiproliferative drugs. However, several complications in infantile hemangiomas are caused even at a low proliferation rate due to the complicated localization. Furthermore, not all antiproliferative drugs are able to induce regression, explaining the risk of the rebound effect after systemic therapy. Therefore, systemic therapy is an adjuvant for complicated infantile hemangiomas or congenital hemangioendotheliomas and requires additional induction of regression, especially by differentiated laser therapy. In endotracheal or periorbital infantile hemangiomas the laser-induced regression sometimes comes too late, necessitating an adjuvant systemic therapy to stop further growth. Furthermore, in kaposiform hemangioendothelioma with KMS an immediately halt to progression is important to stop the coagulopathy [11].

Antiangiogenesis

Inhibitors of vascular growth factors have been well investigated for the therapy of malignancies. The problem in infantile hemangioma is that this tumor forms vessels as a sign of maturation and not as a sign of aggression. So in several investigations a

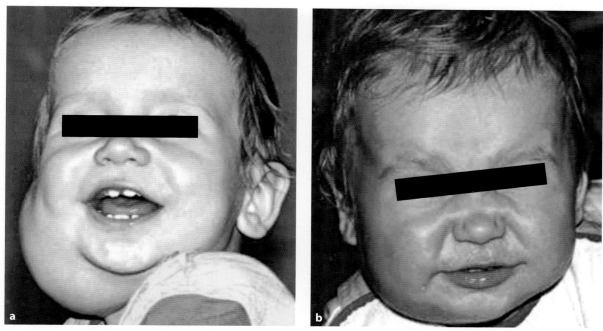

Fig. 8.2. Proliferating hemangioma of the parotis treated with corticosteroids. **a** A 12 month old boy with a proliferating hemangioma of the right parotis. Corticosteroid therapy was started with 2 mg/kg body weight per day for 2 weeks, followed by 1 mg/kg body weight. **b** Four weeks after therapy started the hemangioma had diminished

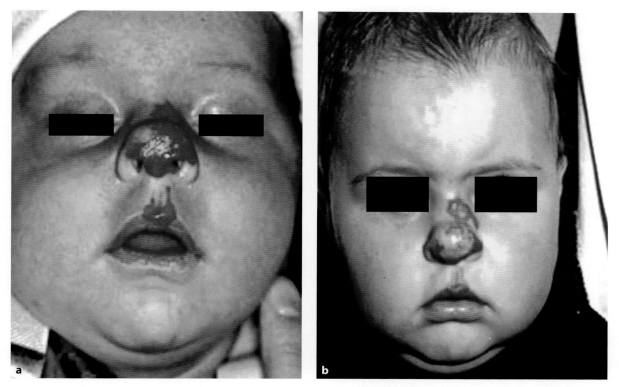

Fig. 8.3. Proliferating hemangioma of the nose tip treated with corticosteroids. **a** A 4 week old girl with proliferating hemangioma of the nose tip. Corticosteroid therapy was started with 2 mg/kg body weight per day for 2 weeks, followed by 1 mg/kg body weight and further tapering. **b** At the age of 10 months corticosteroid therapy was finally stopped. The development of a major soft tissue swelling by the hemangioma was avoided; however, laser treatment was needed to discolor the nose skin

additional pituitary-adrenal axis suppression, secondary diabetes mellitus or immunosuppression with increased susceptibility to infection is extremely rare. During corticosteroid therapy, the child should have a physical examination every 2–4 weeks with monitoring of blood pressure and glucosuria as well as height and weight. Prescription of oral ranitidine or a beta blocker may be necessary. However, all side effects, especially the growth and weight retardation, are reversible [6]. Live attenuated vaccines are contraindicated during the period of corticosteroid treatment while vaccinations with dead vaccines can be performed once the initial high dosage of steroids is reduced.

A unique location for hemangioma is the liver (Fig. 8.4). Recently, three principle categories of liver hemangioma lesions were postulated: focal, multifocal, and diffuse liver hemangioma [14]. A project to institute a web-based international hepatic hemangioma registry was initiated (see www.liverhemangioma.org). In most cases, there are multiple hemangiomas present in the liver, a situation referred to as liver hemangiomatosis.

Children with hemangiomatosis of the liver show an increased abdominal girth, hepatomegaly, or jaundice. Major problems can be seen if high cardiac output failure develops. Furthermore, liver dysfunction or rupture was reported. Therefore, hemangiomatosis of the liver is an indication for medical therapy. First line drugs are corticosteroids. In the past, mortality for liver hemangiomatosis was 70–90%. After the introduction of corticosteroids mortality decreased; however, some reports show that there are cases that do not respond to corticosteroids and may need surgery, embolization or treatment with vincristin or interferon 2 alpha as an ultima ratio.

We cannot complete this chapter without reporting the use of corticosteroids administered intra-lesionally or as topical ointment. During proliferation of well-defined hemangiomas, intralesional injection of corticosteroids can be used [15]. However, in our experience, cryo- or laser-therapy is easier and safer to perform in cases where topical steroid therapy might be possible [16]. A clinical trial comparing spontaneous regression with topical treatment for hemangiomas is needed.

Vincristine

There are some reports on the use of vincristine for the treatment of proliferating, corticosteroid-resistant hemangiomas. It is now recognized as a second line drug to treat function- and life-threatening hemangiomas and vascular tumors [17].

Vincristine is a naturally occurring vinca alkaloid isolated from the leaves of the periwinkle plant *Catharanthus roseus* [18]. It interferes with the mitotic spindle microtubules by binding to tubulin, resulting in inhibition of mitosis. There is considerable experience with the use of vincristine in the treatment of malignancies in children. Vincristine is a vesicant and caution needs to be exercised if given peripherally, due to the risk of extravasation.

Vincristine can be administered if corticosteroid therapy is not efficacious enough. A dose of 1 mg/m^2 (or 0.05 mg/kg body weight in children <10 kg) is generally used intravenously with weekly injections first, and then tapering down by increasing the interval between injections, depending on the clinical response [3]. In one report, a segmental mandibular hemangioma with rapid growth and facial disfigurement in a child with PHACES syndrome showed response to vincristine when the child developed additional obstructive sleep apnea under corticosteroid therapy [19]. In addition, vincristine can be helpful in hemangioma presenting with the Kasabach-Meritt phenomenon (KMP). This phenomenon describes the combination of thrombocytopenia, microangiopathic hemolytic anemia, and a mild consumptive coagulopathy. The vascular lesion that is responsible for the KMP can be a hemangioma; however, vascular tumors such as kaposiform hemangioendothelioma or tufted angioma are more often associated with KMP [20, 21]. A retrospective study on 15 patients with different vascular lesions and KMP shows that vincristine can be a safe and effective drug not only to treat the KMP, but also to decrease the size of the vascular lesion [22].

Neurotoxicity is the dose-limiting side effect of vincristine. A peripheral mixed sensory and motor neuropathy is common. It can also produce an autonomic neuropathy resulting in abdominal pain, constipation and ileus. Hematologic toxicity is rarely encountered with vincristine.

Interferon

The use of interferon alpha has been widely reported for corticosteroid-resistant proliferating hemangiomas [23]. Interferon alpha was initially developed as an antiviral agent and has immunoregulatory, antineoplastic and anti-angiogenic properties [24].

Interferon alpha can be given subcutaneously at a dose of 1–3×10^6 units/m^2 body surface area daily in

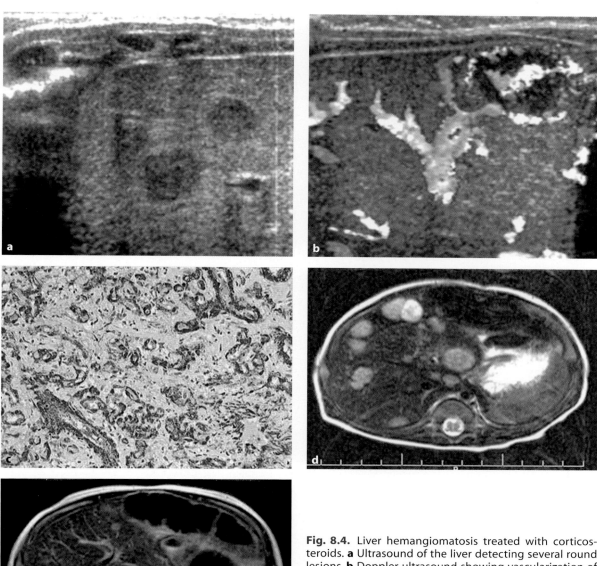

Fig. 8.4. Liver hemangiomatosis treated with corticosteroids. **a** Ultrasound of the liver detecting several round lesions. **b** Doppler ultrasound showing vascularization of the round lesions. **c** Biopsy and immunohistochemistry with alpha actin antibody. Multiple blood vessels are seen, confirming diagnosis of liver hemangiomatosis. **d** Magnetic resonance imaging (MRI) T2 weighted-presenting multiple round lesions involving all liver segments. **e** Result after 8 weeks of therapy with corticosteroids: regression of the lesions

life-threatening hemangiomas. However, this use has now been abandoned because of dangerous side effects. In short term use these include fever, neutropenia and anemia. Of great concern is long term neurotoxicity with development of spastic diplegia in up to 20% of cases [25, 26]. Therefore, we generally do not use interferon alpha in the therapy of hemangioma.

A recent report on intralesional administration of interferon alpha declared this new approach as an effective and safe method of hemangioma treatment [27].

Cyclophosphamide

Some rare reports on alkylating agents used for the treatment of vascular tumors, including hemangioma, are summarized in a review by Hurvitz et al. [4]. Common adverse effects include nausea, vomiting and reversible alopecia. Adequate hydration and alkalization of the urine is to be assured to prevent hemorrhagic cystitis and hyperuricemia. Secondary malignancies have been reported and therefore the use of cyclophosphamide should be reserved for ultima ratio situations.

Bleomycin

Intralesional bleomycin has been used as a method to treat hemangiomas in children and may be particularly helpful for large hemangiomas of the head and neck [28]. However, repeated general anesthetics are required, and scarring with hyperpigmentation may occur.

Perspectives: New Anti-Angiogenic Drugs

The development of drugs targeting angiogenesis, the formation of new blood vessels in solid tumors, has been a focus of cancer research for the last decades. Finally, more and more anti-angiogenic agents are now available and licensed for cancer treatment protocols. Whether these drugs could also be administered in the setting of hemangioma therapy is not yet defined, as toxicity profiles and especially experience in the pediatric age group are still missing. Some pre-clinical data on mouse models of hemangioma are already available and promising. For example, inhibition of Tie-2 signaling with a soluble Tie-2 receptor decreases hemangioma growth in a mouse model [29]. Furthermore, the new tyrosine kinase inhibitors that are now available as oral drugs could have a potential efficacy on hemangioma as expression of tyrosine kinase receptors, such as the vascular endothelial growth factor (VEGF) or the platelet-derived growth factor (PDGF) receptors by endothelial cells in hemangioma have been reported [30, 31].

References

1. Frieden IJ, Haggstrom AN, Drolet BA et al (2005) Infantile hemangiomas: current knowledge, future directions. Proceedings of a research workshop on infantile hemangiomas, April 7–9, Bethesda, Maryland, USA. Pediatr Dermatol 22:383–406
2. Bennett ML, Fleischer AB Jr, Chamlin SL, Frieden IJ (2001) Oral corticosteroid use is effective for cutaneous hemangiomas: an evidence-based evaluation. Arch Dermatol 137:1208–1213
3. Enjolras O, Breviere GM, Roger G et al (2004) [Vincristine treatment for function- and life-threatening infantile hemangioma]. Arch Pediatr 11:99–107
4. Hurvitz SA, Hurvitz CH, Sloninsky L, Sanford MC (2000) Successful treatment with cyclophosphamide of life-threatening diffuse hemangiomatosis involving the liver. J Pediatr Hematol Oncol 22:527–532
5. Dubois J, Hershon L, Carmant L et al (1999) Toxicity profile of interferon alfa-2b in children: A prospective evaluation. J Pediatr 135:782–785
6. Boon LM, MacDonald DM, Mulliken JB (1999) Complications of systemic corticosteroid therapy for problematic hemangioma. Plast Reconstr Surg 104:1616–1623
7. Zarem HA, Edgerton MT (1967) Induced resolution of cavernous hemangiomas following prednisolone therapy. Plast Reconstr Surg 39:76–83
8. Hasan Q, Tan ST, Xu B, Davis PF (2003) Effects of five commonly used glucocorticoids on haemangioma in vitro. Clin Exp Pharmacol Physiol 30:140–144
9. Blei F, Wilson EL, Mignatti P, Rifkin DB (1993) Mechanism of action of angiostatic steroids: suppression of plasminogen activator activity via stimulation of plasminogen activator inhibitor synthesis. J Cell Physiol 155:568–578
10. Bennett ML, Fleischer AB Jr, Chamlin SL, Frieden IJ (2001) Oral corticosteroid use is effective for cutaneous hemangiomas: an evidence-based evaluation. Arch Dermatol 137:1208–1213
11. Sadan N, Wolach B (1996) Treatment of hemangiomas of infants with high doses of prednisone. J Pediatr 128:141–146
12. Rossler J, Wehl G, Niemeyer CM (2007) Evaluating systemic prednisone therapy for proliferating haemangioma in infancy. Eur J Pediatr (Epub ahead of print)
13. Pope E, Krafchik BR, Macarthur C et al (2007) Oral versus high-dose pulse corticosteroids for problematic infantile hemangiomas: a randomized, controlled trial. Pediatrics 119:e1239–e1247
14. Christison-Lagay ER, Burrows PE, Alomari A et al (2007) Hepatic hemangiomas: subtype classification and development of a clinical practice algorithm and registry. J Pediatr Surg 42:62–67
15. Sloan GM, Reinisch JF, Nichter LS et al (1989) Intralesional corticosteroid therapy for infantile hemangiomas. Plast Reconstr Surg 83:459–467
16. Garzon MC, Lucky AW, Hawrot A, Frieden IJ (2005) Ultrapotent topical corticosteroid treatment of hemangiomas of infancy. J Am Acad Dermatol 52:281–286
17. Fawcett SL, Grant I, Hall PN et al (2004) Vincristine as a treatment for a large haemangioma threatening vital functions. Br J Plast Surg 57:168–171
18. Gidding CE, Kellie SJ, Kamps WA, de Graaf SS (1999) Vincristine revisited. Crit Rev Oncol Hematol 29:267–287

19. Herrero HA, Escobosa SO, Acha GT (2007) Successful treatment with vincristine in PHACES syndrome. Clin Transl Oncol 9:262–263

20. Enjolras O, Wassef M, Mazoyer E et al (1997) Infants with Kasabach-Merritt syndrome do not have "true" hemangiomas. J Pediatr 130:631–640

21. Sarkar M, Mulliken JB, Kozakewich HP et al (1997) Thrombocytopenic coagulopathy (Kasabach-Merritt phenomenon) is associated with Kaposiform hemangioendothelioma and not with common infantile hemangioma. Plast Reconstr Surg 100:1377–1386

22. Haisley-Royster C, Enjolras O, Frieden IJ, et al (2002) Kasabach-merritt phenomenon: a retrospective study of treatment with vincristine. J Pediatr Hematol Oncol 24:459–462

23. Ezekowitz RA, Mulliken JB, Folkman J (1992) Interferon alfa-2a therapy for life-threatening hemangiomas of infancy. N Engl J Med 326:1456–1463

24. Sidky YA, Borden EC (1987) Inhibition of angiogenesis by interferons: effects on tumor- and lymphocyte-induced vascular responses. Cancer Res 47:5155–5161

25. Barlow CF, Priebe CJ, Mulliken JB et al (1998) Spastic diplegia as a complication of interferon Alfa-2a treatment of hemangiomas of infancy. J Pediatr 132:527–530

26. Worle H, Maass E, Kohler B, Treuner J (1999) Interferon alpha-2a therapy in haemangiomas of infancy: spastic diplegia as a severe complication. Eur J Pediatr 158:344

27. Kaselas C, Tsikopoulos G, Papouis G, Kaselas V (2007) Intralesional administration of interferon A for the management of severe haemangiomas. Pediatr Surg Int 23:215–218

28. Pienaar C, Graham R, Geldenhuys S, Hudson DA (2006) Intralesional bleomycin for the treatment of hemangiomas. Plast Reconstr Surg 117:221–226

29. Perry BN, Govindarajan B, Bhandarkar SS et al (2006) Pharmacologic blockade of angiopoietin-2 is efficacious against model hemangiomas in mice. J Invest Dermatol 126:2316–2322

30. Berard M, Sordello S, Ortega N et al (1997) Vascular endothelial growth factor confers a growth advantage in vitro and in vivo to stromal cells cultured from neonatal hemangiomas. Am J Pathol 150:1315–1326

31. Takahashi K, Mulliken JB, Kozakewich HP (1994) Cellular markers that distinguish the phases of hemangioma during infancy and childhood. J Clin Invest 93:2357–2364

Laser Therapy of Infantile Hemangiomas and Other Congenital Vascular Tumors of Newborns and Infants

9

Hans Peter Berlien

Abstract

The indications for any therapy of congenital vascular tumors are growing tumors or other complications. Due to specific and calculable reactions, laser offers the best modality for localized therapy because only with laser is it possible to preserve the unaffected epithelial layer. Besides the different wavelengths with their specific absorptions patterns, a great variety of tissue interactions can be achieved by variation of the interaction time and surface protection by cooling and/or compression.

Introduction

Due to the fact that infantile hemangiomas have an especially high capability of spontaneous regression, the indication for active therapy is only in cases where this spontaneous regression occurs too late or there is an excessive growth. The aim of laser therapy is to induce regression – except in cases where an immediate surgical intervention is needed – not a removal of the hemangiomatous tissue. This means that any additional damage of surrounding tissue caused by the laser therapy has to and can be avoided. Laser therapy causes an inflammatory process as a result of intravascular absorption of light and vessel obstruction, and generally does not cause definitive coagulation. This means that for different forms, depths, organs and localizations different lasers and different laser procedures are obligatory.

Laser Therapy

Superselective Laser Systems

The specific absorption is not only a question of the wavelength and the tissue properties: it depends also reciprocally on the exposure time [1]. This means that for superselective absorption the lower the specific absorption, the shorter the exposure time, or the longer the exposure time, the higher the specific absorption. This results in an overlap of indications between the different laser systems. Generally the term "superselective laser systems" is used for laser with an exposure time of less than 100 ms (short pulsed lasers) (Table 9.1) [2].

Table 9.1. Major indications for pulsed laser. Due to the great specific tissue absorption these lasers have only a small band of indications, and are for use by specialists

FLPDL
- flat prodromal phase of IH
- early flat initial phase of IH
- capillary flat residuals in regression phase of IH

KTP
- teleangiectatic prodromal phase of IH
- early punctual initial phase of IH (e.g., eyelid)
- teleangiectatic residuals in regression phase of IH

Pulsed Nd:YAG-Laser
- punctual proliferation phase of IH in endangered regions (e.g., eyelid, ear cartilage, columella, gingiva)
- tuberous residuals in regression phase of IH

R. Mattassi, D.A. Loose, M. Vaghi (eds.), *Hemangiomas and Vascular Malformations*.
© Springer-Verlag Italia 2009

Flash Lamp Pumped Pulsed Dye Laser "FLPD Laser"

The use of flash lamp pulsed dye laser therapy (FLPDL) with wave lengths of 585 or 595 nm and pulse durations of 300 µs to 2 ms is only indicated in the very early stages of infantile hemangiomas not thicker than 2 mm, provided there is no subcutaneous part [3]. Treatment is simple and quick. When the faces of newborn and small children have to be treated, anesthesia is required, while in areas other than the face, local anesthesia (e.g., with EMLA) suffices. Side effects are extremely rare. Occasionally, blisters and scabs are observed, requiring cooling and stabilization of the epidermis by a fluid cooling cuvette. The obligatory bluish-black coloring disappears within 14 days (Fig. 9.1). Scars appear in less than 1% of all cases. Particularly in the anogenital area, there is a danger of ulceration with secondary infection. Early FLPDL therapy of all infantile hemangiomas and their precursor lesions brought no essential advantages compared to an untreated control group [4], but the authors of the study did not differentiate hemangiomas according to their depth nor their various stages of development (Fig. 9.2). Tuberous hemangiomas are no indication for FLPDL, and FLPDL also fails in subcutaneous and endophytically growing hemangiomas [5]. Primary teleangiectatic changes, or residues of mature infantile hemangiomas, also are not suited for the FLPDL (Fig. 9.3). This is an indication for the KTP laser.

Frequency Doubled Nd:YAG Laser ("KTP")

This type of laser must not be mixed up with the pulsed Nd:YAG laser or even with the continuous wave (cw)-ND:YAG laser [6]. Here, the infrared light of the Nd:YAG laser is channeled through a potassium-titanyl-phosphate crystal, which produces from the near infra-red (NIR) of 1064 nm by frequency doubling half the wave length of 532 nm. Thus the biological effect is comparable to that of an argon laser [4]. The advantage of this type of laser is that, due to its higher efficacy, the KTP does not need water cooling, especially when pumped with diodes, unlike the argon laser. This makes it easier to handle. This way small tuberous lesions and telangiectasias can be directly treated under glass spatula compression dot to dot (Fig. 9.4). By short pulse durations of a maximum of 100 ms and avoidance of double exposure or overlapping, absorption only takes place in the hemoglobin of the vessels, so that no thermal side effects are to be expected in the surrounding tissue.

Pulsed Nd:YAG Laser

Unlike in the KTP laser, NIR-radiation is applied directly with the pulsed Nd:YAG laser. The difference compared to the standard cw-Nd:YAG laser is the short pulse rate of 2–10 ms, albeit with high pulse peaks.

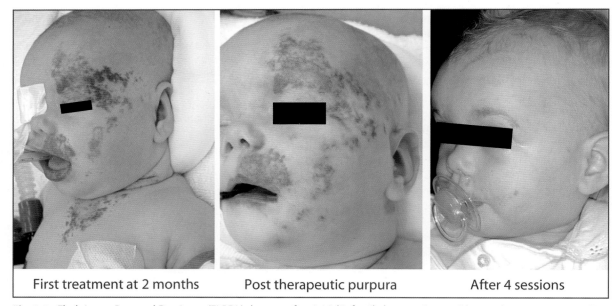

First treatment at 2 months   Post therapeutic purpura   After 4 sessions

Fig. 9.1. Flash Lamp Pumped Dye Laser (FLPDL) therapy of an initial infantile hemangioma with no subcutaneous parts. Due to the risk of complete hair removal the eyebrows were not treated so intensively, so there are more residuals than on the face. Note the pretracheal hemangioma, in such cases routine tracheoscopy to detect early tracheal hemangioma is mandatory

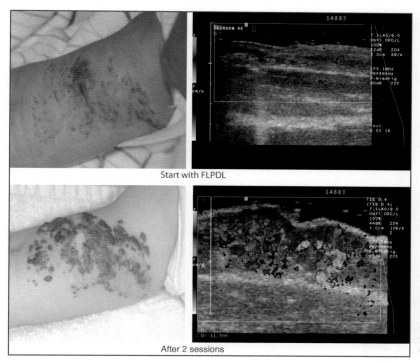

Start with FLPDL

After 2 sessions

Fig. 9.2. FLPDL-therapy of infantile hemangioma. With this therapy a clearance of the intracutaneous parts was obtainable while the therapy failed for the subcutaneous growth

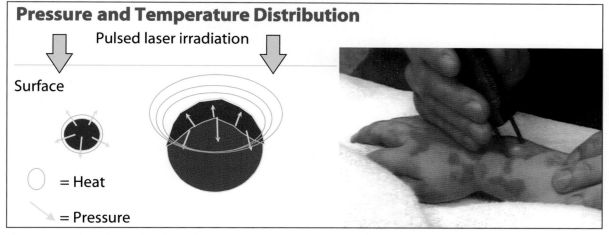

Pressure and Temperature Distribution

Pulsed laser irradiation

Surface

◯ = Heat

↘ = Pressure

Fig. 9.3. Vessel size limits the effect of FLPDL. The shorter the pulse length the smaller the affected volume. This explains why FLPDL is not suitable for larger teleangiectatic vessels

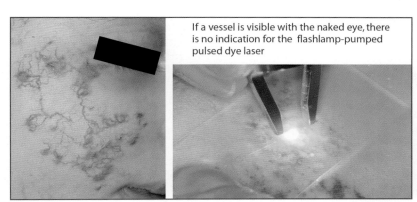

If a vessel is visible with the naked eye, there is no indication for the flashlamp-pumped pulsed dye laser

Fig. 9.4. KTP laser therapy. The glass spatula compression with sodium immersion reduces the size of the vessel, reduces the surface scattering, increases the penetration depth and protects the skin from vaporization

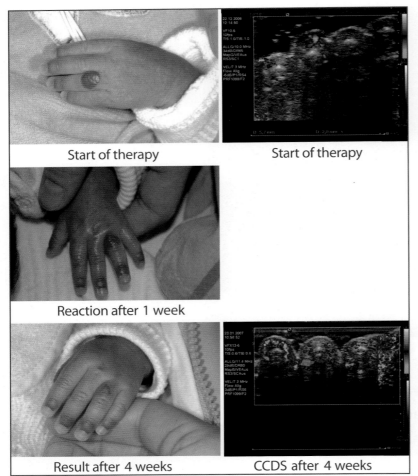

Start of therapy   Start of therapy

Reaction after 1 week

Result after 4 weeks   CCDS after 4 weeks

Fig. 9.5. Pulsed Nd:YAG-laser. Although the near infrared radiation has in principle a great penetration depth, due to the short exposure time in pulsed lasers the reaction depth is limited. This is important in endangered regions, here the finger joint, where the cw-Nd:YAG laser carries the risk of cartilage destruction

While the biophysical penetration is the same as that of the cw-Nd:YAG laser, the actual penetration depth is limited due to the short pulse duration (Fig. 9.5). For this reason, this laser is suited to anatomically endangered regions or larger vein ectasias and tuberous lesions [7]. To avoid secondary damage by scattered radiation or heat conduction, at least one intermittent cooling system by cold air or ice cubes is required, unless the beam is led through the fluid cooling cuvette or the ice cube as with the cw-Nd:YAG laser.

Continuous Wave (cw-Nd:YAG) Lasers

With longer exposure times than 100 ms, thermal conductivity by the laser-heated tissue is a main effect. This means that for the primary reaction a specific absorption is important, but the whole tissue interaction is also triggered by the exposure time (Fig. 9.6). Lasers with a high water absorption, such as Erbium-

or CO_2-lasers, have the same primary effect in all tissues: the real tissue interaction depends only on the exposure time. Besides the argon laser, the cw-Nd:YAG laser is the laser type that has been used for the longest time for the treatment of congenital vascular anomalies. It is the same laser which is used for endoscopic surgery. In addition to the possibility of directing the laser beam via thin glass fibers, the immense biophysical variability has made this laser the "workhorse" for the treatment of congenital vascular anomalies (Table 9.2).

The biophysically determined penetration (drop in photon density to $1/e^2$) of the cw-Nd:YAG laser is 8 mm for most tissues. However, this means that at continuous wave mode at high performance, an effective photon density can still be attained to depths of 20 and 30 mm. On the other hand, the photon density and thus the effective depth can be limited to less than 1 mm by short pulse durations. Suitable cooling procedures protect the penetrated surface enough despite surface absorption so as to allow no tissue reactions

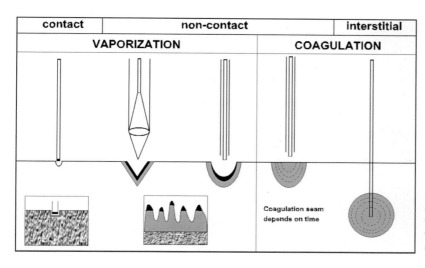

Fig. 9.6. Principle application modes of the cw-Nd:YAG laser. With the different procedure of surface cooling, the variety of tissue interactions increases. Reprinted from [13]

Table 9.2. In cw Nd:YAG laser by changing the application mode and the exposure time a great variety of tissue interactions and therefore a broad range of indications are possible

Direct with intermittent cooling (<100 ms)
– early punctual initial phase of infantile hemangioma (IH)
– tuberous residuals in regression phase of IH

Direct with continuous fluid cooling cuvette (100–200 ms)
– teleangiectatic prodromal phase of IH
– teleangiectatic residuals in regression phase of IH

Transcutaneous with continuous ice cube cooling (cw)
– all stages in IH in all localizations up to 30 mm thickness
– NICH & KHE up to 30 mm thickness (e.g., risk of disseminated intravascular coagulation [DIC])

Impression technique (cw)
– initial/proliferation phase of IH in endangered regions (e.g., eyelid, lip, enoral, urethra, etc.)

Interstitial puncture technique (cw)
– primary subcutaneous, mucous IH all stages
– NICH & KHE thickness >30 mm
– mixed intra-subcutaneous IH >30 mm all stages

Endoscopic application
– n.c.-technique: flat pharyngeal, tracheal IH
– impression: pad-like IH tracheal, vulval, intraanal

n.c., noncontact

there, but only deeper down. Moreover, different absorption coefficients are responsible for the selective effect. Blood and organs rich in blood absorb this NIR-radiation considerably better than connective or fatty tissue. The tissue reaction to the NIR-radiation also differs from tissue to tissue. Collagen shows considerable shrinkage: the endothelium already reacts with a serious vasculitis to power densities which do not yet trigger a reaction in other tissue.

High power densities quickly lead to carbonization, which then fully absorbs the subsequent laser radiation. Thus, vaporization sets in with two consequences: if one wants to ablate or cut, this process must occur very quickly in order to avoid unwanted thermal effects in the vicinity. If coagulation is intended especially in the deep regions, this process must be avoided, as no radiation gets down deep enough. The direction of these processes determines the wide usage of the cw-Nd:YAG laser [8].

Transcutaneous Direct Application

Small tuberous lesions and telangiectasias may also be treated with the cw-Nd:YAG laser, analogous to the pulsed Nd:YAG laser and the KTP laser. To avoid thermal damage, short pulse rates of maximum 100 ms, an output of 25 W and small spot diameter of up to 0.5 mm are required, using a focusing hand piece. Besides, intermittent and post cooling with ice cubes has to take place to avoid thermal damage by heat blockage.

Transcutaneous Application with Fluid Cooling Cuvette

If intermittent cooling is not sufficient, continuous cooling is required. The heat capacity of spray or cold air cooling is not sufficient for the heat blockage caused by the cw-Nd:YAG laser. Various contact cooling systems are on the market. Cooled sapphire plates are easy to handle, but have a series of disadvantages. The metal frame of the cooling Peltier element may lead to frostbite in cases of direct skin contact. The biggest disadvantage, however, is that their plane surface cannot adapt to the anatomic situation, especially in children's faces, so that they either do not have full con-

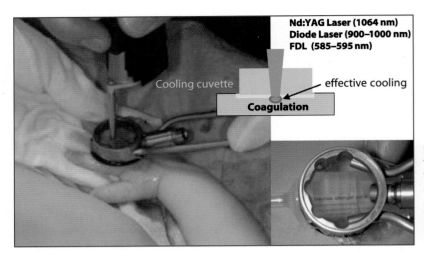

Fig. 9.7. Cooling chamber, principle of the fluid colling cuvette. The high transparent flexible latex-membrane allows a continuous control of the laser process and follows any anatomical structure without uncontrolled compression. However, the heat capacity is limited for pulsed applications

tact with the surface or are too heavily compressed at the edges, causing not only frostbite, but also changes in the microcirculation. Thus, they can actually be used only for large plane areas. The fluid cooling cuvette with a 40% refrigerated glycol solution (side of the patient) has a highly flexible, highly transparent latex membrane which, through changes in the outlet valve, can adapt even to difficult anatomic silhouettes (Fig. 9.7). An additional advantage is that this pre-stressing makes it possible to adjust the compression pressure and the blood flow to vary the tissue absorption [9]. With maximum compression, the overlying tissue can be made transparent for the Nd:YAG laser radiation. With negative pressure (suction), the tiniest capillary vessels can be expanded, boosting the specific absorption. The cooling capacity has been calculated to have a reaction in the center of the laser beam given the necessary absorption, while adverse events by scattering and thermal conduction are avoided in the surrounding areas. In case of vein ectasias, this procedure is better suited than the KTP.

Transcutaneous Application with Continuous Ice Cube Cooling

If subcutaneous lesions are to be treated transcutaneously, a continuous Nd:YAG laser application would create so much heat that none of the above mentioned cooling systems would be able to completely protect the transient tissue from unwanted coagulation. Deep freezing systems such as liquid nitrogen or deep-temperature Peltier elements cannot be directed sufficiently, so that frostbite would result. Here, radiation through a transparent ice cube without air bubbles seems to be the solution. The

melting of ice to water is one of the most energy-consuming processes. This high heat capacity is capable of completely rerouting the heat that builds up in the transient tissue by basic absorption, so there are no reactions on the surface. On the other hand, natural law prevents the temperature from dropping below 0 degrees Celsius, avoiding frostbite. Since meltwater always guarantees good tissue contact, contact gels etc. are superfluous. This cooling effect is limited to 2 mm due to the thermal conductivity properties of the tissue, so that laser radiation can treat subcutaneous lesions thanks to its greater penetration, without causing any defects on the surface. Prerequisites are the use of a focusing hand piece with a focus diameter of 0.5–1 mm. This focus has to be positioned on the tissue surface through an ice cube, as otherwise sufficient penetration will not be attained because of diffraction scattering. As the ice cube has its own absorption for this laser radiation, a prolonged exposition would drill a hole in the ice cube ("chimney effect"), letting radiation get directly to the tissue surface. Therefore, the ice cube has to be moved above the hemangioma under laser exposition, the ray itself moving in small spiral motions with a radius of about 5 mm to avoid too high a load for a single spot. If only the laser beam could be moved above the ice cube, with the ice cube remaining still, the chimney effect could be avoided, but the developing heat on the surface of the hemangioma would melt the ice cube so much that there would be no more direct tissue contact between ice cube and hemangioma ("igloo effect"). By compression with the ice cube – especially in large hemangiomas – the depth of penetration can be increased and by pressure on the surface the absorption decreased, boosting the protection (Fig. 9.8).

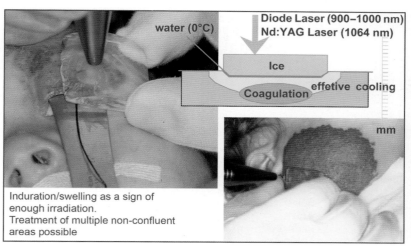

Induration/swelling as a sign of enough irradiation.
Treatment of multiple non-confluent areas possible

Fig. 9.8. Transcutaneous Nd:YAG-laser treatment with ice cube cooling. For continuous laser application, a greater heat capacity is required to save the overlying skin. Irradiation through a clear ice cube allows a deep laser reaction without any damage to the overlying skin. The protection is so perfect that in eyelid treatment it is possible to carry out a transpalpebral coagulation without noticing. Therefore, the cornea in this case must be protected with a metal spatula

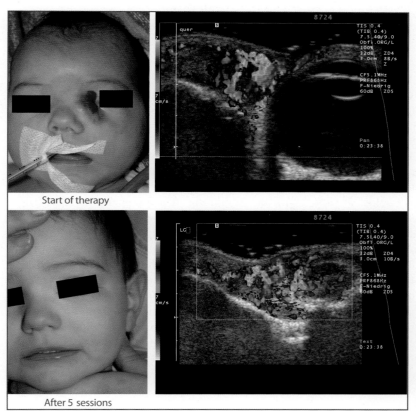

Start of therapy

After 5 sessions

Fig. 9.9. Transcutaneous Nd:YAG-laser treatment with ice cube cooling. Even in parabulbar hemangioma a safe induction of regression is possible without any risk of burn scars. The beam has to be directed away from the bulb to avoid secondary damage due to scattering

This procedure is only recommended under anesthesia because of the associated pain. Besides, this is also necessary because of laser safety, because most hemangiomas are located in the face near the eyes. For the exact positioning of the laser parameters intraoperative color-coded duplex sonography (CCDS) is required, as this alone enables determi-nation of activity and exact stage, dimension and, where applicable, involvement of various layers (Fig. 9.9). To choose the laser output, the following rules apply: the more active and aggressive the growth, and the earlier the stage, the smaller the output to avoid an overreaction. The more vessels that are already visible, the higher the output needed to

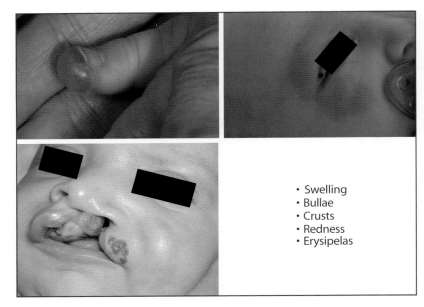

- Swelling
- Bullae
- Crusts
- Redness
- Erysipelas

Fig. 9.10. Side effects after transcutaneous ice cube cooled Nd:YAG-laser. Blebs can result not as burning bleb but due to the secondary swelling as a late bleb. Furthermore, after a latency of 24–48 hours in the lymph drainage vincinity a lymphangitis can occur. In these cases immediately antibiotic treatment can cure this erysipelas

attain involution. Moreover, the stronger the intracutaneous lesion, the smaller the output. However, in exclusive subcutaneous lesions, the output is higher. Treatment next to the eyes necessitates protection from forward scattered radiation. Metal spatulas ("eye spatulas") are suited for this purpose. These float on a kanamycin-ointment bed in such a way that the back side never touches the cornea. For this reason, the customary "eye shields" are obsolete, as they lie directly on the cornea and may lead to secondary burns. Despite these precautions, the direction of the laser beam should always be away from the eyeball. At the columella, attention should be paid to the cartilage structure of the nose. In case of hemangiomas on the lips, the laser also has to be turned away from the gingiva, to avoid destruction of the dental germ. A hemangioma of the gingiva itself can then be treated with the FLPD laser. The aim is not a definite coagulation of the infantile hemangioma but the induction of a vasculitis. A visible blanching or even an involution during laser treatment should be avoided as this would be equivalent to overdosing. The optimal total dose has been reached when during laser treatment the hemangioma starts to show a swelling, is bulging, and the surrounding area turns red, which lasts for up to 12 hours. Occasionally, 6–24 hours postoperatively, subcutaneous blue indurations develop as an expression of the vasculitis with vessel breakdown. This reaction is common in very active infantile hemangiomas in the early proliferation phase. As the overlaying epidermis is easily

damaged, postoperatively enough ointment should be applied and the area should be protected against scratches with suitable measures such as the wearing of gloves. A bandage is rarely necessary, except in case of heavy mechanical abrasions. Although this treatment does not cause injuries on the surface of the skin, about 2% of the children, 12–48 hours after the operation, develop erysipelas with the beginning of a lymphangitis (Fig. 9.10). This is seen frequently in the face. Erysipelas does not develop in the hemangioma itself or around it, but occasionally a few centimeters away draining into the lymph. This inflammation can be differentiated from the direct postoperative laser-induced inflammation as this region is sensitive to touch and hardened. In already exulcerated or even secondarily infected hemangiomas, this reaction has never been noted, nor in interstitial treatment when puncturing. It thus is not a nosocomial infection. An immediate treatment with oral antibiotics with a broad spectrum cephalosporin will cause the clinical symptoms to subside within a few hours. Fever and symptoms do not exist at that time, but the infiltrate may persist for a few days. As a regression in hemangioendotheliomas cannot be attained as easily as in infantile hemangiomas (Fig. 9.11), clearly increased output up to 50 W is required as is normally only used for the treatment of vascular malformations. In contrast to the interstitial puncture technique, uniform coagulation can be achieved, so that fibrosis will not be as pronounced after healing is completed.

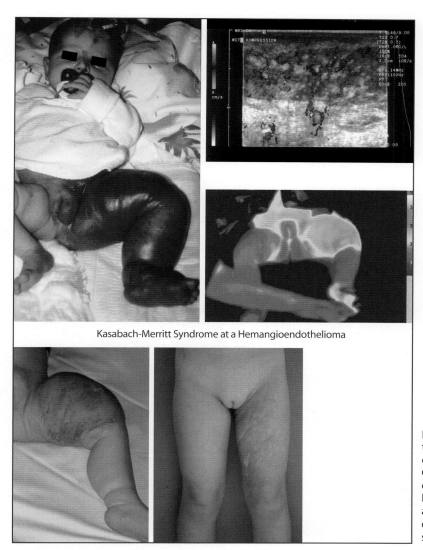

Kasabach-Merritt Syndrome at a Hemangioendothelioma

Fig. 9.11. Disseminated intravasal thrombopaty "DIC". Full clinical course of a Kasabach-Merrit Syndrome. The CCDS shows the typical interstitial edema, the thermography shows the hyperthermia. The clinical outcome in all cases of congenital hemangioenditheliomas is the same: chalasia of the skin and atrophy of subcutis and fascia

Impression Technique

Unlike in interstitial puncturing, the fiber in the impression technique is placed on the surface and pressed into the hemangioma. This way, a shift of the laser effect below the surface is also attained, without triggering coagulation on the surface of the hemangioma (except for the fiber contact area). Therefore, this technique should be used for the skin only in limited cases, as it may cause small scars. However, it is an ideal technique for hemangiomas reachable from the mucosa, including the conjunctiva (Fig. 9.12), as it leads to a "restitutio ad integrum" even in the contact area. With a laser output of a maximum of 5 W, the in-depth effect can be adjusted by length of exposition. This way, laser application becomes possible even near critical structures. In hemangiomas on the upper as well as the lower eyelid, a curved fiber holder is used for laser application from the conjunctiva to the outside. The skin temperature above the hemangioma is constantly being controlled with a finger (Fig. 9.12), the position of the fiber tip can be controlled with the CCDS (Fig. 9.13). In lip hemangiomas, likewise, the laser can be applied intraorally. The technique thus closes the gap between direct application, even with the pulsed Nd:YAG laser which operates only on the surface, and the transcutaneous ice cube application which reaches large volumes.

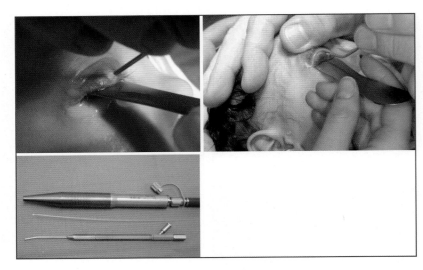

Fig. 9.12. The impression technique allows a precise application of laser energy to subcutaneous volumes. Even when no scattering can occur, near the eye the bulb and the cornea must be protected with a metal spatula

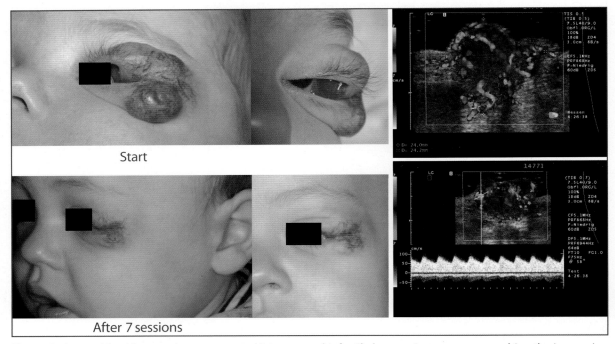

Fig. 9.13. In combined intra-, subcutaneous and intramucosal infantile hemangioma you can combine the impression technique with the transcutaneous ice cube cooled Nd:YAG laser technique in one session to treat larger areas without any additional damage to the skin

Interstitial Puncture Technique

In very large, deep and particularly in purely subcutaneous hemangiomas, neither the impression technique nor the transcutaneous ice cube method can totally avoid thermal damage to the surface. In these cases, the hemangioma is punctured with a teflon vein catheter and the fiber is inserted (Fig. 9.14). Output should be between 4 and 5 W. As with higher out-

puts, there are immediate carbonizations at the fiber tip which for one thing would burn the tissue and for another would prevent a uniform distribution of the laser radiation. Intraoperative CCDS control is obligatory [10] to avoid erroneous puncturing and to monitor the adequate laser reaction via the color bruit. Skin temperature above the laser area must be monitored continually with a finger – just as in the impression technique – when the distance from the fiber tip to

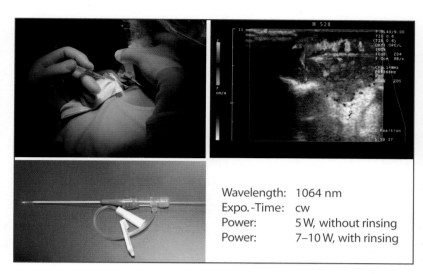

Fig. 9.14. Interstitial Nd:YAG-laser treatment (ITT). For more deeply located or thicker lesions the interstitial puncture technique allows any localization to be reached. The point of puncture should be a minimum of 1 cm away from the edges of the lesion to prevent any postoperative bleeding by this tunnel. CCDS control is mandatory to detect any endangered anatomical structure and to control the laser process by the color bruit. In larger lesions one has to perform multiple puncture with afterloading technique before initiating lasering, in order to avoid disturbances of the ultrasound image by the gas reaction during the laser

Wavelength: 1064 nm
Expo.-Time: cw
Power: 5 W, without rinsing
Power: 7–10 W, with rinsing

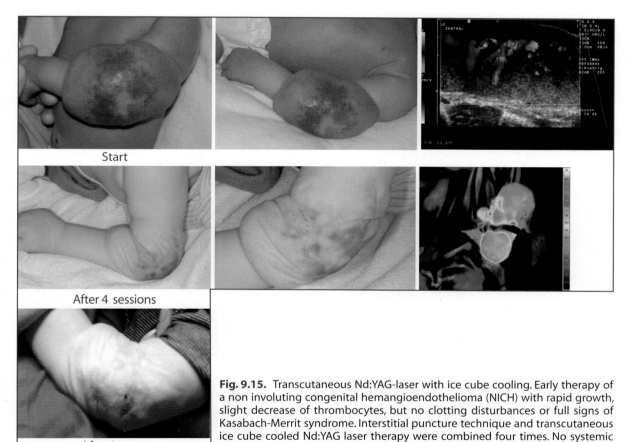

Start

After 4 sessions

After 1 year

Fig. 9.15. Transcutaneous Nd:YAG-laser with ice cube cooling. Early therapy of a non involuting congenital hemangioendothelioma (NICH) with rapid growth, slight decrease of thrombocytes, but no clotting disturbances or full signs of Kasabach-Merrit syndrome. Interstitial puncture technique and transcutaneous ice cube cooled Nd:YAG laser therapy were combined four times. No systemic prednisolone or chemotherapy

the surface is less than 10 mm. Thermal damage of the surface thus can safely be avoided, but when nerves are being directly aimed for, for instance, with the fiber tip, they may be damaged. This can be excluded by the transcutaneous ice cube technique. By optimizing the laser parameters and the ice cube quality, the indication for the interstitial technique for infantile hemangiomas therefore has clearly dropped. Even vast parotid hemangiomas are only rarely treated this way. For large hemangioendotheliomas (Fig. 9.15), be it the Kaposi-like (KHE) or the non-involuting congenital hemangioma (NICH), this technique represents an expansion of the transcutaneous ice cube technique, as by direct application subcutaneously an immediate coagulation of the hemangioendotheliomas can be achieved. In patients with a Kasabach-Merritt syndrome along with a coagulopathy, however, the bleeding risk through puncturing has to be avoided. In such cases, small coagulations of the dermis should be accepted and the ice cube technique with a high output of 60 W applied.

Endoscopy

In infantile hemangiomas, there is an indication for endoscopic treatment, primarily in subglottal and tracheal infantile hemangiomas [11] as well as in the urethra and the anal canal. While an involvement of the male urethra by an infantile hemangioma is rare, and by differential diagnosis a vascular malformation should be considered, in girls, vulvar and perineal infantile hemangiomas are clearly more common. To exclude further lesions at the bladder neck, which can also be affected by a vascular malformation, a cysto-urethroscopy should always be performed. The endoscope is entered through the working canal and in flat disseminated hemangiomas a punctual coagulation is achieved by non-contact of the fiber tip with the tissue with an output of 10 W, pulsed, and with exposures lasting a maximum of 100 ms. Confluent coagulation definitely has to be avoided. In case of pad-like hemangiomas, the impression technique is performed over the endoscope as described above with a maximum output of only 5 W.

Especially in subglottal and tracheal hemangiomas, the hemangioma must not be coagulated completely, as scarred strictures may remain [12]. Circular applications should be avoided as well (Fig. 9.16). In infantile hemangiomas one has to be particularly careful of the vocal cords themselves. Only short, single punctual applications are permissible, to avoid fibrosis, and thus limiting function of the vocal cords. In no case should it be attempted to remove the hemangioma in one session (Fig. 9.17). For this procedure, a postoperative intubation for safety reasons is usually not necessary. In infantile hemangiomas of the larynx and the trachea, simultaneous short-interval high-dose prednisone therapy is essential. With this regimen we were able to avoid primary tracheotomy for more than 20 years in patients with infantile hemangiomas. In children who underwent tracheotomy in emergency situations elsewhere and who then came to us, the tracheostoma could be closed after a maximum of two sessions.

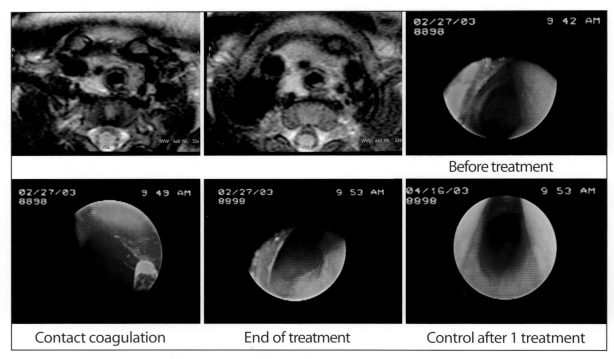

Before treatment

Contact coagulation   End of treatment   Control after 1 treatment

Fig. 9.16. Subglottic infantile hemangioma in a child with facial hemangioma. Only a routine tracheoscopy allowed this hemangioma to be detected and treated so early that a tracheotomy could be avoided

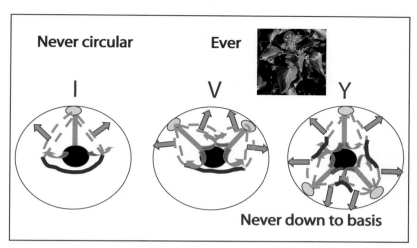

Fig. 9.17. Nd:YAG-laser contact-incision. Even in circular lesions, tracheal laser should not be carried out circularly or down to the base. In infantile hemangioma, especially in early stages, an introduction of regression is enough to prevent airway obstruction

References

1. Anderson RR, Parish JA (1981) The optics of human skin. J Invest Dermatol 77:9–13
2. Tong AKF, Tan OT, Boll J et al (1987) Ultrastructure: effects of melanin pigment on target specificity using a pulsed dye laser (577 nm). J Invest Dermatol 88:747–752
3. Poetke M, Philipp C, Berlien HP (2000) Flashlamp-pumped pulsed dye laser for hemangiomas in infancy. Arch Dermatol 136:628–632
4. Achauer BM, Vander Kam VM (1989) Capillary hemangiomas (strawberry mark) of infancy: comparison of argon and Nd:YAG laser treatment. Plast Reconstr Surg 84(1):60–69
5. Ashinoff R, Geronemus RG (1993) Failure of the flashlamp-pumped pulsed dye laser to prevent progression to deep hemangioma. Pediatr Dermatol 10:77–80
6. Poetke M, Urban P, Philipp C, Berlien HP (2004) Laserbehandlung bei Hämangiomen – Technische Grundlagen und Möglichkeiten. Monatsschr Kinderheilkunde 152:7–15
7. AWMF online (2007) Empfehlungen zur Behandlung mit Laser und hochenergetischen Blitzlampen (HBL) in der Dermatologie, Empfehlungen der Deutschen Dermatologischen Gesellschaft
8. Berlien HP, Waldschmidt J, Müller G (1988) Laser treatment of cutaneous and deep vessel anomalies. In: Waidelich W (ed) Laser optoelectronics in medicine. Springer Verlag, Berlin-Heidelberg-New York, pp 526–528
9. Poetke M, Philipp C, Berlien HP (1997) Ten years of laser treatment of hemangiomas and vascular malformations: techniques and results. In: Berlien HP, Schmittenbecher PP (ed) Laser surgery in children. Springer Verlag Berlin, pp 82–91
10. Urban P, Philipp CM, Poetke M, Berlien HP (2005) Value of colour coded duplex sonography in the assessment of haemangiomas and vascular malformations. Medical Laser Application 20(4):267–278
11. Cholewa D, Waldschmidt J (1998) Laser treatment of hemangiomas of the larynx and trachea. Lasers in Surgery and Medicine 23:221–232
12. Apfelberg DB, Maser MF, Lash H, White DN (1985) Benefits of CO_2 laser in oral hemangioma excision. Plast Reconstr Surg 75:46
13. Berlien HP, Müller GJ (2003) Applied laser medicine. Springer-Verlag Berlin Heidelberg p 69

Surgery of Hemangiomas

10

Gianni Vercellio, Vittoria Baraldini

Abstract

Surgical management of infantile hemangiomas (Hm) usually consists of late correction of contour deformities after completed spontaneous involution with excision of remaining fibrofatty tissue and exuberant skin. The range of indications to early surgical excision of Hm during the proliferating phase or after partial involution has been recently enlarged with the introduction of particular techniques adopted in order to minimize intra-operative bleeding and optimize scarring. On the basis of our experience, early surgical excision can be considered in the following situations: rapidly growing Hm with expectance of relevant fibrofatty remnants after involution; voluminous tuberous Hm anatomically located in barely exposed areas where scars are easily concealed; pedunculated Hm with a narrow implantation base; non involutive congenital Hm (NICH type); palpebral Hm with secondary functional impairment of palpebral motility not responding to corticosteroids and/or laser treatment; ulcerated and bleeding Hm not responding to corticosteroids and/or laser treatment; and Hm of the nose producing secondary cartilage deformity.

Introduction

Among the different therapeutic options for common hemangiomas (Hm) a marginal role has traditionally been reserved for surgery. This is for multiple reasons: the natural tendency of Hm to spontaneously involute, the good response of Hm to corticosteroids and laser treatment, and the high incidence of bad cosmetic results after surgical excision with hypertrophic surgical scars compared to the persistent fibro-fatty remnants remaining after completed spontaneous involution [1, 2].

Furthermore, the main challenge for the surgeon when approaching large Hm in the proliferative phase is intraoperative bleeding control: a few specific techniques have been developed in order to reduce bleeding during the operation.

Although parents are normally reluctant to consider surgery because it requires general anesthesia and occasionally blood transfusion, they often ask for an early excision of the mass, particularly when it affects exposed anatomical areas.

As for other vascular anomalies, the assessment of indications to early surgical excision of Hm requires an evaluation of different parameters: anatomical areas involved, Hm type and size, past complications, Hm life cycle phase, functional implications and the level of response to alternative treatments [3].

Indications and Timing for Surgical Treatment

Indications and timing for surgical treatment are strictly related to each other. There is a general agreement about postponing surgical treatment of Hm in the expectation of a complete spontaneous involution. Therefore indications to surgery are normally restricted to the treatment of fibro-fatty remnants with different techniques: excision of exuberant fibro-fatty tissue (liposuction can be employed) and correction of contour deformities [1–3].

Indications to early surgical excision of Hm in the proliferative phase are more controversial [4] and can be listed as follows:

1. Rapidly growing Hm with expectance of relevant fibrofatty residuum after involution.

R. Mattassi, D.A. Loose, M. Vaghi (eds.), *Hemangiomas and Vascular Malformations*.
© Springer-Verlag Italia 2009

2. Voluminous tuberous Hm affecting anatomical sites where scars would be easily hidden (i.e. neck, scalp).
3. Pedicled tuberous Hm with a narrow implantation base (excisable using the "round block" technique).
4. Non involutive congenital Hm (NICH type – Fig. 10.1).
5. Palpebral Hm with secondary functional impairment of palpebral motility scarcely or not responding to corticosteroids and/or laser treatment.
6. Hm of the nose producing secondary cartilages deformity.
7. Ulcered and bleeding Hm not responding to corticosteroids and/or laser treatment.

Techniques

The main purpose of surgery for removing Hm, regardless the life-cycle phase (proliferative or involutive), is to optimize the final cosmetic result [5]. When approaching large Hm in the proliferating phase, intraoperative bleeding control is the main challenge for the surgeon: a few surgical tricks can be employed in order to minimize intra-operative bleeding. Two different surgical techniques for partial or total excision of a critical Hm can be used: 1) the lenticular shaped incision and linear closure technique; and 2) the circular excision and purse-string closure technique, which had been previously reported as the "round-block technique" [6–9].

The first method is traditionally used for removing skin masses with a lenticular shaped incision and linear closure: this technique is proposed for lesions larger than 3 cm in diameter at the base. Skin incision must be oriented with the axis of the relaxed skin tension lines and must be drawn along the border between affected tissue and normal skin [10, 11]. In this kind of surgery blood losses are not great in volume but their amount may be considered relevant when the patient's low weight is taken into consideration.

In order to minimize bleeding by reducing the lesion's vascular supply, a technique of hemostatic "squeezing" at the tumor's base can be employed to remove the most voluminous tumors. A special clamp has been designed (Fig. 10.2). This is manufactured in such a way that it can be disassembled into two parts by removing a screw that acts as a hinge. Reinsertion of the screw enables reassembly of the two parts as a clamp. The two parts of this disassembled clamp are blindly inserted under the skin through a small skin incision adjacent to the Hm and passed into the subcutaneous tissue on opposite sides of the mass. The two parts are then reassembled after insertion of the screw and the clamp is closed underneath the Hm base thus compressing its blood supply (Fig. 10.3).

In order to make the clamp blind insertion easier and reduce vascularity, a variable volume of epinephrine solution in normal saline (0.1% dilution) is injected within the subcutaneous tissue underlying the Hm and circumferentially to the lesion [3].

Detachment of the vascular tumour from the underlying and surrounding tissues is then obtained using monopolar diathermy. After resection the clamp is released and complete bleeding control is accomplished using bipolar diathermy on the residual afferent vessels that normally present a radial distribution.

Linear closure by side-to-side approximation of the wound edges is finally obtained: an intradermal

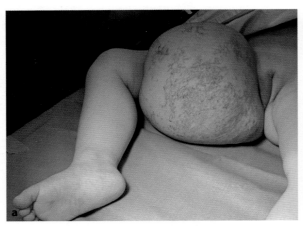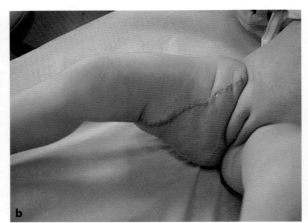

Fig. 10.1. Giant non involuting congenital hemangioma in the thigh with functional gait impairment. **a** Excision by lenticular incision and linear closure technique. **b** Postoperative results

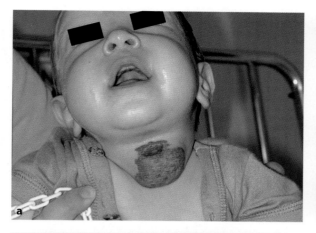

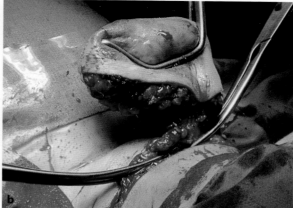

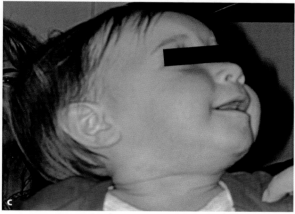

Fig. 10.2. Hemangioma in a 9 month old girl. **a** Large cervical hemangioma. **b** Lenticular incision and linear closure technique for excision. An original clamp with de-joined branches is blindly inserted under the skin for hemostatic squeezing at the base of the vascular tumour. **c** Follow-up control 6 months after surgery

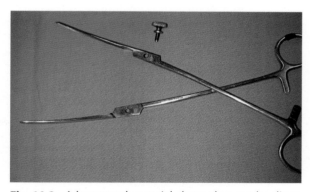

Fig. 10.3. A homemade special clamp that can be disassembled into two parts by removing a screw that acts as a hinge

absorbable running suture is tailored to close the skin. Sometimes it is necessary to lengthen the skin incision along its main axis up to one third of its original size from each end in order to avoid "dog ears" at the wound extremities.

The round-block technique, described by Mulliken [12] and more recently adopted by the authors is indicated for excision of the smaller lesions, sized less than 30 mm in diameter (Fig. 10.4).

The advantages of using the purse-string closure technique for removing localized Hm are due to the minimization of the subsequent scar length (up to 50% shorter compared with results obtained with the traditional linear closure technique) and in minimizing the adjacent structure distortion, since tension is equally applied along multiple radial lines with a symmetrical concentric distribution pattern rather than along a main axis perpendicular to the linear wound.

In our experience, preliminary hydrostatic undermining by saline injection is always useful before performing the circular skin incision in order to detach the vascular tumour from the underlying and surrounding tissues and to encourage a symmetrical distortion of adjacent structures by concentric distribution of tension lines.

When conspicuous blood losses are expected, a running Polypropylene or Nylon 2/0 non traumatic suture is temporarily placed around the lesion base. This suture is fixed on a Silicon tourniquet (Vessel loop®) achieving in this way at the same time either

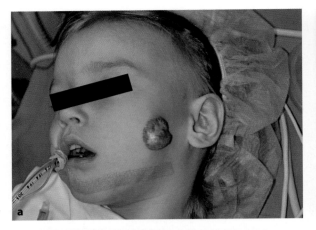

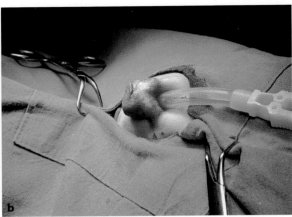

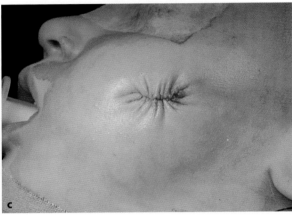

Fig. 10.4. Facial hemangioma. **a** "Round-block" technique in a partially involuted facial hemangioma. **b** After temporary positioning of a hemostatic circular suture at the lesion base, a round block excision is performed with circular skin incision. Concentric purse-string sutures in the subcutaneous and intradermic layers are then tailored. **c** Tightening first the subcutaneous purse-string suture and then the intradermal one apposes the wound margins. This procedure produces multiple radial gathered ridges which usually flatten in a few weeks

hemostatic squeezing of the Hm or radial recruiting of surrounding healthy skin [3].

After having completed the Hm removal and accurate hemostasis using bipolar diathermy the temporary hemostatic running Nylon suture is removed. The circular defect is then closed with a double purse-string suture: a 3/0 Vicril running circular suture within the subcutis and a 3/0 running absorbable monofilament for skin intra-dermal suture. If a small opening remains, one or two percutaneous additional sutures can be placed to approximate the wound edges [3].

After circular excision of a giant Hm in selected cases the large circular skin defect can be closed, combining a linear closure technique centrally with purse string closures at the wound extremities in order to reduce the scar length. A drain is not normally needed.

Postoperative Care

An occlusive dressing with an Iodopovidone gauze is left unchanged for 48 hours to prevent postoperative bacterial wound contamination after both techniques. Further subsequent medication is planned after ten days. The running absorbable sutures are left in situ until they dissolve.

Infection, delayed wound healing and scar widening occur with a relevant incidence after Hm excision with the round block technique (20%).

Parents need to be very well prepared and informed about the possible moderate scar widening: the eventual need of a second surgery a few months later to correct the scar if it is not cosmetically acceptable should be always discussed before the first operation.

Conclusion

On the basis of the authors' experience, the range of indications for surgical removal of Hm can be enlarged to the proliferative phase using particular surgical techniques in order to achieve good bleeding control and to optimize the final cosmetic result. Early excision might prevent psychological stigmatization of the affected children and parents [13, 14].

However, even for the largest tumours early surgical removal of Hm should be always evaluated by the surgeon as a treatment option after having considered the chance of obtaining a rapid improvement with less invasive treatments such as corticosteroids administration and/or laser photocoagulation techniques.

References

1. Margileth AM, Museles M (1965) Cutaneous hemangiomas in children: diagnosis and conservative management. 194(5):523–526
2. Enjolras O, Mulliken JB (1993) The current management of vascular birthmarks. Pediatr Dermatol 10(4):311–313
3. Baraldini V, Coletti M, Cigognetti F, Vercellio G (2007) Haemostatic squeezing and purse-string sutures: optimising surgical techniques for early excision of critical infantile haemangiomas. J Pediatr Surg 42:381–385
4. Frieden IJ et al (2005) Infantile hemangiomas: Current knowledge, future directions. Proceedings of research Workshop on Infantile Hemangiomas. Pediatr Dermatol 22(5):384–406
5. Demiri EC, Pelissier P, Genin-Etcheberry T et al (2001) Treatment of facial haemangiomas: the present status of surgery. Br J Plast Surg 54(8):665–674
6. Peled IJ, Zagher U, Wexler MR (1985) Purse-string suture for reduction and closure of skin defects. Ann Plast Surg 14:465
7. Tremolada C, Blandini D, Beretta M et al (1997) The "round block" purse-string suture: a simple method to close skin defects with minimal scarring. Plast Reconstr Surg 100(1):126–131
8. Patel KK, Telfer MR, Southee R (2003) A "round block" purse-string suture in facial reconstruction after operations for skin cancer surgery. Br J Oral Maxillofac Surg 41(3):151–156
9. Weisberg NK, Greenbaum SS (2003) Revisiting the purse-string closure: some new methods and modifications. Dermatol Surg 29(6):672–676
10. Gillespie PH, Banwell PE, Hormbrey EL et al (2000) A new model for assessment in plastic surgery: knowledge of relaxed skin tension lines. Br J Plast Surg 53(3):243–244
11. Gibson T, Kenedi RM (1967) Biomechanical properties of the skin. Surg Clin North Am 47:279
12. Mulliken JB, Rogers GF, Marler JJ (2002) Circular excision of hemangioma and purse-string closure: the smallest possible scar. Plast Recontr Surg 109(5):1544–1554
13. Dieterich-Miler CA, Cohen BA, Ligget J (1992) Behaviour adjustment and self-concept of young children with haemangiomas. Pediatr Dermatol 9:241
14. Tanner JL, Dechert MP, Frieden IJ (1998) Growing up with a facial hemangioma: parent and child coping and adaptation. Pediatrics 101(3):446–452

Facial Hemangiomas

11

Paul Rieu

Abstract

Facial hemangiomas present a special challenge for the medical profession. Nowadays parents are better informed via the world wide web and through patient support groups, leading them to demand the greatest attention and state of the art treatment for their child. Parents are faced with their children's disfigurement daily and they experience the "rapid growing" vascular tumor as an increasing problem in their interactions with each other, their child and the community. In this chapter we address the different presentations of facial hemangiomas and the diagnostics and different state of the art treatment modalities available.

Face

In general the face is the first thing people look at when addressing a person. The face is important in verbal as well as in non verbal communication. Disfigurement of the face seriously influences social contact. Parents become upset when they discover their newborn baby has a growing tumor, such as an infantile hemangioma, and they have many questions and concerns about the future of their child. In fact, they have only one major question for the medical field (general practitioner, health care doctor, pediatrician, pediatric dermatologist, pediatric surgeon, plastic surgeon, etc.): can you stop the growth and/or remove the hemangioma as soon as possible?

Unfortunately, there is still not enough knowledge about the etiology of these tumors, and basic scientific research is hampered by lack of an animal model, leaving us to rely upon clinical empirical treatments by experienced specialists [1]. Nevertheless, progress is being made in ongoing research, and well designed and properly conducted prospective clinical trials should be encouraged.

Nowadays people are aware of their right to optimal medical counseling, and they have access to a lot of information through the world wide web and are informed by patient support groups. Uniformity in diagnosis and treatment is important in order to avoid miscommunication, misunderstanding and medical shopping.

Diagnosis

In most cases the diagnosis of hemangioma can be made by knowledge of clinical history and physical examination. In the immediate postnatal period it is difficult even for experienced specialists to tell whether a birthmark is a hemangioma precursor lesion, capillary malformation or developing hemangioma. Usually within a few weeks it becomes clear if there is a developing hemangioma. However, it may be difficult to distinguish a flat hemangioma until, for example, ulceration is seen, which never occurs in a true capillary malformation (port wine stain) (Fig. 11.1).

Subcutaneous or more deeply localized hemangiomas present themselves at a later stage unless they occur in areas with bony structure with thin subcutis such as the skull, frontal, peri-orbital, jugular, glabella and nasal area. If the skin is not involved, progressive growth and bulging overlying skin and sometimes a bluish teint may raise the suspicion of a developing subcutaneously localized hemangioma. Parotid hemangiomas can grow quite large, may not be visible in the first weeks and will not always show skin changes. Ultrasound quickly confirms a suspected deep hemangioma.

R. Mattassi, D.A. Loose, M. Vaghi (eds.), *Hemangiomas and Vascular Malformations*.
© Springer-Verlag Italia 2009

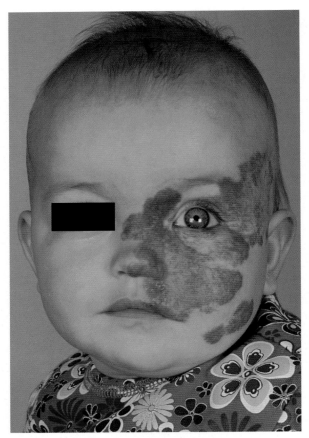

Fig. 11.1. Flat hemangioma. Sometimes there are difficulties with accurate diagnosis

Treatment

Treatment of facial hemangioma is a challenge for all of those who are involved in the care of affected children. The tumor either arises soon after birth or is already visible. All facial hemangiomas should be examined by an experienced doctor as soon as they appear because there is a great variety in presentation at several delicate localizations and because there are some very special subtypes. Precursor lesions are often not recognized. Midwifes, obstetricians, pediatricians, doctors and nurses in community healthcare centers should be trained to distinguish the various birthmarks, including precursor lesions of hemangioma, and should learn when to consult an experienced specialist.

It is most important to first distinguish between a hemangioma and a vascular malformation [2]. Next, it is necessary to distinguish between a localized or a segmental form and determine whether it is superficial (dermal), deep (subcutaneous) or a combination of the two. In the case of a heman-

gioma, it is important to consider the phase of growth (proliferative/plateau/involutive) at the first consultation.

There are several facial localizations that are problematic or even life-threatening. These include peri-orbital or beard-like presentation with subglottic involvement or very large segmental distribution. In these cases, immediate expert consultation and treatment is necessary. Segmental forms present more complications than localized forms, and may give additional insight into facial hemangioma development [3]. Large segmental hemangiomas may be recognized as part of an association designated PHACE (for posterior fossa brain malformations, hemangiomas, arterial anomalies, coarctation of the aorta and cardiac defects, and eye abnormalities) [4]. Other forms such as rapid involuting congenital hemangioma (RICH) or non involuting congenital hemangioma (NICH) can be encountered and should be recognized as variant forms of hemangioma, even though application of the term hemangioma to these forms is not strictly correct. Sometimes there may be confusion with tumors such as infantile fibrosarcoma [5, 6].

The wait-and-see policy for small localized hemangioma is still our standard approach, but medical treatment with corticosteroids has to be considered more liberally when facial hemangiomas are concerned [7]. Corticosteroid injection therapy is an option; however, we are still reluctant to use this treatment in the case of periorbital hemangioma, where we favor systemic corticosteroids [8]. In difficult cases (i.e., large segmental hemangiomas, refractive to corticosteroids) treatment with Vincristine is justified [9]. Interferon therapy has been discarded because of the necessity of long-term subcutaneous injections and serious neurological sequelae [10]. Although Pulsed Dye laser initially seemed promising, a scientifically reliable study did not show a significant difference when early laser intervention was used [11]. The early treatment of hemangioma with Pulsed Dye laser remains controversial. Nd:Yag laser needs special instrumentation, skill and has to be performed under general anesthesia [12]. Surgery in the active, proliferative stage is acceptable when there are serious threats such as deprivation amblyopia, large ulcerations and bleeding and/or in case of serious psychosocial problems. When corrective surgery is needed for cosmetic reasons we prefer surgery in a late(r) stage when involution has occurred, the child has grown and the result of surgery is more predictable.

Eye

Hemangiomas in and around the orbita present a special challenge because they interfere with visual development during early childhood and therefore need immediate action. The critical period for binocularity is 3 months to 2 years [13]. A growing hemangioma in the upper eyelid or in the orbita changes the form of the eyeball and interferes with the normal curvation of the cornea, causing anisometropic astigmatism and refractive amblyopia, while complete occlusion leads to stimulus deprivation amblyopia. Early treatment is indicated in order to prevent long-term sequelae of visual impairment. Medical treatment with corticosteroids is the first choice in order to stop growth and induce an accelerated involution. This is usually combined with patching, i.e., occlusion of the unaffected eye for at least one hour daily. However an exact evidence-based treatment protocol still has to be defined. Some authors, including ourselves, prefer systemic corticosteroid therapy [8], while others advocate intralesional injection therapy (Fig. 11.2) [13, 14].

Nasal Tip

Hemangiomas of the tip of the nose are a notorious problem. They involute slowly and often serious ulceration destroys the cartilaginous septum. While there are advocates of early treatment for these hemangiomas, others adhere to a delayed treatment when the hemangioma has markedly involuted. The proponents of delayed treatment argue that better cosmetic results can be achieved after involution. On the other hand, a very disfigured nasal tip is a psychosocial burden for the patient and for parents and often early correction is desirable [15]. Again, experience guides the balance between early treatment, ranging from intralesional corticosteroids to surgery, and a more conservative policy, such as a course of systemic corticosteroids and/or a wait-and-see policy. Vincristine may have a place, but there are no prospective studies that support this treatment (Fig. 11.3).

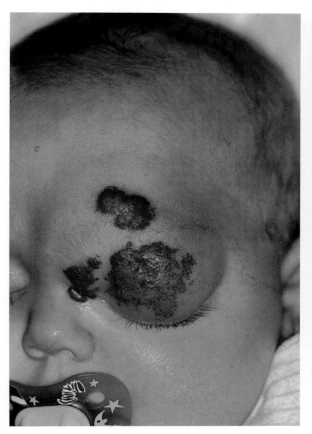

Fig. 11.2. Large hemangioma of the upper eyelid causing complete visual obstruction

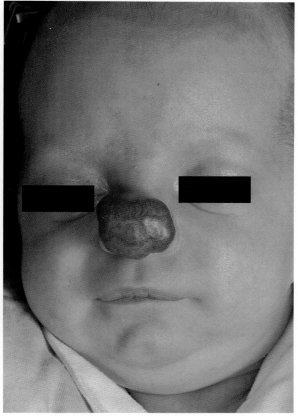

Fig. 11.3. Awkward tip of the nose hemangioma

Filtrum and Lips

In case of larger hemangiomas in the area of the filtrum or upper lip, we prefer intralesional corticosteroid injection therapy and to wait as long as possible for reduction and involution before performing corrective surgery. The boundaries of the anatomical structures are often easier to delineate at a later stage, and there is a serious risk of destroying them with early surgical intervention. In exceptional cases a careful reductive surgical intervention without removing the total hemangioma may be necessary.

Parotid

We have not yet encountered a hemangioma in the parotid region that needed early surgery. Very large hemangiomas may obstruct the acoustic meatus, or extend internally and compress the trachea. In fact, we have always been able to deal with these hemangiomas by systemic corticosteroid therapy, or with a wait-and-see policy in the case of smaller hemangiomas. Others have the same experience [16]. Hearing development is not hampered by temporary occlusion of the meatus (in contrast with visual impairment by occlusion of the pupil). However, cleaning or drainage of the outer ear maybe difficult for a period of time and may need extra attention. A large hemangioma located in the preauricular area mainly in the cutis and subcutis may need secondary surgical reduction, but again this condition represents an exceptional situation (Fig. 11.4).

Segmental Forms and PHACES

Special attention needs to be paid to segmental presentations, such as a beard-like hemangioma. In this instance, further investigation by magnetic resonance imaging (MRI) and ear nose and throat (ENT) laryngo-tracheoscopy is obligatory, especially when a stridor develops. However, general practitioners, health care professionals, pediatricians and pediatric dermatologists should be aware of the risk of developing subglottic obstruction by a hemangioma developing in the tracheal area. Our treatment consists of an intralesional corticosteroid injection in the subglottic hemangioma, followed by a 7 day intubation at the intensive care unit and detubation under direct vision by the ENT specialist [17]. When neccessary, this is followed by a course of systemic corticosteroids.

Large segmental hemangiomas of half the face or head and neck region are rarely treatable by surgery, and disfigurement is a serious threat. Recent studies show that intensive diagnostic investigation needs to be done in these segmental hemangiomas, because there may be other underlying developmental malformations, such as posterior brain cysts, microphtalmia, large brain vessel abnormalities, etc., all of which are brought together under the acronym PHACES [4]. The main therapy is early systemic corticosteroid therapy and, where possible or feasible, surgical reduction of the hemangioma. However, in these cases Vincristine is increasingly used as first choice as an alternative therapy. Again, good prospective studies are needed to support this policy.

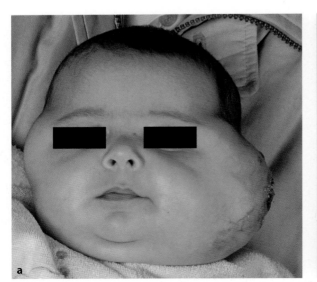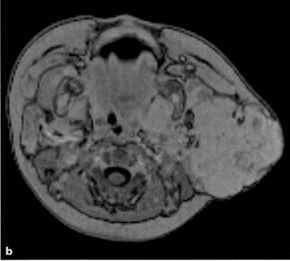

Fig. 11.4. Parotid hemangioma. **a** Huge hemangioma of the parotid gland. Clinically no airway obstruction. **b** MRI shows deviation of the trachea but no compression. Complete regression without therapy

Rapid Involuting Hemangioma/Non Involuting Hemangioma

Rapid involuting hemangioma (RICH) and non involuting hemangioma (NICH) are possibly variations of hemangioma, which have some clinical aspects of juvenile hemangioma, but in other ways seem to be closer to vascular malformations [5, 6]. The endothelium does not express glucose transporter-1 (Glut-1). In general, RICH rapidly regresses within the first year of life, while NICH does not regress at all. The latter has more dilated venous vessels and a very typical blue halo. We have seen two cases of retroauricular NICH and have removed them surgically.

Kaposiform Hemangioendothelioma/ Tufted Angioma

Giant hemangioma in connection with deep thrombocytopenia in combination with consumption coagulopathy called Kasabach Merritt phenomenon was formerly thought to be a special form of juvenile hemangioma. However, it appears that this form is not a normal hemangioma, but a vascular tumor such as kaposiform hemangioendothelioma (KHE) or tufted angioma (TA) [18]. The clinical aspect is totally different from a normal developing hemangioma. The vascular swelling has a purple bluish aspect, is tender and quite diffuse. Life-threatening bleeding may develop. Suspected cases should be referred to specialised centers because treatment is notoriously difficult. Nowadays, medical treatment by Vincristine is considered state of the art [19]. Some cases show the clinical aspects as described but do not develop deep thrombocytopenia; however, D-Dimer elevation is a sign of consumption coagulopathy. In all these cases biopsy of the tumor is a prerequisite to underscore clinical diagnosis and to justify Vincristine therapy. Over time these tumors regress, thrombocytopenia and coagulopathy are restored, but remnants of the tumor may remain life long (Fig. 11.5).

Psycho-Social Impact

In a short retrospective study we investigated the psychological and social impact of facial hemangiomas on parents and children. In a cohort of 19 patients, 10–16 years old, functional health and social-emo-

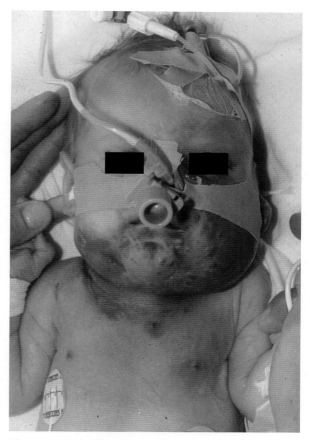

Fig. 11.5. Kaposiform hemangioendothelioma (KHE). Failure to stabilize coagulopathy and platelet consumption resulted in serious bleeding and patient's death

tional development was measured by validated questionaires. We used the Illness Cognition Questionnaire (ICQ) to assess the meaning of hemangioma for parents, the Dartmouth COOP Functional Health Assessments Charts (COOP/WONCA) to assess functional health, and the Self Perception Profile for Children (SPPC) and Adolescents (SPPA) to assess self-esteem. The results demonstrated normal coping strategies by parents, with global self-worth and physical appearance comparable to normal; however, adolescents scored below average concerning close friendship. These data suggest good adjustment to facial hemangiomas. However, in our opinion children and parents deserve psychological support and treatment when facial hemangiomas cause serious distress (Fig. 11.6) [20].

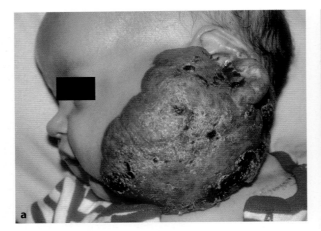
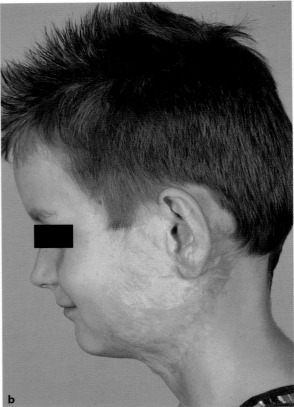

Fig. 11.6. Cutaneous hemangioma. **a** Large cutaneous hemangioma with ulceration. **b** Late result after resection of superfluous fibrofatty residue and partially scarred skin

References

1. Bauland CG, Steensel van MA, Steijlen PM et al (2006) The pathogenesis of hemangiomas: a review. Plas Reconstr Surg 117:29e–35e
2. Mulliken JB, Glowacki J (1982) Hemangioma and vascular malformations in infants and children: A classification based on endothelial characteristics. Plast Reconstr Surg 69(3):412–422
3. Haggstrom A, Lammer EJ, Schneider RA et al (2006) Patterns of infantile hemangiomas: new clues to hemangioma pathogenesis and embryonic facial development. Pediatrics 117:698–703
4. Frieden IJ, Reese V, Cohen D (1996) PHACE syndrome: the association of posterior fossa brain malformations, hemangiomas, arterial anomalies, coarctation of the aorta and cardiac defects, and eye abnormalities. Arch Dermatol 132(3):307–311
5. Konez O, Burrows PE, Mulliken JB et al (2003) Angiographic features of rapidly involuting congenital hemangioma (RICH). Pediatr Radiol 34(1):15–19
6. Enjolras O, Mulliken JB, Boon LM et al (2001) Non-involuting congenital hemangiomas: a rare cutaneous vascular anomaly. Plast Reconstr Surg 107:1647–1654
7. Pope E, Krafchik BR, Macarthur C et al (2007) Oral versus high-dose pulse corticosteroids for problematic infantile hemangiomas: a randomised, controlled trial. Pediatrics 119:e1239–e1247
8. Enjolras O, Riché MC, Merland JJ, Escande JP (1990) Management of alarming hemangiomas in infancy: a review of 25 cases. Pediatrics 85:491–498
9. Enjolras O, Brevière GM, Roger G (2004) Vincristine treatment for function- and life-threatening infantile hemangioma. Archives de Pédiatrie 11:99–107
10. Barlow CF, Priebe CJ, Mulliken JB et al (1998) Spastic diplegia as a complication of interferon alfa-2a treatment of hemangiomas of infancy. J Pediatr 132(3):517–530
11. Batta K, Goodyear HM, Moss C et al (2002) Randomised controlled study of early pulsed dye laser treatment of uncomplicated childhood hemangiomas: results of a 1-year analysis. Lancet 360:521–527
12. Stier MF, Glick SA, Hirsch RJ (2008) Laser treatment of pediatric vascular lesions: Port wine stains and hemangiomas. J Am Acad Dermatol 58:261–285
13. Weiss AH, Kelly JP (2008) Reappraisal of astigmatism induced by periocular capillary hemangioma and treatment with intralesional corticosteroid injection. Ophthalmology 115(2):390–397
14. Ranchod TM, Frieden IJ, Frederick DR (2005) Corticosteroid treatment of periorbital hemangioma of

infancy: a review of the evidence. Br J Ophthalmol 89:1134–1138

15. Faguer K, Dompmartin A, Labbe D et al (2002) Early surgical treatment of Cyrano-nose haemangiomas with Rethi incision. Br J Plast Surg 55(6):498–503

16. Greene AK, Rogers GF, Mulliken JB (2004) Management of parotid hemangioma in 100 children. Plast Reconstr Surg 113(1):53–60

17. Meeuwis J, Bos CE, Hoeve LJ, Voort van der E (1990) Subglottic hemangiomas in infants: treatment with intralesional corticosteroid injection and intubation. Int J Pediatr Otorhinolaryngol 19:145–150

18. Enjolras O, Wassef M, Mazoyer E et al (1997) Infants with Kasabach-Merritt syndrome do not have "true" hemangioma. J Pediatr 130(4):631–640

19. Haisley-Royster C, Enjolras O, Frieden IJ et al (2002) Kasabach-Merritt phenomenon: a retrospective study of treatment with Vincristine. J Pediatr Hematol Oncol 24(6):459–462

20. Rieu PN, Mepschen M, Verhaak C, Spauwen PHM (2006) Facial hemangiomas: functional status and self-esteem of the child. Oral presentation during the 16th International Workshop on Vascular Anomalies of the International Society for the Study of Vascular Anomalies (ISSVA), Milan, June, pp 14–17

Anogenital Hemangiomas

12

Rainer Grantzow, Kathrin Schäffer

Abstract

Only 1% of hemangiomas are in the anogenital region. Their main complication is ulceration due to the macerating influence of urine and stool. Ulcerated hemangiomas are painful, may become infected or cause systemic infection, and have a tendency to heal slowly. Prevention of ulceration is the most important aim in these cases. Active therapy with laser is possible, but may induce ulceration. Due to this serious side effect, a wait-and-see policy should be considered as an alternative. Ulcerated hemangiomas have to be treated like other chronic wounds, with hydrocolloid dressings or with barrier creams to prevent contact with stool and urine. Healed ulcerated hemangiomas eventually develop flat scars with hypopigmentation.

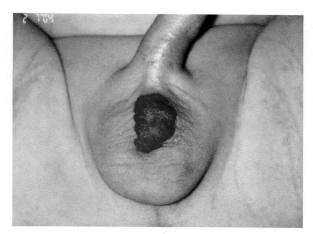

Fig. 12.1. Flat scrotal hemangioma

Diagnosis

Hemangiomas in the anogenital region are rare and comprise about 1% of all hemangiomas. They are seen at the perineum, the labia and the scrotum (Figs. 12.1, 12.2). Due to their localisation, there are no optical or aesthetic problems as found with facial localisation. Ano-genital hemangiomas show the same development as other hemangiomas, including the well-known phases of proliferation and regression. They can be classified into intracutaneous, subcutaneous and combined types.

The diagnosis is visual except in the case of the subcutaneous type. In these cases duplex sonography must be carried out to verify the diagnosis and thereby exclude other soft tissue tumours, in particular malignant tumours such as rhabdomyosarcomas.

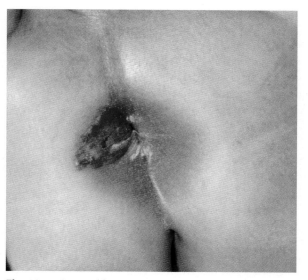

Fig. 12.2. Perianal hemangioma with a small ulceration

R. Mattassi, D.A. Loose, M. Vaghi (eds.), *Hemangiomas and Vascular Malformations.*
© Springer-Verlag Italia 2009

Sometimes it can be difficult to distinguish a hemangioma from a nevus flammeus or another form of vascular malformation. Occasionally the appearance of labial venous malformations can imitate subcutaneous hemangioma, but duplex sonography will usually lead to the correct diagnosis. Magnetic resonance imaging (MRI) investigations are not necessary to evaluate ano-genital hemangiomas; however, MRI is mandatory to detect further pelvic malformations in case of venous malformation.

Perineal hemangiomas can be associated with defects such as anorectal, neurologic, renal or urinary tract and genital malformations. Acronyms such as SACRAL Syndrome [1] or PELVIS Syndrome [2] are proposed in such rare cases.

Complications

The major problem of perineal hemangiomas is their tendency to ulcerate. Normally ulceration occurs in the phase of strong proliferation and is seen only in the first 4–5 months of life; ulceration is uncommon after this stage. Reasons for this complication are numerous. Despite the hyperperfusion of a hemangioma, the skin can be underperfused due to micro arteriovenous (AV) fistulas in the centre of the hemangioma that have a steal effect at the surface and can lead to skin necrosis. Secondly, the moisture under a nappy can macerate and damage the skin and reduce its function as a barrier against bacterial invasion. These two mechanisms in combination result in ulceration occasionally with secondary bacterial infection. Unfortunately, these ulcerations require a long time to heal because of the negative influence of stool and urine. Furthermore, they are very painful and present a challenge in wound management.

Prevention and Therapy

The avoidance of ulceration should be the main aim, and the target of all interventions is to minimise extrinsic factors such as moisture and extended contact with urine and stool. In this situation it is very important to advise the parents of the necessity to change nappies frequently. Additionally the hemangioma should be covered with a barrier cream such as zinc oxide paste.

In principle, the possibilities of hemangioma treatment in the anogenital region are the same as in other regions. According to size, volume and shape of the lesion, dye, Nd-YAG laser or surgical interventions can be performed. In contrast to facial hemangiomas, aesthetic problems are irrelevant and therefore indications to active treatment are rare. Furthermore, the main problem in the therapy of perianal and genital hemangiomas is that such therapy can initiate ulceration (Fig. 12.3a) and result in deterioration [3]. In particular, swelling and thermal damage to the skin after laser therapy (dye- and Nd-YAG laser) can trigger ulceration of the vulnerable skin, the avoidance of which is the main aim of all therapy. In addition, deeper parts of the hemangioma can grow despite dye laser treatment because the depth of dye laser effect is only 0.8 mm [4]. This dilemma should be considered seriously before any laser application. Due to these complications, the traditional wait-and-see policy has many advantages for hemangiomas at this localisation. The relative merits of the dye laser versus the wait-and-see approach are discussed in the only existing randomised and controlled study [5].

In case of ulceration, different aspects of therapy have to be noted. A crucial point is the dressing of the local wound, which should protect against stool and urine, accelerating wound healing and make the painless change of wound dressings possible. Hydrocolloids are standard, if localisation enables their application (Fig. 12.3b, c). Changing of the dressing should be painless and is necessary only twice weekly. If this is not possible (beneath the anus or female genitalia), vaseline-impregnated gauze can be used, but must be changed more frequently than hydrocolloids. Small defects can be treated with barrier creams such as zinc oxide paste. Additionally, topical antibiotics can be applied, but the effects of such a treatment are uncertain. However, gentle cleaning of the wound (shower, bath), or application of painless antiseptic liquids (Octenisept®) are the basic treatment for secondary wound healing. Systemic therapy with antibiotics may be necessary, if signs of infection such as fever or leucocytosis are present. Impairment of wound healing after dye laser application in ulcerated hemangiomas has been reported [6, 7], but there are no controlled and randomised studies about the effect of dye laser treatment on wound healing. Unfortunately, the report of David et al. [6] concerns only 4.4% of cases treated (n = 7) with an anogenital localisation, while that of Kim et al. [7] concerns 14 of 22 cases.

Systemic steroid therapy is a further option for hemangioma treatment, but its serious side effects have to be weighed in view of the low efficacy of this kind of treatment. Furthermore, the immuno-

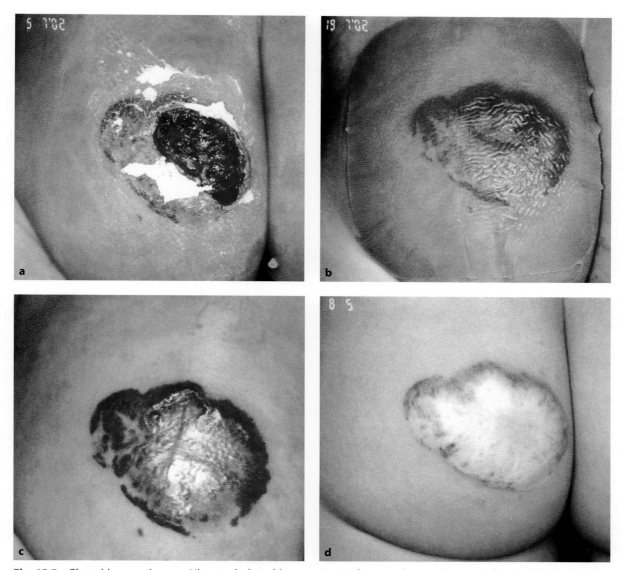

Fig. 12.3. Gluteal hemangioma. **a** Ulcerated gluteal hemangioma after cryotherapy (wrong indication). **b** Twelve days later with hydrocolloid dressing and reduction of the wound size. **c** Closed wound after 6 weeks wound management with hydrocolloid dressing. **d** Residuals 2 years later with typical flat scar and hypopigmented skin

suppressive effect of steroids may have a negative influence in cases of infected ulcers. Furthermore, steroids can inhibit wound healing and prolong the time to wound healing.

The last option for the treatment of anogenital hemangiom is surgical excision. This procedure is possible only for small hemangiomas, when primary closure of the wound is possible. However, these hemangiomas are usually harmless and do not need any therapy.

After healing and remission of ulcerated hemangiomas, a flat scar with typical hypopigmentation will appear (Fig. 12.3d). This scar is robust and there is no danger of further ulceration.

References

1. Stockman A, Boralevi F, Taieb A, Léauté-Labrèze C (2007) SACRAL Syndrome: Spinal dysraphism, anogenital, cutaneous, renal and urologic anomalies, associated with an angioma of lumbosacral localisation. Dermatology 214:40–45
2. Girard C, Bigorre M, Guillot B, Bessis D (2006) PELVIS Syndrome. Arch Dermatol 142:884–888
3. Witman PM, Wagner AM, Scherer K, Waner M (2006) Complications following pulsed dye laser treatment of superficial hemangiomas. Lasers Surg Med 38:116–123
4. Poetke M, Philipp C, Berlien HP (2000) Flashlamp pulsed dye laser for hemangiomas in infancy. Arch Dermatol 136:628–632
5. Batta K, Goodyear HM, Moss C et al (2002) Randomised controlled study of early pulsed dye laser treatment of uncomplicated childhood haemangiomas: results of 1-year analysis. Lancet 360:521–527
6. David LR, Malek MM, Argenta LC (2003) Efficacy of pulse dye laser therapy for the treatment of ulcerated hemangiomas: a review of 78 patients. Br J Plast Surg 56:317–327
7. Kim HJ, Colombo M, Friede IJ (2001) Ulcerated hemangiomas: Clinical characteristics and response to therapy. J Am Acad Dermatol 44:962–972

Part III
VASCULAR MALFORMATIONS

Genetic Aspects of Vascular Malformations

13

Nisha Limaye, Miikka Vikkula

Abstract

Vascular malformations are comprised of a variety of developmental defects of the vasculature. Typically sporadic in nature, they can sometimes occur as incompletely penetrant, inherited traits. The genetic bases of several of these anomalies have been identified, and are described in this review. This has had a hugely beneficial impact in terms of the precise diagnosis and appropriate, effective treatment of different disease entities; it has also revealed potential therapeutic targets for the future. The advances made thus far, however, are largely confined to the rare, familial forms, and much remains to be uncovered about the genes that mediate common sporadic versions of vascular malformations. Moreover, the pathogenic pathways and molecular mechanisms by which the aberrant genes cause these defined, often heterogeneous lesions, remain to be thoroughly dissected. Previous studies have largely focused on the analysis of blood samples, as these are more accessible. Further progress in identifying the somatic events that cause sporadic lesions or locally exacerbate the pathogenic effects of germline-heterozygous mutant alleles, will require the additional assessment of irregularities of gene expression and function at the level of lesion-derived tissue.

Introduction

Vascular malformations are localized, structural irregularities of the vasculature, which occur due to developmental defects during vasculogenesis, angiogenesis, and lymphangiogenesis: the major processes that give rise to and maintain the mature, adult vascular system [1]. They are distinguished from vascular tumors, which consist mainly of hemangiomas, by a variety of biological, histological, and clinical features [2]: unlike the far more common hemangiomas (10–12% of infants), vascular malformations are present at birth, grow proportionately with the individual, and do not spontaneously regress. The inherited forms can result in the appearance of new lesions, which typically stay small, later in life. They show no sex-preponderance, and have normal endothelial cell turnover, in contrast to hemangiomas in their proliferative phase.

Vascular malformations are quite rare, with an estimated incidence of about 0.3% [3]. They are further subdivided on the basis of the particular vascular component involved, and their flow characteristics, as detected by techniques such as Doppler ultrasound. Thus, they include the slow-flow capillary, venous, and lymphatic malformations, and the fast-flow arterial malformations, as well as combinations of these (Table 13.1). Lesions vary widely in terms of their number (single or multiple, the latter more commonly observed in hereditary forms), extent (isolated or large and diffuse), and localization (cutaneous, muco-cutaneous, or deep, involving the viscera, nerve, bone or muscle). They can sometimes occur in association with other signs and symptoms, i.e., in syndromes (for a detailed review see [3]).

Major advances have been made in identifying the genetic bases of several of the vascular malformations (Table 13.1; reviewed in [4]). As we will further describe, this has already had a hugely beneficial effect on the accurate diagnosis and appropriate management of certain anomalies, such as glomuvenous malformations (GVMs), which can sometimes be hard to distinguish from venous malformations (VMs), while warranting different approaches to treatment. In certain cases, identification of causative genes has even allowed for the precise

R. Mattassi, D.A. Loose, M. Vaghi (eds.), *Hemangiomas and Vascular Malformations*.
© Springer-Verlag Italia 2009

Table 13.1. Genes and loci implicated in the pathogenesis of vascular malformations, classified by component vasculature

Malformation	Locus	Locus (Gene)	Name
Capillary anomalies			
Capillary malformations (CM)	–	–	(?)
Cerebral cavernous malformation (CCM)	7q11-22	CCM1	(KRIT1)
	7p13	CCM2	(malcavernin)
	3q26.1	CCM3	(PDCD10)
	3q26.3-27.2	CCM4	(?)
Capillary malformation-arteriovenous malformation (CM-AVM)	5q13-22	CMC1	(RASA1)
Venous anomalies			
Venous malformations (VM)	–	–	(?)
Cutaneomucosal venous malformation (VMCM)	9p21	VMCM1	(TIE2/TEK)
Glomuvenous malformation (GVM)	1p21-22	VMGLOM	(GLMN)
Lymphatic anomalies			
Lymphatic malformations (LM)	–	–	(?)
Primary lymphedema (LE)			
Primary congenital LE (Milroy disease)	5q35.3	PCL1	(FLT4/VEGFR3)
LE-distichiasis/ptosis/yellow nail	16q24.3	LD	(FOXC2)
Hypotrichosis-LE-telangiectasia (HLT)	20q13.33	HLT	(SOX18)
Osteoporosis-LE-anhydrotic ectodermal--dysplasia-immunodeficiency (OLEDAID)	Xq28	IP2	(NEMO)
LE-hereditary cholestasis (Aagenaes syndrome)	15q	LCS1	(?)
Combined (with arterial) malformations			
Arteriovenous malformations (AVM)	–	–	(?)
Hereditary hemorrhagic telangiectasia or	9q33-34	HHT1	(ENG)
Rendu-Osler-Weber (HHT/ROW)	12q11-14	HHT2	(ALK1)
	5q31.3-32	HHT3	(?)
	7p14	HHT4	(?)
Juvenile polyposis-HHT (JPHT)	18q21.1	JPHT	(SMAD4/MADH4)
Ataxia-telangiectasia (AT)	11q23	AT1	(ATM)
PTEN hamartoma tumor syndrome (PHTS) (including Cowden; Bannayan-Riley-Ruvalcaba; Proteus syndromes)	10q23.3	PHTS	(PTEN)

delineation of new disease entities, as in the case of capillary malformation-arteriovenous malformation (CM-AVM). In addition to aiding diagnosis, knowledge of the genetic bases of pathology can yield useful information on the pathways and mechanisms mediating disease, therefore also shedding light on the role of these molecules in normal development and function, and providing us with potentially useful therapeutic targets. Towards this end, *in vitro* and *in vivo* animal models are being extensively employed to study the various genes implicated in vascular malformations.

Capillary Malformation (CM)

CMs (OMIM 163000; detailed review in [3]) are the most frequently occurring vascular malformations, with an incidence of about 0.3% in the population. These slow flow cutaneous lesions appear

flat, reddish to purple, and irregular, giving them the name "port-wine stain". Sometimes quite extensive, they are most frequently found in the face and neck regions, but can also occur on the trunk and limbs. Histologically, they consist of dilated capillary-like channels, combined with areas of increased but normal-looking capillaries, usually within the dermis. The endothelial cell lining is flat and normal, but there is a decrease in the level of neuronal markers, indicative of a paucity of innervation. CMs are predominantly sporadic in nature, although rare autosomal-dominant hereditary forms such as capillary malformation-arteriovenous malformation (CM-AVMs) have been observed in some families. While the etiology of the former remains unknown, the identification of the RasGT-Pase *RASA1* as the causative gene in CM-AVM [5] may help shed some light on the pathways likely to be involved in the common sporadic form as well.

Capillary Malformation-Arteriovenous Malformation (CM-AVM)

CM-AVM (OMIM 608354; reviewed in [6, 7]) is characterized by small, multifocal, pink-red CMs, often with a pale halo. In about a third of cases, these are accompanied by AVMs, arteriovenous fistulas (AVFs), or Parkes Weber syndrome (PWS; OMIM 608355), characterized by large cutaneous stains on an extremity, which also shows soft tissue and skeletal hypertrophy, and AV micro-fistulas. Mutations in the molecule p120RasGAP (*RASA1*), a RasGTPase activating protein (RasGAP) that inhibits Ras, have been identified to cause the autosomal-dominant disorder [5]. Mutations in the gene, located on *5q13–22*, primarily cause premature truncation and loss of function, which would be expected to lead to chronic Ras activation. Given the importance of Ras in a variety of pathways important in endothelial cell (EC) proliferation, survival, and function (including those stimulated by VEGF, TIE2, and Ephrin), this chronic activation could be what causes the CM-AVM phenotype. RASA1 may also be able to act in a Ras-independent manner, through its interaction with p190RhoGAP, which seems to play a role in cell movement, or its ability to promote pro-survival Akt activation [6].

It is extremely important to rule out the presence of deeper vascular anomalies that are sometimes associated with CMs, as when they occur in the context of CM-AVM, or as part of sporadic syndromes, such as Sturge-Weber syndrome (SWS; characterized in addition by leptomeningeal and ocular vascular malformations), Klippel-Trenaunay syndrome (KTS; in which an affected extremity shows, in addition, hypertrophy of soft tissue and bone, varicose veins, deep venous defects, lymphatic malformations) and others, all of which have an unknown etiology.

Cerebral Cavernous Malformation (CCM)

CCM (OMIM 116860; reviewed in [8]) occurs as a sporadic or autosomal-dominantly inherited cerebral vascular anomaly with incomplete penetrance. It is characterized by enlarged capillary-like channels lined with a single layer of endothelial cells lacking tight junctions, within a dense collagenous matrix with no intervening brain parenchyma. Lesions occur predominantly in the brain, but have also been observed in the retina, spinal cord, and skin as crimson, irregular hyperkeratotic cutaneous capillary-venous mal-

formations (HCCVMs). Symptoms of CCM include headaches, seizures, and cerebral hemorrhage; however, while the anomaly has an estimated prevalence of 0.5% based on large-scale magnetic resonance imaging (MRI) and autopsies, the clinical incidence is much lower, since it is often asymptomatic. Truncating mutations and/or large genomic deletions in three different genes have so far been identified to cause the disease: *CCM1* (*KRIT1* on *7q21–22*; [9, 10]), *CCM2* (*malcavernin* or *MGC4607* on *7p13–15*; [11]), and *CCM3* (*PDCD10* on *3q26.1*; [12]), with a fourth locus suggested on *3q26.3–27.2* [13]. The truncating nature of the hundreds of mutations identified in these genes shows that loss of function caused by haploinsufficiency is central to disease mediation. It is likely, however, that an additional somatic "second-hit" mutation may be required to cause complete, localized loss of function resulting in lesion-formation, as borne out by two somatic mutations identified in a single sporadic CCM patient, and a double-hit mutation identified in a patient carrying a known, inherited *KRIT1* mutation [14, 15].

While the precise functions of the three known CCM genes remain to be unraveled, studies have begun to give us some insight into their nature (reviewed extensively in [8]). *KRIT1* mRNA is expressed primarily in neurons, astrocytes and epithelial cells, while the protein has been detected in vascular endothelial cells (vECs) early in angiogenesis, and in capillaries and arterioles in the adult. It consists of various protein- and cytoskeletal-interaction domains including an NPXY motif, ankyrin repeats, and a C-terminal FERM domain. It has been found to bind the sorting nexin protein SNX17, as well as integrin cytoplasmic domain-associated protein-1 α (ICAP-1α), which in turn plays a role in cell adhesion and migration by binding β1-integrin. KRIT1 may compete with ICAP-1α's interaction with β1-integrin, thereby affecting EC structure and function downstream of integrin signaling. Since ICAP-1α and KRIT1 can both shuttle between the nucleus and cytoplasm, with the former able to sequester the latter in the nucleus, KRIT1 could also be acting as a transcription factor. *KRIT1*$^{-/-}$ mice die at mid-gestation, with abnormal differentiation of arteries. This raises the possibility that it is important in arterial development, failing which, a default venous phenotype results in the CCM sinusoids. *KRIT1*$^{+/-}$ mice, on the other hand, fail to show any CCM-like vascular lesions, perhaps because they lack a local second-hit.

CCM2 is a scaffold-protein involved in MEKK3 kinase-dependent activation of the p38 MAPK pathway, and it interacts with both actin and the small

GTPase RAC1, important in actin organization. It shows very similar, overlapping distribution with CCM1, and indeed has been shown to be able to interact with the latter and sequester it in the cytoplasm. The interaction probably occurs through the CCM2 phosphotyrosine binding (PTB) domain, similar to that of ICAP-1α, and the three molecules have been found to form a complex. CCM1 and 2 have also been found to complex with MEKK3, thus placing the two proteins squarely within the same (likely the integrin signaling) pathway, as suggested by the similarity in phenotype between patients with causative mutations. One potential difference may be the presence of HCCVMs, which have been reported only in familial cases with *KRIT1* mutations. Given the low prevalence of these cutaneous lesions, however (only seven such families, each with multiple affected members, have so far been described [16–18]), a firm correlation will require more extensive studies. Homozygous *CCM2* deletion, as in the case of *CCM1*, causes embryonic lethality in mice, and morpholino-mediated inactivation of either CCM gene results in dilation of the heart and embryonic death. Finally, the *CCM3* gene *PDCD10* has a very similar expression pattern to CCM1 and 2, and this, in light of the similarity in phenotype, again suggests that it too may be functionally linked to the other CCM genes. However, not much else is known about the protein and its functions.

Venous Anomalies

Venous anomalies [3] are a group of slow-flow malformations, with an estimated incidence of about 1 in 10,000, primarily comprising venous malformations (VMs), which account for about 95% of patients. These are primarily sporadic in nature (sporadic venous malformation or VM) but can also occur in the autosomal dominantly-inherited form, cutaneomucosal venous malformation (VMCM; about 1%). About 5% of venous anomalies are typically dominantly-inherited glomuvenous malformations (GVM).

Venous Malformation (VM)

VMs (reviewed in detail by [3, 19]) consist of expanded venous-like channels, with a thin, flat endothelial cell layer, and sparse, patchy areas of vascular smooth muscle cells (vSMCs). They are usually located in the skin or mucosa, but very often infiltrate deeper into muscles, nerves and bones. Visceral VMs can affect different organs including the liver, spleen, gastrointestinal (GI) tract and central nervous system (CNS), and rarely, vertebral bodies. They are usually congenital, and the cutaneous and mucosal forms can be flat or raised and bluish-purple, ranging from small blebs to much more extensive lesions, with single, large lesions being more common in the sporadic form. Localized intravascular coagulation (LIC) in VMs causes increased D-dimer products in 40% of patients, and soluble fibrin and decreased fibrinogen are associated with more extreme lesions [20]. The etiology of these sporadic malformations is currently unknown, although the gene for the familial form, VMCM, has been identified, and may give us important clues as to the (potentially overlapping) pathways and molecules that may be involved. VMs can occur in the context of more complex syndromes, also of unknown etiology, such as KTS, described earlier; Maffucci syndrome, in which multiple enchondromas are also observed; and blue rubber bleb nevus (BRBN) syndrome, in which both cutaneous blebs as well as GI tract VMs occur.

Cutaneomucosal Venous Malformation (VMCM)

The autosomal dominant VMCM (OMIM 600195; reviewed in detail by [4, 19]) is characterized by multiple small, raised cutaneous lesions that seldom infiltrate deeply. The presence of oral mucosal lesions along with family history is typical, although the anomaly can often be asymptomatic. Activating mutations in *TIE2* (*TEK*), the endothelial cell-specific tyrosine kinase receptor for the angiopoietins (*ANG-1, 2*, and *4* in human or *3* in mouse) located on *9p21*, have been found to mediate the disease [21].

TIE2 plays an important role in microvascular sprouting, maturity, stability, and integrity (reviewed in [4, 19]). Upon ligand binding with multimeric forms of its activating ligand ANG-1, TIE2 forms homodimers and undergoes phosphorylation. ANG-2, on the other hand, is generally considered to be an antagonist; its effects, however, seem to be strongly context-dependent. TIE2 has also been found to be able to heterodimerize with TIE1, a close paralog, with the latter being able to modulate TIE2 signaling, again in certain contexts.

Deletions of the *TIE1*, *TIE2* or *ANG-1* or *2* genes all result in severe defects in vascular development and embryonic lethality in mice. *TIE2^{-/-}* mice have defects in primary capillary plexus formation due to a deficiency of ECs, as well as incomplete cardiac development, and hemorrhage. While *Ang1*$^{-/-}$ mice show a similar, overlapping phenotype, *Ang2*-overexpressing transgenics are similar to *TIE2*-defective mice. TIE2 activation results in the phosphorylation and activation of a variety of downstream signaling intermediates, including PI3K and Akt, which have an anti-apoptotic effect. PI3K can also activate focal adhesion kinase (FAK*)* and the endothelial-specific nitric oxide synthase (eNOS*)*, which participate in cell migration and sprouting. Other signaling molecules that can interact with TIE2 include Dok-R, which can affect cell migration, Grb2, 7, and 14, and the protein tyrosine phosphatase Shp2, which can in turn associate with FAK and activate the MAPK pathway, influencing EC migration and survival. By interacting with ABIN-2, a novel inhibitor of NF-κB, TIE2 may exert its anti-inflammatory effects on ECs, reducing leukocyte extravasation and promoting vessel stability and integrity [22].

As reviewed in [19], two *TIE2* mutations have so far been reported in VMCM (R849W and Y897S), both of which lie within the kinase domain. Both of these cause ligand-independent TIE2 hyperphosphorylation when overexpressed in vitro. TIE2 phosphorylation in ECs from normal and VM lesion vessels, on the other hand, seem to be comparable. The R849W mutation has been found to have a strong anti-apoptotic effect, which is dependent on pAkt and p52Shc [23, 24], but does not cause proliferation. While overexpression of TIE2 causes activation of the transcriptional regulators STAT-3 and 5, the mutant form is able, in addition, to activate STAT-1 and cause an increased induction of the p21 cell cycle inhibitor. The mutations could be hypothesized to contribute to reducing EC apoptosis in the absence of adequate SMCs; however, the mechanism by which they contribute to the paucity of the latter remains unknown. We recently identified six VMCM families with novel inherited hyperphosphorylating *TIE2* mutations, all but one of which also lie within the kinase domain. Six additional families carrying the R849W mutation. We also identified a somatic second-hit mutation in one patient, indicating that, as in the case of CCM, VMCM may have a paradominant mode of inheritance [25]. Significantly, somatic mutations in TIE2 were also identified in sporadic VM [25]. This illustrates the utility of screens to detect somatic changes responsible for common, sporadic anomalies, in the genes (or pathways) implicated in their rare, inherited counterparts.

Glomuvenous Malformation (GVM)

GVMs (OMIM 138000; detailed review in [4, 26]) consist of raised, nodular, pink to blue-purple cutaneous lesions, often multifocal and hyperkeratotic. Histologically, they appear as distended venous channels, their hallmark being the presence of rounded "glomus" mural cells, which are abnormally differentiated SMCs, lacking their spindle shape as well as certain developmental markers. Unlike VMs, these malformations do not infiltrate deeply, are often painful upon palpation, cannot be completely emptied upon compression, and do not cause the coagulation abnormalities that can be observed in VMs. It is important to differentiate GVMs from VMs, as they entail different modes of treatment: the main therapy for GVM is surgical resection, or, in some cases, sclerotherapy. Most GVMs (about 70%) are autosomal-dominantly inherited, showing incomplete penetrance that increases with age, and wide heterogeneity even amongst members of the same family. Mutations in the *glomulin* (*GLMN*) gene on *1p21–22* mediate the anomaly [27], with about 30 different loss of function changes identified so far in about 100 families. Only eight of these mutations are common, allowing for relatively efficient screening of the gene. The mutations occur across the entire gene, with no genotype-phenotype correlations. The glomus cells in GVMs seem to lack expression of *GLMN*. Added to the identification of a somatic second-hit [27], this would suggest a paradominant mode of inheritance for this malformation as well.

GLMN (reviewed in [4, 26]) is expressed primarily in, and is very specific to, vascular SMCs, which fail to differentiate appropriately in its absence. It appears after most other SMC differentiation markers, but precedes smoothelin-B. GLMN has been found to be able to bind FKBP12, which in turn impairs TGF-β signaling by binding TGFβ RI and inhibiting its phosphorylation by TGFβ RII. Thus, by competing for binding with FKBP12, GLMN could play a role in promoting TGF-β signaling, which is known to be important in SMC development, and which, in the absence of GLMN, may be profoundly hampered. GLMN can also bind the inactive form of c-MET, the tyrosine kinase receptor for HGF, which participates in cell proliferation, tube formation by ECs, as well as SMC migration. Upon ligand-binding and phosphorylation of c-MET by HGF, GLMN undergoes phosphorylation and is released, accompanied by activation of the kinase p70S6K and its downstream target PI3-K. In addition, c-MET expression is itself upregulated by TGF-β, and thus, GLMN may be acting synergistically in both signaling pathways. By its ability to interact with Cul7, GLMN may also participate in the regulation of ubiquitin-mediated protein degradation.

Lymphatic Malformations (LM)

LMs [3] are defects in lymphatic structure characterized by no-flow microcystic or macrocystic lesions, lacking connections with the lymphatic vessel system. They consist of dilated channels lined by a flat endothelium filled with a clear fluid, but no blood except when intracystic bleeding occurs. This can cause the malformations, which otherwise appear to be of normal skin color, to appear bluish-purple to red. LMs can be secondary, due to infection or trauma, or primary, in which case they are usually congenital or appear in infancy, growing with the individual. Depending on the size and location of these structures, they can cause a variety of problems including pain, anatomic distortion and overgrowth, obstruction, skeletal hypertrophy and abdominal chylous ascites. The etiology of these sporadic malformations remains unknown, with major controllers of lymphatic development, such as VEGFR3 and PROX1, remaining good candidates.

Lymphedema

Lymphedema [3] is a diffuse lymphatic anomaly, characterized by swelling caused by fluid accumulation due to defective lymphatic drainage, usually of the lower extremities. Lymphedema can be primary or secondary due to infection or trauma. Primary lymphedema, which can occur in sporadic as well as incompletely penetrant, inherited forms, can either be isolated, or form part of syndromes, such as Turner syndrome (short stature, estrogen deficiency, and cardiac and other problems caused by partial or complete chromosome X-monosomy), Noonan syndrome (short stature, facial dysmorphisms, and cardiac defects, for which gain-of-function mutations in genes in the MAPK kinase pathway including *PTPN11, KRAS, SOS1,* and *RAF1,* have been identified), or Hennekam syndrome (an autosomal recessive syndrome with LMs in the intestine and extremities, dysmorphia, and mental retardation). Primary lymphedema is further subdivided according to age of onset of the disease, into: type I congenital lymphedema, usually present at birth, which can sometimes cause pre-

natal pleural effusion and hydrops-fetalis; type II praecox lymphedema or Meige disease (OMIM 153200), which occurs between puberty and 35 years of age; and lymphedema tarda, which occurs later in life.

An autosomal-dominant inherited form of congenital primary lymphedema called Milroy disease (OMIM 153100) can be caused by phosphorylation-inhibitory mutations in the tyrosine-kinase domain of the vascular endothelial growth factor receptor 3 (*VEGFR-3* or *FLT-4* on *5q35.3*) [28, 29]. *De novo* mutations in the gene have also been recently identified in a few sporadic cases [30]. VEGFR3 expression is found to be elevated in lymphatic ECs; *VEGFR3*-mutant (*Chy*), as well as receptor-deficient mice, show a very similar phenotype to the human, supporting its role in lymphangiogenesis and lymphedema pathogenesis [4].

Loss of function and missense mutations in the forkhead transcription factor *FOXC2* on *16q24.3* have been identified as the cause for some inherited cases of lymphedema associated with distichiasis (OMIM 153400), ptosis (OMIM 153000), and yellow nail syndrome (OMIM 153300) [31–33]. The causative gene in some inherited cases of hypotrichosis-lymphedema-telangiectasia syndrome (HLTS; OMIM 607823), characterized by sparse hair and lymphedema and, sometimes, cutaneous telangiectasias, has been identified as the transcription factor *SOX18* ([34]; detailed review in [35]). Mutations that act in both a dominant and a recessive manner have been identified. *Ragged* (*Ra*) mice have a very similar phenotype to the human, caused by four different (probably dominant-negative) mutations in *Sox-18*, which impair its trans-activation and interaction with partner MEF2C. *Sox-18*-deficient mice, on the other hand, have a normal phenotype, perhaps due to functional redundancy with *Sox7* and/or *17*. SOX-18 has been shown to activate VCAM-1 expression, which in turn has an important role in EC activation, inflammation, and lymphatic physiology.

The rare osteoporosis, lymphedema, anhydrotic ectodermal dysplasia with immunodeficiency (OLEDAID; OMIM 308300) syndrome, in which lymphedema occurs in early childhood, has been found to be caused by mutations in *NF-κB essential modulator* (*NEMO*) on *Xq28* [36], causing reduced NF-κB activation. Autosomal recessive Aagenaes syndrome or hereditary cholestasis with lymphedema (OMIM 214900), which shows, amongst other symptoms, growth retardation, rickets, jaundice and lymphedema, has been linked to an as yet unidentified gene on 15q [37].

Arteriovenous Malformation (AVM)

AVMs (reviewed in detail in [6]) are fast-slow lesions in which a direct connection is made between the arteries and veins (AV fistulas), or the capillary bed interconnecting them is replaced by a "nidus", in which many arteries connect with and empty directly into draining veins, accompanied by fibrosis and thickened muscle walls. Cutaneous AVMs appear red-purple, and are warm, with a thrill. AVMs can be present at birth or appear later. They are sometimes asymptomatic, but can also, depending on their size and location, or expansion due to trauma, hormonal changes or incomplete treatment, cause various problems including dysmorphism, and CNS or cardiac symptoms. AVMs can be the most complex anomalies to treat, as inappropriate treatment can exacerbate the condition. The genetic bases of sporadic AVM are currently unknown, and molecules that participate in AV-differentiation, such as those involved in the Notch signaling pathway, are considered to be good candidates. As described previously for CM-AVM, in which cutaneous capillary malformations are associated with arteriovenous malformations, genes for the inherited forms of various syndromes associated with AVMs have on the other hand been successfully identified.

Hereditary Hemorrhagic Telangiectasia (HHT)

HHT (Rendu-Osler-Weber or ROW; OMIM 187300, reviewed in detail in [6, 38]), an autosomal dominant disorder characterized by epistaxis, telangiectasias and AVMs in the brain, lung, or liver, has an estimated incidence of about 1–2 in 10,000. Telangiectasias, which are local dilations of post-capillary venules with increased SMC layers, are also observed in other syndromes including ataxia-telangiectasia (Louis Bar syndrome; OMIM 208900), a recessive disorder with neurovascular symptoms including cerebellar ataxia and multiple telangiectasias, caused by inactivating mutations in the nuclear protein kinase *ATM* on *11q23* [39], which activates cellular responses to double-stranded breaks in DNA.

At least four different genes can mediate the disease: HHT1 is caused by mutations in the *Endoglin* (*ENG*) gene on *9q33–34* [40], and HHT2 by those in *activin receptor-like kinase 1* (*ALK1*) on *12q11–14* [41]. The hundreds of mutations identified in both genes seem to cause haploinsufficiency. Loci on *5q31.3–32* and *7p14* are linked to HHT3 and 4 respectively [42, 43], although the causative genes remain to be identified. HHT1 and 2 have similar phenotypes, although cerebral and pulmonary AVMs are more common in HHT1, which shows earlier onset and a lower penetrance than HHT2, in which hepatic AVMs are more frequent [6]. Autosomal-dominant juvenile (gastrointestinal) polyposis-HHT syndrome (JPHT; OMIM 175050) is caused by *MADH4/SMAD4* [44].

Both the HHT1 and 2 genes, as well as *SMAD4*, belong to the TGF-β pathway, known to be extremely important in regulating cell proliferation, migration and differentiation, as well as the extracellular matrix in the vascular (and many other) systems. Both ALK1 and ENG are expressed mainly on vECs. ALK1 is a type I serine-threonine kinase receptor for the TGF-β superfamily, which is recruited and activated upon ligand binding by the type II receptors for these proteins. ENG is a homodimeric transmembrane glycoprotein that interacts with heteromeric receptors (including ALK-1 in vECs) for the TGF-β superfamily, modulating cellular responses to these ligands. It has also been found to play a role in actin skeletal organization. In vECs, TGF-β signaling through ALK1 is mediated by the receptor regulated R-Smads SMAD 1, 5, and 8. Ubiquitously expressed SMAD4 hetero-oligomerizes with activated R-Smads, and they translocate to the nucleus where, depending on a variety of other co-factors, they can transcriptionally activate the expression of many different genes (reviewed in [6, 38]).

Alk1$^{-/-}$ mice die at mid-gestation, with few capillaries, AVMs between major vessels, and defective vSMC recruitment. *Alk1*$^{+/-}$ heterozygous deletion-mutants do have an HHT-like phenotype, with mucocutaneous and visceral lesions. *Eng*$^{-/-}$ mice also show embryonic lethality, with vascular and cardiac defects, and the presence of AVMs between major vessels with *Eng*$^{+/-}$ mice showing HHT phenotypes like cerebral AVMs and telangiectasias. Deletion of the murine SMAD4 version *Dpc4* causes embryonic death, with significantly smaller size, low levels of proliferation, lack of a mesoderm, and disorganized endoderm; heterozygous mutants, however, seem normal (reviewed in [4, 6, 38]).

PTEN Hamartoma Tumor Syndrome (PHTS)

Mutations in the tumor suppressor gene *PTEN* on *10q23.3* have been identified in a group of complex tumor-susceptibility syndromes often associated with fast-flow vascular anomalies, and the *PTEN*-associated subsets of these are collectively termed

PHTS [6]. They include Cowden syndrome (CS; OMIM 158350), with mucocutaneous lesions, gastrointestinal (GI) hamartomas, and increased risk of carcinomas; Bannayan-Riley-Ruvalcaba syndrome (BRRS; OMIM 153480) which shows macrocephaly, lipomas, GI polyps, thyroiditis, and vascular malformations; and Proteus syndrome (PLS; OMIM 176920), with hand and foot overgrowth, limb asymmetry, and cranial hyperostosis. PTEN, a lipid and protein (tyrosine and serine-threonine) phosphatase, inhibits the PI3K/Akt survival pathway. It can also inhibit the vascular growth factor VEGF, Shc and Ras activity, as well as FAK, downregulating integrin-stimulated cell migration. Interestingly, its mRNA level can in turn be modulated by TGF-β. EC-specific deletion of PTEN is embryonic lethal due to cardiac and vascular abnormalities, increased EC proliferation, drop in the number of vessels, which are dilated, and defective vSMC recruitment. Heterozygous PTEN-deleted ECs exhibit increased proliferation and response to a variety of growth factors, all of which support its important role in vascular regulation and tumor suppression [6, 38, 45].

Conclusion

The genetic etiology and pathogenic mechanisms underlying the wide variety of vascular malformations that occur in humans represent a complex problem, and much remains to be learnt. However, studies have begun to reveal certain common themes. While they are more commonly sporadic than inherited, factors such as incomplete penetrance and the presence of small or asymptomatic lesions can make it difficult to actually rule out any family history of these anomalies. The genes identified to mediate the rare inherited counterparts of vascular malformations generally carry loss of function mutations that cause haploinsufficiency, the exception being the activating mutations in TIE2-mediated VMCM. It is probable that the same, or functionally related genes and

pathways, also participate in the predominant, sporadic forms, the etiologies of many of which remain to be dissected. Most of these gene defects seem to act primarily in the EC compartment, with the exception of GVM, in which vSMCs are abnormally differentiated.

There is mounting evidence that paradominant inheritance or a second somatic hit model of causation is a feature of many anomalies. Such a model would account for certain features common to vascular malformations: incomplete penetrance, and the localized and heterogeneous nature of lesions, which can vary widely in terms of age at incidence, number, location, and size, even within families, with sporadic forms tending to show single, and familial forms multiple lesions. This is supported by data from animal models, in which homozygous gene-deletions typically cause profound vascular defects and embryonic lethality, while the heterozygous deletion-mutants often do not have phenotypes similar to that seen in humans, appearing normal instead. The use of conditional, cell-specific mutants would therefore be of great use in recapitulating and unraveling the effects of disease-mutations.

The identification of second-hits may be hampered by tissue heterogeneity in lesions, or by inadequate sensitivity of screening methods, and enrichment for the right cell type (lesion vs. normal or vEC vs. vSMC) can be accomplished by laser microdissection. Alternatively, trans-heterozygosity, in which a germline mutation in one allele of a gene is accompanied by local loss of an allele of a functionally related gene, could be hypothesized to occur at the site of a malformation, although no examples of this have yet been reported. Finally, pathways involved in or overlapping with signaling downstream of the integrins, TGF-β, and VEGF are dysregulated in multiple anomalies. This underlines their prominence in vascular development and function, and suggests that they warrant close attention in future attempts to decipher the etiopathogenesis of other malformations as well.

References

1. Adams RH, Alitalo K (2007) Molecular regulation of angiogenesis and lymphangiogenesis. Nat Rev Mol Cell Biol 8:464–478
2. Mulliken JB, Glowacki J (1982) Hemangiomas and vascular malformations in infants and children: a classification based on endothelial characteristics. Plast Reconstr Surg 69:412–422
3. Boon LM, Vikkula M (2007) Vascular malformations. In: Fitzpatrick's dermatology in general medicine, 7th edn. McGraw-Hill Professional Publishing
4. Brouillard P, Vikkula M (2007) Genetic causes of vascular malformations. Hum Mol Genet 16 Spec No 2:R140–R149
5. Eerola I, Boon LM, Mulliken JB et al (2003) Capillary

malformation-arteriovenous malformation, a new clinical and genetic disorder caused by RASA1 mutations. Am J Hum Genet 73:1240–1249

6. Revencu N, Boon LM, Vikkula M (2007) Arteriovenous malformation in mice and men. In: Marmé D, Fusenig N (eds) Tumor angiogenesis: Mechanisms and cancer therapy. Springer-Verlag, Heidelberg, pp 363–374

7. Revencu N, Boon LM, Mulliken JB, Vikkula M (in press) RASA1 and capillary malformation-arteriovenous malformation. In: Epstein CJ, Erickson RP, Wynshaw-Boris A (eds) Inborn errors of development. Oxford University Press, Oxford

8. Revencu N, Vikkula M (2006) Cerebral cavernous malformation: new molecular and clinical insights. J Med Genet 43:716–721

9. Laberge-le Couteulx S, Jung HH, Labauge P et al (1999) Truncating mutations in CCM1, encoding KRIT1, cause hereditary cavernous angiomas. Nat Genet 23:189–193

10. Sahoo T, Johnson EW, Thomas JW et al (1999) Mutations in the gene encoding KRIT1, a Krev-1/rap1a binding protein, cause cerebral cavernous malformations (CCM1). Hum Mol Genet 8:2325–2333

11. Liquori CL, Berg MJ, Siegel AM et al (2003) Mutations in a gene encoding a novel protein containing a phosphotyrosine-binding domain cause type 2 cerebral cavernous malformations. Am J Hum Genet 73:1459–1464

12. Bergametti F, Denier C, Labauge P et al (2005) Mutations within the programmed cell death 10 gene cause cerebral cavernous malformations. Am J Hum Genet 76:42–51

13. Liquori CL, Berg MJ, Squitieri F et al (2005) Low frequency of PDCD10 mutations in a panel of CCM3 probands: potential for a fourth CCM locus. Hum Mutat 27:118

14. Kehrer-Sawatzki H, Wilda M, Braun VM et al (2002) Mutation and expression analysis of the KRIT1 gene associated with cerebral cavernous malformations (CCM1). Acta Neuropathol (Berl) 104:231–240

15. Gault J, Shenkar R, Recksiek P, Awad IA (2005) Biallelic somatic and germ line CCM1 truncating mutations in a cerebral cavernous malformation lesion. Stroke 36:872–874

16. Labauge P, Enjolras O, Bonerandi JJ et al (1999) An association between autosomal dominant cerebral cavernomas and a distinctive hyperkeratotic cutaneous vascular malformation in 4 families. Ann Neurol 45:250–254

17. Eerola I, Plate KH, Spiegel R et al (2000) KRIT1 is mutated in hyperkeratotic cutaneous capillary-venous malformation associated with cerebral capillary malformation. Hum Mol Genet 9:1351–1355

18. Limaye N, Revencu N, Van Regemorter N et al (in preparation) Novel KRIT1 mutations mediating cerebral cavernous malformations (CCMs)

19. Wouters V, Boon LM, Vikkula M (in press) TIE2 and cutaneomucosal venous malformation. In: Epstein CJ,

Erickson RP, Wynshaw-Boris A (eds) Inborn errors of development. Oxford University Press, Oxford

20. Dompmartin A, Archer A, Thibon P et al (in press) Consumptive coagulopathy associated with venous malformations is frequent: need for treatment? Arch Dermatol

21. Vikkula M, Boon LM, Carraway KL et al (1996) Vascular dysmorphogenesis caused by an activating mutation in the receptor tyrosine kinase TIE2. Cell 87:1181–1190

22. Hughes DP, Marron MB, Brindle NP (2003) The antiinflammatory endothelial tyrosine kinase Tie2 interacts with a novel nuclear factor-kappaB inhibitor ABIN-2. Circ Res 92:630–636

23. Morris PN, Dunmore BJ, Brindle NP (2006) Mutant Tie2 causing venous malformation signals through Shc. Biochem Biophys Res Commun 346:335–338

24. Morris PN, Dunmore BJ, Tadros A et al (2005) Functional analysis of a mutant form of the receptor tyrosine kinase Tie2 causing venous malformations. J Mol Med 83:58–63

25. Limaye N, Wouters V, Uebelhoer M et al (2008) Somatic mutations in the Angioprotein-Receptor TIE2 can cause both solitary and multiple sporadic venous malformation. Nat Genet (in press)

26. Brouillard P, Enjolras O, Boon LM, Vikkula M (in press) GLMN and glomuvenous malformation. In: Epstein CJ, Erickson RP, Wynshaw-Boris A (eds) Inborn errors of development. Oxford University Press, Oxford

27. Brouillard P, Boon LM, Mulliken JB et al (2002) Mutations in a novel factor, glomulin, are responsible for glomuvenous malformations ("glomangiomas"). Am J Hum Genet 70:866–874

28. Irrthum A, Karkkainen MJ, Devriendt K et al (2000) Congenital hereditary lymphedema caused by a mutation that inactivates VEGFR3 tyrosine kinase. Am J Hum Genet 67:295–301

29. Karkkainen MJ, Ferrell RE, Lawrence EC et al (2000) Missense mutations interfere with VEGFR-3 signalling in primary lymphoedema. Nat Genet 25:153–159

30. Ghalamkarpour A, Morlot S, Raas-Rothschild A et al (2006) Hereditary lymphedema type I associated with VEGFR3 mutation: the first de novo case and atypical presentations. Clin Genet 70:330–335

31. Finegold DN, Kimak MA, Lawrence EC et al (2001) Truncating mutations in FOXC2 cause multiple lymphedema syndromes. Hum Mol Genet 10:1185–1189

32. Bell R, Brice G, Child AH et al (2001) Analysis of lymphoedema-distichiasis families for FOXC2 mutations reveals small insertions and deletions throughout the gene. Hum Genet 108:546–551

33. Fang J, Dagenais SL, Erickson RP, Arlt MF et al (2000) Mutations in FOXC2 (MFH-1), a forkhead family transcription factor, are responsible for the hereditary lymphedema-distichiasis syndrome. Am J Hum Genet 67:1382–1388

34. Irrthum A, Devriendt K, Chitayat D et al (2003) Mutations in the transcription factor gene SOX18

underlie recessive and dominant forms of hypotrichosis-lymphedema-telangiectasia. Am J Hum Genet 72:1470–1478

35. Ghalamkarpour A, Devriendt K, Vikkula M (in press) SOX18 and the Hypotrichosis-Lymphedema-Telangiectasia Syndrome. In: Epstein CJ, Erickson RP, Wynshaw-Boris A (eds) Inborn errors of development. Oxford University Press, Oxford

36. Smahi A, Courtois G, Vabres P et al (2000) Genomic rearrangement in NEMO impairs NF-kappaB activation and is a cause of incontinentia pigmenti. The International Incontinentia Pigmenti (IP) Consortium. Nature 405:466–472

37. Bull LN, Roche E, Song EJ et al (2000) Mapping of the locus for cholestasis-lymphedema syndrome (Aagenaes syndrome) to a 6.6-cM interval on chromosome 15q. Am J Hum Genet 67:994–999

38. Abdalla SA, Letarte M (2006) Hereditary haemorrhagic telangiectasia: current views on genetics and mechanisms of disease. J Med Genet 43:97–110

39. Savitsky K, Bar-Shira A, Gilad S et al (1995) A single ataxia telangiectasia gene with a product similar to PI-3 kinase. Science 268:1749–1753

40. McAllister KA, Grogg KM, Johnson DW et al (1994) Endoglin, a TGF-beta binding protein of endothelial cells, is the gene for hereditary haemorrhagic telangiectasia type 1. Nat Genet 8:345–351

41. Johnson DW, Berg JN, Baldwin MA et al (1996) Mutations in the activin receptor-like kinase 1 gene in hereditary haemorrhagic telangiectasia type 2. Nat Genet 13:189–195

42. Cole SG, Begbie ME, Wallace GM, Shovlin CL (2005) A new locus for hereditary haemorrhagic telangiectasia (HHT3) maps to chromosome 5. J Med Genet 42:577–582

43. Bayrak-Toydemir P, McDonald J, Akarsu N et al (2006) A fourth locus for hereditary hemorrhagic telangiectasia maps to chromosome 7. Am J Med Genet 140:2155–2162

44. Gallione CJ, Repetto GM, Legius E et al (2004) A combined syndrome of juvenile polyposis and hereditary haemorrhagic telangiectasia associated with mutations in MADH4 (SMAD4). Lancet 363:852–859

45. Marchuk DA, Srinivasan S, Squire TL, Zawistowski JS (2003) Vascular morphogenesis: tales of two syndromes. Hum Mol Genet 12 Spec 1:R97–R112

Epidemiology of Vascular Malformations

14

Géza Tasnádi

Abstract

There are few reports on the epidemiology of congenital vascular malformations (CVM). We performed a study on 3,573 3 year old children and found 43 cases of CVM or related symptoms: an incidence of 1.2%. Infiltrating or localized venous and/or arteriovenous (AV) defects were noticed in 16 cases (37%), port wine stain in 15 cases (35%), lymphedema, lymphatic defects in 5 (12%), phlebectasia with nevus and limb length discrepancy in 5 (12%) and phlebectasia in 2 cases (4%).

Vascular malformations (VM) arise from an error in morphogenesis in any combination of arterial, venous and lymphatic vascular networks. These vascular anomalies are present at birth, grow proportionally to the size of the child and do not exhibit any tendency to involute spontaneously. Hormonal factors, such as the gestational hormonal reaction by infants, puberty, or pregnancy, may influence the growth of these vascular lesions, causing acceleration in size during these periods. Physical (hemodynamic) exercise, direct trauma or infection may also trigger a rapid expansion [1]. Genetic loci [2] and related syndromes [3] have also been discovered and have shed new light on the clinical behavior of vascular malformations.

Incidence of Vascular Malformations

The great majority of CVMs are recognizable in childhood. Pratt studied VMs in neonates. In his series, only five of 1,096 neonates showed a VM, indicating that such anomalies are rare [4].

Tasnádi examined 3,573 3 year old children, and found 43 cases of congenital vascular defects or related symptoms (1.2%). Nevi were noticed in 15 cases (0.43%), phlebectasia in two cases (0.05%), phlebectasia with nevus and hypertrophy or hypotrophy in an extremity in five cases (0.14%), infiltrating or localized venous and/or arteriovenous (AV) defects in 16 cases (0.44%) and lymphedema or lymphangiectasia in five cases (0.14%) [5].

Compared with other inborn errors, such as congenital heart defect (0.88%) or spina bifida (0.2%), the incidence of CVM is rather high [6, 7].

By far the most common type of VM are portwine stains (nevi) that occur in an estimated three children per 1,000 births [8].

Distribution of Vascular Malformations

Close to half of the vascular defects in children were venous malformations (48.5%), more than one third had arterial and AV shunting defects (35.8%), lymphatic malformations were found in 10%, and combined defects were found in 5.7% of cases.

The number of extratruncular forms was very high. Ninety-seven percent of AV and capillary defects and 57% of venous malformations were extratruncular.

Distribution by Gender

The sex distribution in children with venous malformations was roughly even, with a boy to girl ratio of 1:1.2. However, AV shunt defects were close to four times more frequent in girls than in boys. For lymphatic malformations the boy to girl ratio was 1:1.

R. Mattassi, D.A. Loose, M. Vaghi (eds.), *Hemangiomas and Vascular Malformations*.
© Springer-Verlag Italia 2009

Time of Appearance

Arterial-capillary malformations were mainly noticed at birth. Venous malformations were often visible at birth, but symptoms appear only later. Lymphatic malformations appeared at birth, in puberty and also later. AV defects were rarely noticed at birth. They appeared mainly in childhood and adolescence.

Body Location of VMs

In general, truncular forms appeared most frequently in the extremities, whereas extratruncular forms, both infiltrating and limited, were most commonly located in the head and neck [9].

References

1. Tasnádi G, Osztovics M (1977) Pathogenesis of angiodysplasias. Acta Paediatr Acad Sc Hung 18:301–309
2. Vikkula M, Boon LM, Mulliken JB (2001) Molecular genetics of vascular malformations. Matrix Biol 20:327–335
3. Mueller-Lessman V, Behrendt A, Wetzel WE et al (2001) Orofacial findings in the Klippel-Trenaunay syndrome. Int J Paediatr Dent 11:225–229
4. Pratt AG (1967) Birthmarks in infants. Arch Dermatol Syph 67:302
5. Tasnádi G (1993) Epidemiology and etiology of congenital vascular malformations. Semin Vasc Surg 6:200–203
6. Lilienfeld AM (1969) Population differences in frequency of malformations at birth. In: Fraser FC, Mc Kusick VA (eds) Congenital malformations. Proceedings of the third international conference. The Hague, The Netherlands, 7–13 Sept, Excerpta Medica, Amsterdam/New York, p 251
7. Smith DW (1970) Recognizable patterns of human malformations. WB Saunders, Philadelphia
8. Miller AC, Pit-Ten Cate IM, Watson HS (1999) Stress and family satisfaction in parents of children with facial port-wine stains. Pediatr Dermatol 16:190–197
9. Geronemus RG, Ashinoff R (1991) The medical necessity of evaluation and treatment of portwine stains. J Dermatol Surg Oncol 17:76–79

Classification of Vascular Malformations

15

Raul Mattassi, Dirk A. Loose, Massimo Vaghi

Abstract

As congenital vascular malformations (CVM) are a complex mixture of different vessels, classification is difficult. In the past, different descriptions, syndromes with common names and complex classifications have been used to define these diseases. Only recently, two main classifications, more or less accepted, have been proposed: the Mulliken Classification, based on flow velocity in the defect, and the Hamburg Classification, based on the vessels' embryological development. Both of these classifications are imperfect. A combination of both may offer the best option to define these pathologies clearly.

Introduction

The history of classification of congenital vascular malformations (CVM) reflects the great difficulties encountered in understanding these pathologies. Few diseases have generated such a large number of different names and syndromes. Before the introduction of angiography, only description of the clinical picture was possible; in the literature at this time, a list of case presentations is found. In 1863 Rudolf Virchow, the father of cellular pathology, divided vascular birthmarks in "angioma simplex", "angioma cavernosum" and "angioma racemosus" [1]. At that time and until much later, the difference between hemangioma and vascular malformation was not clear and many descriptions included one or the other disease or both in the same series. The term "angioma" was also the cause of much misunderstanding because many authors used this term to describe both hemangiomas and CVMs. As John Mulliken very clearly said, "this terminology con-fusion is responsible, in no small way, for improper diagnosis, illogical treatment and misdirected research effort" [2].

Besides the term "angioma", many other expressions were used, including nevus angiectoides, varice aneurysm, cirsoid aneurysm, hemangioma cavernosum, arteriovenous angioma and red angioma telangiectaticum. Some well known descriptions, like the papers of Klippel-Trenaunay (K-T) and of Parkes-Weber (P-W) led to the definition of "syndromes". Other authors described combinations of CVM with other diseases, like Maffucci syndrome, or cases with CVM in different locations, like Sturge-Weber syndrome. After these publications, CVMs were often defined as syndromes, such as K-T or P-W; and although some attempt was made to distinguish between arteriovenous (AV) malformations (P-W syndrome) and venous CVM (K-T syndrome), confusion remained and frequently cases were defined as K-T-P-W.

With the advent of angiography there were better options for studying CVM and different classifications were proposed, although not widely accepted. Some were too complex, including long lists of syndromes, while others did not cover all types of CVM. The existence of mixed forms contributed to difficulty in achieving a simple and complete classification.

A main step along the difficult path to clarity was the publication of Mulliken and Glowacky [3] in 1982, which definitively distinguished hemangiomas from vascular malformations, based on cellular kinetics, physical examination and natural history. Another step was the decision, taken during a consensus session at the 7th Meeting of the International Workshop on Vascular Malformations in Hamburg in 1988, to abolish the term "angioma", which had been the cause of much confusion [4].

R. Mattassi, D.A. Loose, M. Vaghi (eds.), *Hemangiomas and Vascular Malformations*.
© Springer-Verlag Italia 2009

After these clarifications, the goal was to find a common classification in order to have a common language. The International Society for the Study of Vascular Anomalies (ISSVA) established a commission of experts who presented their conclusion during the 11th International Workshop held in Rome in 1996. The effort of the commission was to propose a classification as simple as possible without confusing "common named syndromes". The classification proposed divided the malformations into basic categories, as "single vessel type or simple" and "combined" forms [8] (Table 15.1).

However, there is still need for a more detailed differentiation within the single groups in order to achieve greater clinical impact, as a guide for diagnosis process, a treatment schema and for outcome evaluation.

The most widely accepted classifications today that offer better options are those of Mulliken and Glowacky [3] and the modified Hamburg classification [5]. These are completely different from each other, as each is based on a different concept.

Mulliken and Glowacky proposed a classification based on flow characteristics, dividing CVM into

high-flow and low-flow lesions, adding syndromes of complex cases and identification with alphabetic letters (Table 15.2).

The main advantage of this classification is that it includes all types of vascular anomalies and introduces a very effective and simple system of letters to define the class of defect. Combination of two or more malformations can be expressed simply with this system; the predominant defect is indicated by the first letters of the compete diagnosis. The main disadvantage is that it neglects defining subgroups for better clinical work, as indicated earlier.

The Hamburg Classification is based on the vessel's embryological development (Table 15.3). According to embryological data [6, 7], a CVM

Table 15.1. Vascular anomaly classification (ISSVA) (1996)

Single vessel type
- capillary
- venous
- lymphatic
- arterials

Combined malformations
- arteriovenous
- lymphaticovenous
- capillary-venous
- capillary-lymphaticovenous

Table 15.2. Classification of vascular malformations according to Mulliken and Glowacky

Slow flow
- Capillary (CM)
- Lymphatic (LM)
- Venous (VM)

Fast flow
- Arterial (AM): aneurysm, coarctation, ectasia
- Arteriovenous fistulas (AVF)
- Arteriovenous (AVM)

Complex combined (often with associated skeletal overgrowth)
- Regional syndromes
  Sturge Weber: facial CM, intracranial CM, VM, AVM
  Klippel-Trenaunay: limb-truncal capillary lymphaticovenous (CLVM)
  Parkes-Weber: limb CLVM with AVF
- Diffuse syndromes
  Maffucci: LVM, enchondromas
  Solomon: CM, VM, intracranial AVM, epidermal nevi, etc.
  Proteus: CM, VM, macrodactyly, hemihypertrophy, lipomas, pigmented nevi, scoliosis

Table 15.3. Classification of vascular malformations according to the Hamburg Classification [5]

Types	Forms	
	Truncular	**Extratruncular**
Predominantly arterial defects	Aplasia or obstruction Dilatation	Infiltrating Limited
Predominantly venous defects	Aplasia or obstruction Dilatation	Infiltrating Limited
Predominantly lymphatic defects	Aplasia or obstruction, Dilatation	Infiltrating Limited
Predominantly AV shunting defects	Deep Superficial	Infiltrating Limited
Combined/mixed defects	Arterial and venous without shunt	Infiltrating hemolymphatic
	Hemolymphatic with or without shunt	Limited hemolymphatic

may take a specific form depending on the stage of embryological development. Pathologic effects at an early stage, the retiform stage, produce areas of dysplastic vessels inside the tissues, while a late effect, during the truncular phase, may result in anomalies of main vessels, such as aplasia, stenosis or aneurysm.

The advantage of this classification is the clear division into embryological based subgroups that have been widely appreciated for clinical application.

A good example is to consider a goal of a diagnostic process to classify a malformation according to this system which means to have an helpful guideline.

The main defect of the Hamburg Classification is that it does not address capillary malformations.

Addition of capillary malformations as a separate group to the system would complete it.

Unfortunately, both classifications are not universally accepted. Moreover, some authors use other less known classifications or even simply the old Klippel-Trenaunay-Parkes-Weber syndrome denomination, with which a clear diagnosis is very often not achieved.

A good compromise could be a combination of both classifications with the Hamburg Classification as a basis because of its advantage of subgroup classifications, completed with the capillary malformation group and the system of alphabetic letters from the Mulliken Classification in order to define the defect.

Some pictures of different CVM with examples of classification are demonstrated (Figs. 15.1–15.5).

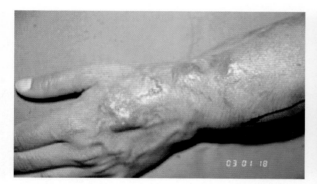
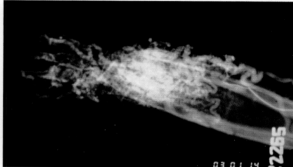

Fig. 15.1. AV malformation of the left arm. Clinical aspect (*left*); angiography (*right*). According to the ISSVA this would be an AV malformation; according to the Mulliken Classification, a fast flow, AV malformation, *AVM*; and according to the Hamburg classification, an extratruncular, infiltrating, AV malformation

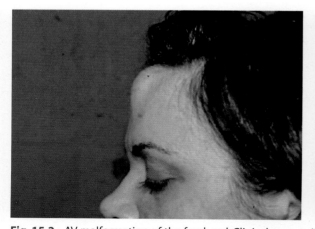
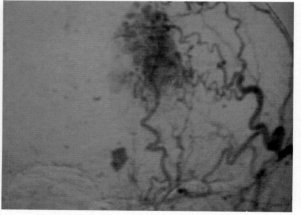

Fig. 15.2. AV malformation of the forehead. Clinical aspect (*left*), angiography (*right*). According to the ISSVA this would be an AV malformation; according to the Mulliken Classification, a fast flow, AV malformation, *AVM*; and according to the Hamburg classification, an extratruncular, limited, AV malformation

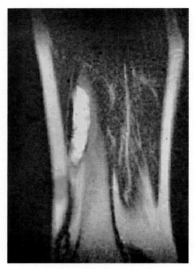 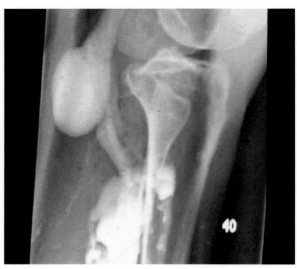

Fig. 15.3. Intramuscular venous malformation of the thigh. According to the ISSVA Classification this is a venous malformation; according to the Mulliken Classification, a low flow, venous malformation, *VM*; and according to the Hamburg classification, an extratruncular, limited, venous malformation

Fig. 15.4. Aneurysm of a popliteal vein. According to the ISSVA Classification this would be a venous malformation; according to the Mulliken Classification, a low flow, venous malformation, *VM*; and according to the Hamburg classification, a venous malformation, truncular, dilatation

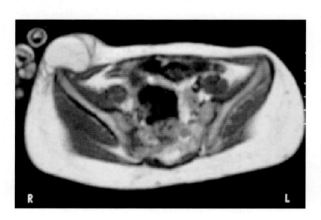

Fig. 15.5. Superficial hygroma. According to the ISSVA Classification this would be a lymphatic malformation; according to the Mulliken Classification, a low flow, lymphatic malformation, *LM*; according to the Hamburg classification, an extratruncular, limited, lymphatic malformation

References

1. Irchow R (1863) Angiome. In: Die Krankhaften Geschwülste. Hischwald, Berlin
2. Mulliken J (1993) Cutaneous vascular anomalies. Seminars in Vasc Surg 6:204–218
3. Mulliken J, Glowacky J (1982) Hemangiomas and vascular malformations in infants and children: A classification based on endothelial characteristics. Plast Reconstruct Surg 69:412–422
4. Belov S, Loose DA, Weber J (1989) Vascular malformations. Einhorn Presse, Reinbek, p 29
5. Belov S (1993) Anatomopathological classification of congenital vascular defects. Seminars in Vasc Surg 6:219–224
6. Woolard HH (1922) The development of the principal arteries stem in the forelimb of the pig. Contr to Embryol Carnegie Inst 4:141–154
7. Rienhoff WF (1924) Congenital arteriovenous fistula. Bull John Hopkins Hosp 35:271–284
8. Enjolras O, Mulliken JB (1997) Vascular tumors and vascular malformations (new issues). Adv Dermatol 13:375–423
9. Rutherford RB (1995) Classification of peripheral congenital vascular malformations. In: Ernst CB, Stanley JC (eds) Current therapy in vascular surgery. Mosby, St. Louis, pp 834–834

Non Invasive Diagnostics of Congenital Vascular Malformations

16

Massimo Vaghi

Abstract

Non invasive diagnostic methods include functional tests, morphofunctional tests and imaging. Functional tests include pressure measurement and volume measurement. Morphofunctional tests are given by duplex scan, which is also used successfully during treatment. Imaging methods are mainly computed tomography (CT) and magnetic resonance (MR).

Introduction

The aim of a correct diagnosis is to define the type, the localization, and the hemodynamic alterations of a pathology. Two other important advantages of a correct diagnosis are the possibility of guiding the therapy and sampling numerical data useful for follow-up.

Diagnostic tools can be divided into three categories: 1) functional tests; 2) morphofunctional tests; and 3) imaging.

Functional Tests

Functional tests are useful for physiological measurements and evaluation of the hemodynamics of a whole limb. Usually they give quantitative measures which are very important for the follow-up of the patients.

The most important measurements are pressure measurements obtained by the use of continuous wave (CW) Doppler and plethysmographic devices and volume measurements, which are very important in the evaluation of venous diseases.

Hand held CW Doppler devices can give qualitative data during physical examination of the type of arterial flow and the presence and length of venous refluxes.

Morphofunctional Tests

Morphofunctional tests are represented by duplex scanning, which is the main non invasive examination method for congenital vascular malformations.

Duplex scanning allows a segmental examination of the vascular tree in axial and transverse planes. The blood flow alterations are located with precision and important numerical data can be obtained from the Doppler curve: blood flow determination; pulsatility index, resistance index and reflux time.

The ultrasound image is able to localize extratruncular malformations in surrounding tissues and to detect the infiltration of bones, nerves and joints.

Real time sonography is effective for detecting functional impairments in skeletal muscles (Fig. 16.1).

Real time color Doppler investigation is often important in detecting the hemodynamics of arteriovenous AV shunts (Fig. 16.2).

High flow vessels in bones can be detected using transcranial settings (Figs. 16.3, 16.4).

In venous malformations it is very important to detect segmental and long refluxes in the deep and superficial vein systems (Fig. 16.5). The lateral side of the lower limb should be investigated in all patients in order to detect a marginal vein and to study its course.

An emerging problem is represented by nerve compression and infiltration caused by the vascular malformation itself and related tissue pathology such as phlebitis and tissue scarring secondary to treatments (Fig. 16.6).

R. Mattassi, D.A. Loose, M. Vaghi (eds.), *Hemangiomas and Vascular Malformations*.
© Springer-Verlag Italia 2009

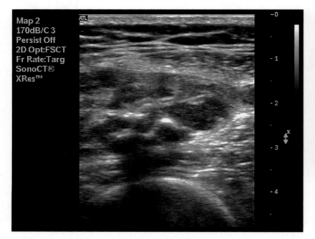

Fig. 16.1. Structural alteration of muscle localized at the left thigh secondary to vein infiltration, demonstrated by ultrasound

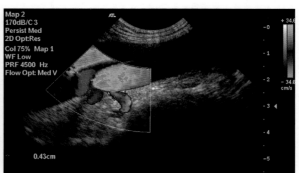

Fig. 16.2. AV shunts demonstrated by color Doppler

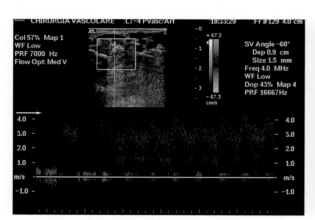

Fig. 16.3. Diffuse intra and extraosseous AV shunts (note *arrow* and the peak frequency ratio (PFR) value in the duplex scan)

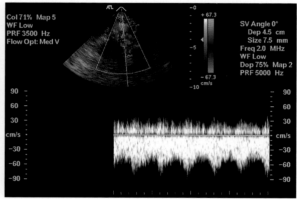

Fig. 16.4. Demonstration of an intratibial high flow malformation by color Doppler equipment set for transcranial examination

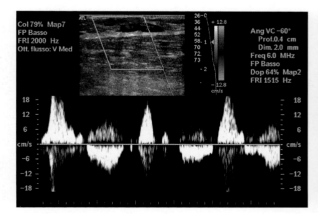

Fig. 16.5. Venous valve incompetence

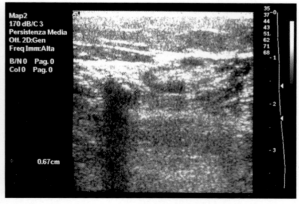

Fig. 16.6. Phleboliths demonstrated by ultrasound

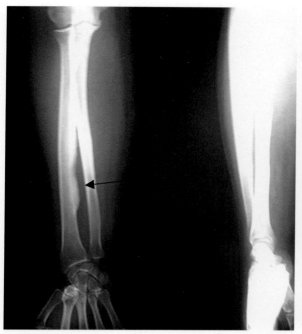

Fig. 16.7. X-ray of the right forearm: interosseous membrane calcification in a case of venous dysplasia (*arrow*)

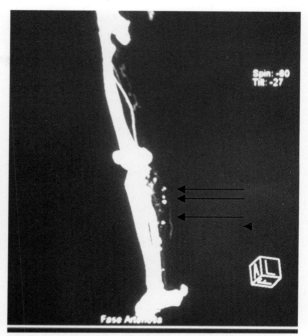

Fig. 16.8. CT scan of multiple phleboliths in the leg (*arrows*)

In cases of lymphatic malformations, ultrasound can detect edema and the presence of cysts.

Ultrasound of the limbs to study congenital vascular anomalies is a time-consuming but extremely useful procedure. Two types of investigations should be performed. Diagnostic oriented investigations define the type and the extension of the pathology, while treatment oriented investigations are segmentary studies to define the localization and extension of AV shunts, the connections of the venous malformations with the deep and superficial veins, bone, joints and involvement of nerves.

Ultrasound is also extremely useful as a guide during treatment: in case of surgical treatment to localize the malformation; and in case of injective treatment as a guide to reach and correctly puncture the vessels to be treated. In case of foam injection it is possible to follow the distribution of the sclerosing agent only by ultrasound.

Imaging

Imaging includes conventional radiological imaging, computed tomography (CT) and magnetic resonance (MR).

Conventional radiological imaging is useful in detecting the secondary effects of vascular malformations on soft tissues and bones. Calcifications in soft tissues are very easy to detect on plain films (Figs. 16.7, 16.8). Vascular bone syndromes, characterized by bone elongation or shortening are evident in comparative limb films (Fig. 16.9).

Thickening or thinning of bones are signs of possible infiltrations of malformed vessels.

A rare form of bone infiltration and destruction is represented by Gorham's syndrome, which is also known as vanishing bone syndrome. This disease is characterized by progressive bone resorption of the epiphysis and metaphysis of long bones (humerus and femur). The cause of this syndrome is not well known but it seems to be related to venous and lymphatic infiltrations (Figs. 16.10, 16.11).

CT and MR scans give important data about the anatomic extension of vascular malformations. This information is of great value in the cases of extratruncular vascular malformations which may be considered as similar to an organ pathology.

The intrinsic difference between these two kinds of investigations is their capability of contrast visualization of soft tissues and vessels.

MRI allows a correct intrinsic contrast representation of soft tissues and vascular vessels with the

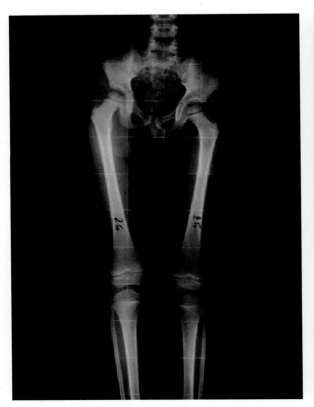

Fig. 16.9. Right lower limb elongation

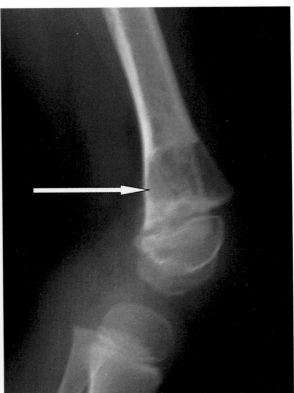

Fig. 16.10. X-ray of the right femoral bone in Gorham syndrome. Notice the large cyst (*arrow*)

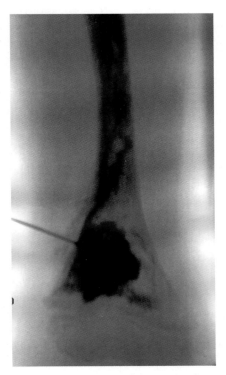

Fig. 16.11. Puncture of the cyst and contrast medium injection

possibility of getting important data about the quality of flow in the vessels (differentiation between high and low flow vessels according to the presence or absence of flow voids in the vessels). Venous malformations give a hypo- or isointense signal to the muscles in T1 weighted sequences. Otherwise, in T2 weighted sequences with fat saturation, veins give a high signal intensity (Figs. 16.12–16.15). In MRI the use of contrast media is limited to the distinction between venous and lymphatic malformations and sarcomas. Lymphatic malformations do not have any enhancement after gadolinium injection.

CT has an intrinsic contrast for air and bone and no intrinsic contrast capability to highlight the vessels. To visualize vessels, contrast medium is necessary (Fig. 16.16).

Computer aided reconstruction of CT and MRI images may help in the planning of interventional and surgical activities.

It should not be forgotten that not all vascularized lesions in soft tissues are vascular anomalies. Soft tissue tumors misdiagnosed as vascular malformations are not uncommon. The diagnostic efficacy of each non invasive procedure is indicated in Table 16.1.

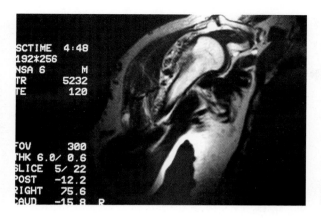

Fig. 16.12. MRI of diffuse AV shunt in the right shoulder

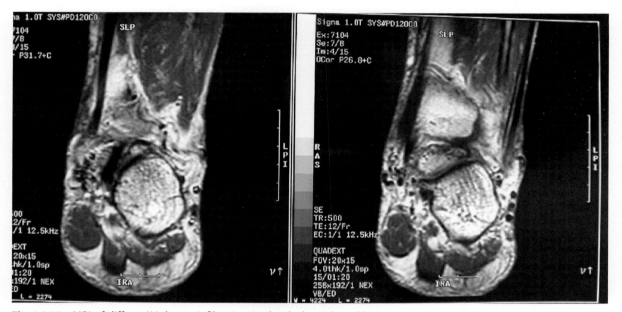

Fig. 16.13. MRI of diffuse AV shunts infiltrating in depth the right ankle

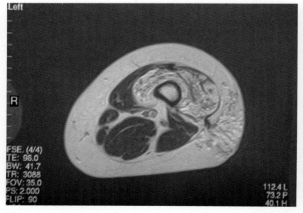

Fig. 16.14. MRI of diffuse venous malformation of the left quadriceps

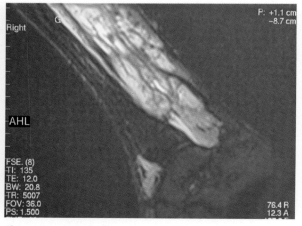

Fig. 16.15. MRI of diffuse venous infiltration of the left triceps

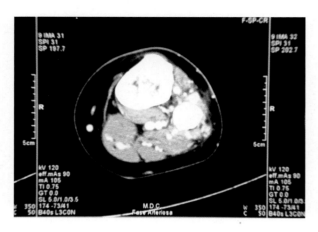

Fig. 16.16. CT scan of an AV shunt in the peroneal bone

Table 16.1. Diagnostic utility of different non invasive procedures

Type of defect	Axial resolution	Transversal resolution	Doppler CW	Plethysmographic studies	Pressure measurements	Duplex scanning	CT	MRI
Truncular	+	−	+	+	+	+	+/−[2]	−
Extratruncular	−	+	+/−[1]	−	+/−[1]	+	+[2]	+

[1] According to the size of the malformations: large extratruncular malformations can give significant alterations in the hemodynamics of a limb

[2] CT with the use of contrast media is very useful in the imaging process in case of bone involvement in truncular and extratruncular vascular malformations

References

1. Paltiel HJ, Burrows PE, Kozalewich HP et al (2000) Soft tissue vascular anomalies: utility of US for diagnosis. Radiology 214:747–754
2. Dubois J, Garel L, Grignon A et al (1998) Imaging of haemangiomas and vascular malformations in children. Acad Radiol 5:390–400
3. Dubois J, Soulez G, Oliva VL et al (2001) Soft tissue venous malformations in adult patients: imaging and therapeutic issues. Radiographics 21:1519–1531
4. Burrows PE, Laor T, Paltiel H, Robertson RL (1998) Diagnostic imaging in the evaluation of vascular birthmarks. Dermatol Clin 16:674–682
5. Rutherford RB (1993) Non invasive testing in the diagnosis and assessment of arterio-venous fistula. In: Bernstein EF (ed) Vascular diagnosis. Mosby, Saint Louis, pp 608–609
6. Wu JK, Bisdorff A, Gelbert F et al (2005) Auricular arteriovenous malformation: evaluation, management and outcome. Plast Reconstr Surg 115:985–995

Nuclear Medicine in Diagnostics of Vascular Malformations

17

Roberto Dentici

Abstract

Three nuclear imaging techniques can be used for the study of congenital vascular malformations (CVM): whole body blood pool scintigraphy (WBBPS), lymphoscintigraphy and transarterial lung perfusion scintigraphy (TLPS). WBBPS is able to demonstrate the whole vascular system and to recognize truncular and extratruncular vessel malformations. High flow malformations are indicated by the form of the activity-time curves. Lymphoscintigraphy for the study of CVM is best performed by a separate demonstration of the deep and superficial lymphatic systems. TLPS is effective to confirm or rule out the presence of an arteriovenous (AV) shunt.

Introduction

Nuclear imaging technique may have a more important role in the evaluation of angiodysplastic malformations, where tissue structure subversion, unpredictability of the morphological picture, frequent multifocality and, in a few cases, the remarkable extent of the corporeal districts cannot be unequivocally answered with the use of more traditional methods.

The frequent lack of a recognized anatomic and structural consideration and the difficult distinction between masses generically defined as "liquid" may result in ambiguous nuclear magnetic resonance (NMR) patterns, while the presence of an anomalous escape course, of segregated vascular districts, low recirculation speed or the pathological mixture typical of lymph-venous abnormalities represent an impasse for angiographic interpretation.

In this corner of "diagnostic half-light" nuclear investigations make a useful contribution, albeit with the intrinsic limitations of a discipline that founds its methodology more on functional than on morphological aspects [1].

While there are some procedures that have been made obsolete by the technical and diagnostic refining of radiological studies, the nuclear methods that have resisted represent a real complementary diagnostic tool for the evaluation of angiodysplasia, thanks to their procedural simplicity, lack of invasiveness, high tolerability and low biological cost from a dosimetric point of view [2].

Whole Body Blood Pool Scintigraphy (WBBPS)

WBBPS (Fig. 17.1) is valuable for the initial screening of malformations and as an intermediate evaluation parameter for partial corrective procedures (post-interventional and/or post-embolization control). On the other hand, therapeutic or conservative treatments must be attempted several times in the instrumental follow-up of suspicious recidivism.

WBBPS, a simple procedure from a technical point of view, makes red blood cells visible through the use of physiological contrast medium. This allows the vascular tree to be visualized in its entirety, as if a radiological contrast medium had been used. In this way, areas of high and/or altered "haematic" signal indicate the presence of the vascular malformation (Fig. 17.2).

As an example, in the truncular forms of vascular malformation it is possible to distinguish anomalies of both arterial and venous course, stenotic occlusions and expansions of the vessels. The

R. Mattassi, D.A. Loose, M. Vaghi (eds.), *Hemangiomas and Vascular Malformations*.
© Springer-Verlag Italia 2009

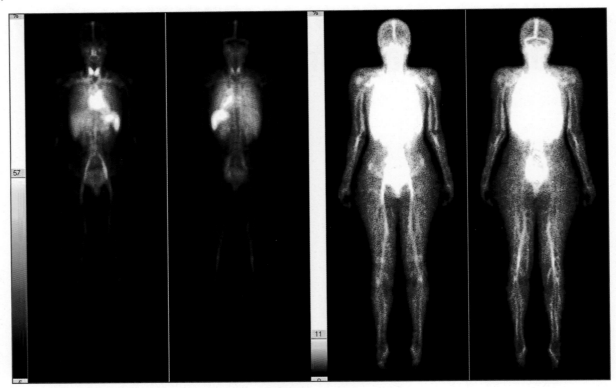

Fig. 17.1. Whole body blood pool scintigraphy (WBBPS): normal whole body scan

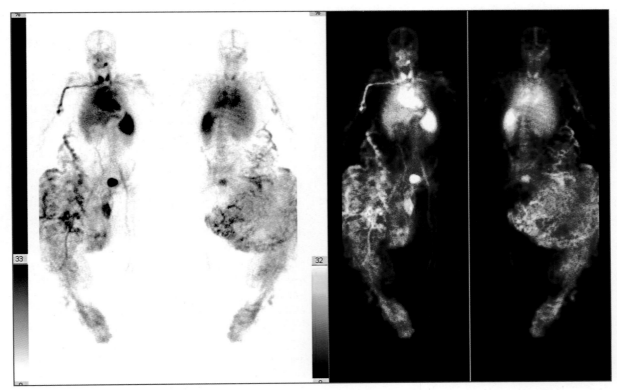

Fig. 17.2. Young patient with right lower limb overgrowth. WBBPS study demonstrates a total subversion of the vascular tree of the right leg. The dysplastic mass is spreading to the abdominal wall, partially surrounding the splanchnic tissues. The tomographic three-dimensional reconstruction emphasizes the chaotic structural complexity of this malformation

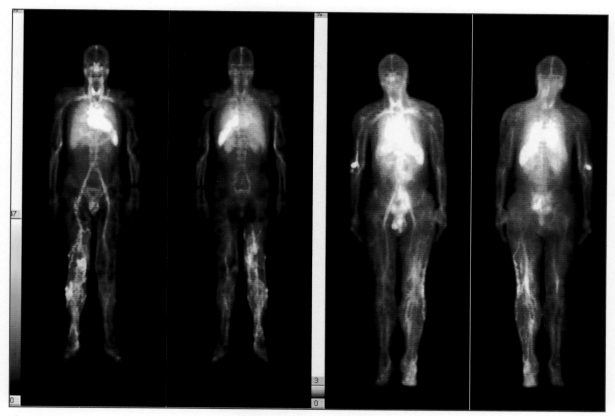

Fig. 17.3. Two cases of marginal vein of the inferior limb. Deep venous trunks are faintly visualized

poor or absent evidence of an artery or vein section, such as the slowing down or the absence of downstream flow, demonstrate hypoplasia or aplasia of the vessel, respectively (Fig. 17.3). Aneurysms are also recognizable with a typical and irregular increase in calibre.

In the extratruncular forms of vascular malformation, the tracer "accumulates" in pathological areas, providing a clear vision of the extent of the dysplasia. With images acquired in mutually orthogonal projections and especially with the three-dimensional tomographic reconstruction, it is also possible to better define and locate the lesion.

Of great interest is the possibility of identifying vascular malformations that, because of their liquid or mucinous aspect, can deceive sophisticated methods such as computer tomography (CT) and NMR: areas already catalogued as "angiomatous" but that are "cold" (not vascularised) according to scintigraphy should be carefully re-examined. Finally, in some cases, whole body acquisition can reveal hidden abnormalities.

Furthermore, the study can be extended to the following day: this is possible because the biological contrast medium, represented by radiolabelled erythrocytes, remains active throughout its radioisotope decay. This is particularly suitable for the evaluation of lymphovenous abnormalities in which the slow recirculation time and mixture among the two pathological circuits does not allow an immediate evaluation using the most traditional radiological techniques, which are limited by the rapid elimination of contrast medium (Fig. 17.4).

It is possible to view the "discharge" or the "effusion" of the autologous cells from the intravascular compartment to the lymphatic one, achieving results of absolute diagnostic value. The main limitation of this method is the poorly detailed image, which does not allow discrimination between venous and arterial structures.

It is possible to differentiate between high flow malformations (arteriovenous malformations [AVM]) and low flow masses (prevailing venous component) by the comparative analysis of the transit time of the

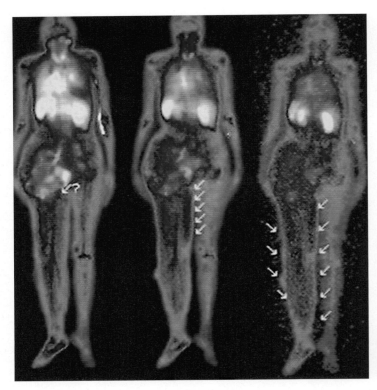

Fig. 17.4. Lymphovenous shunt, detected by WBBPS. At the second day scan, a progressive subdermal haematic spillage is observed (*arrows*). Reproduced from [3]

tracer in the pathological and corresponding healthy districts: the presence of an AVM is almost always revealed by activity-time curves obtained by the acquired dynamic sequence during the intravenous administering of radiotracer. The estimation of intralesional haemodynamics is essential in determining the appropriate treatment: surgical resection, arterial embolisation or sclerotherapy (Fig. 17.5).

Flow study (with the analysis of transit time or with direct puncture into the intravascular space of the lesion) provides a quantitative indicator of intralesional haemodynamics in low-flow lesions, in addition to accurate distinction between high-flow and low-flow lesions. For the percutaneous injection of sclerosing agents, the estimation of the flow characteristics of soft-tissue vascular anomalies is essential for determining appropriate patient management. The last promising methodological aspect of great interest is represented by whole body tomographic study, which can be extended to any corporeal district.

The tomographic approach in nuclear medicine has been used for the study of cerebral and myocardial perfusion (with ad hoc radiolabelled tracers) and for the evaluation of hemangioma (preva-

lently hepatic), thanks to the possibility of revealing the "vascular nature" of lesions, not seen with methods such as echography, CT-angiogram and NMR.

The most recent generation of nuclear equipment and the availability of iterative rebuilding algorithms allow images of higher definition and total body images in three-dimensional rotation to be obtained; these can help to better define the highlighted lesions and their topographical relationships.

The availability of updated image-fusion software allows exams acquired with radiological methods to be imported and nuclear medicine imaging (NMI), CT and NMR images to be melted, obtaining an iconography of high diagnostic content, in which structural and functional aspects of primary importance are merged in areas not accessible for clinical or sonographic exams; for instance, angiomatous intracranial or facial malformations (Fig. 17.6).

This new gold standard is today within the reach of nuclear equipment supplemented with a single "hybrid" diagnostic position, a multihead gamma camera and a multislice CT.

The integration of NMI and NMR is anticipated in the near future.

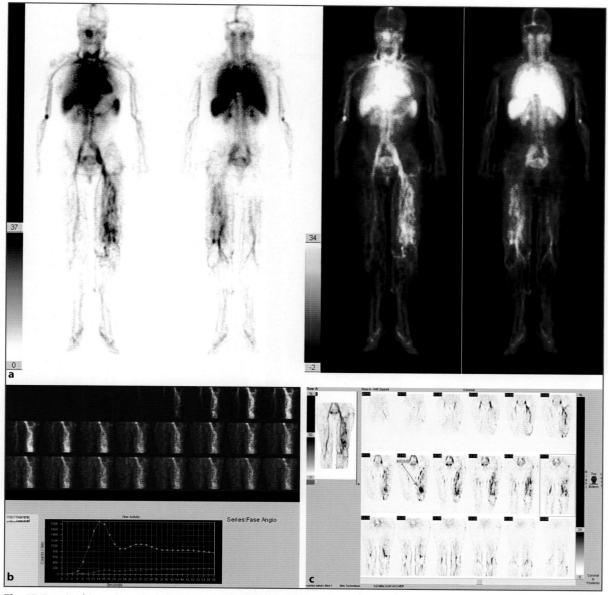

Fig. 17.5. a In this patient the whole body scan demonstrates a complex intra and extratruncular malformation. **b** Study of the tracer's transit time is barely suggestive of an arteriovenous shunt. **c** At tomographic reconstruction, the AVM nidus is visible above the knee joint and in front of femoral artery (*arrow*)

Lymphoscintigraphy

Historically, the instrumental approach to the alterations of the lymphatic system was carried out by radiological lymphangiography with a contrast medium. This method represents the gold standard for the study of a series of alterations and compromises of the lymphatic system, from the simple lymphoedema to the staging of neoplasia involving the pelvis and the abdominal area [4].

While this method is able to reveal every detail of the lymphatic grid, escape routes, the presence of morphological alterations and the calibre of vessels, it does have some drawbacks, which relegate it as an historical instrument of the radiologist rather than as one of the active tools of diagnostic practice. Radiological lymphangiography is technically very difficult, requiring a microsurgical approach to the inter-digital lymphatic capillaries; it also employs an oily contrast medium that remains in cir-

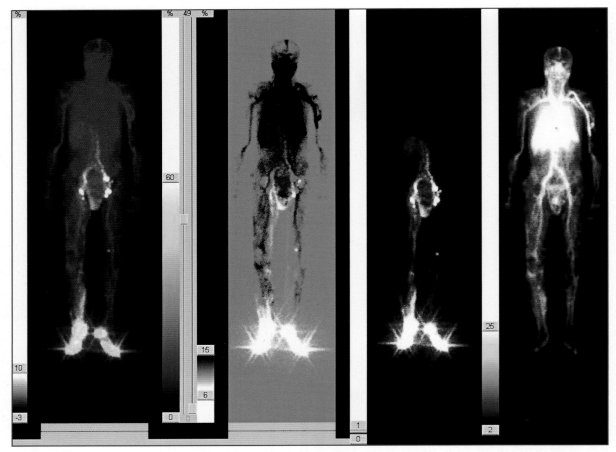

Fig. 17.6. Fusion imaging of a complex composite malformation involving the right inferior limb and the pelvis. The venous dysplasia mainly includes the calf and the lateral side of the knee and thigh. The lymphatic defect involves dermal effusion of the calf, the internal side of the thigh, the scrotum and the peritoneal space, configuring a picture of probable lymphocele complicated by abdominal spillage. No evidence of lymphovenous shunt

culation and which may cause local complications at the injection point (to the point of tissutal necrosis), may be the cause of lymphangitis (in some cases worsening the clinical picture and causing functional damage that may exacerbate lymphoedema) and, in extreme situations, may cause distant oily emboli, with the passage of the contrast medium into the blood stream. Taking into consideration these quite major problems, scintigraphy provides an alternative that is able to provide high quality information and requires no special training. In addition, scintigraphy is not invasive, harmless to the lymphatic endothelium, devoid of collateral adverse effects (and therefore well tolerated by the patient), economic, repeatable and especially reproducible (Fig. 17.7).

The investigation consists of administering a preparation of micelles of purified human albumin, with very low immunogenic power, in colloidal form, radiolabelled with an artificial radioisotope with a low energy and a reduced half-life, intradermally or subcutaneously. The substance has a very high biocompatibility, and is filtered and degraded at the hepatic level and removed by urinary course in the hours immediately following administration. Furthermore, the very low dose of radioactivity makes its use absolutely safe, even for the study of congenital pathologies in infants [5–7]. This test is repeatable, and can be prolonged for another 24 hours, allowing lymphovenous shunt evaluation.

From a methodological point of view, various approaches have been proposed: most of them aim to evaluate the capacity of the lymphatic circulation to transport the radiolabelled substance (and then, indirectly, the lymph) in a centripetal sense; to verify

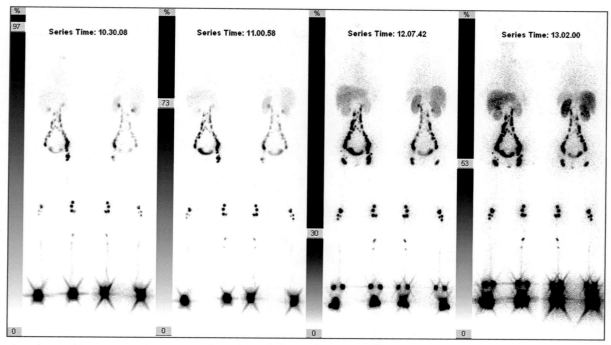

Fig. 17.7. Lymphangioscintigraphy with colloidal albumin: study of inferior limbs. Normal whole body scan

transit times and the percent of substance "purified" from the injection point (a rather liberally understood concept of clearance); the maintenance of a "throbbing" flow inside the manifolds; the display; the number and percent quantification of lymph node captation and the passage in the main blood stream.

There are several trends of thought about the "type" of circulation that can be analysed: deep or superficial.

The investigation represents the necessary complement of an evaluation of "lymphoedema without further exploration"; diagnosis is itself already within the reach of the clinical exam and of a careful anamnesis.

Independent of the type of evaluation, we have found that for the evaluation of malformative alterations it is preferable to distinguish between the deep and the superficial circulation, as frequently alterations in the deep circulation are totally offset by a superficial circulation that functionally corrects any insufficiencies, of primary or secondary nature.

In fact, only about 20% of the lymphatic circulation starts in the muscle-fasciae compartment, in continuity with the deep lymph nodes. This explains why it difficult to see a normal alteration of the deep manifold, as it is masked or hidden by a superficially normal or differently pathological lymphoscintigraphic pattern (Fig. 17.8) [8].

This is even more true in the study of the complex alterations where subversion of the normal vascular anatomy frequently results in somatic alterations, such as corporeal segment gigantism, alterations in the number and morphology of skeleton segments, secondary cardiac and circulation alterations, or, on the contrary, hypotrophy and hypoplasia as a consequence of a growth defect (Fig. 17.9) [9].

Such alterations often involve the formation of anomalous ectasias of the lymphatic trunks, of preferential escape courses, or the development of "lymphatic lakes" dependent on the presence of concomitant muscular alterations or on aberrant dysplastic venous masses and, finally, shunting in the venous circulation [10]. Therefore it is preferable to evaluate the draining capacity of deep manifolds using a single deep injection at the level of the plantar arc (or palmar, in the case of a superior limb study), followed by an early scintigraphic scanning (within 10 minutes) to highlight the main deep lymphatic trunk and the deep lymph nodal stations. In normal situations, after a few minutes, the high capacity of extraction of the radioactive tracer from the injection point allows a clear visualisation of the intermediate (popliteal, inguinal, iliac, para-aortical) lymph nodal stations.

In the case of a lack of conformity of the highlighted pattern with respect to the normal picture,

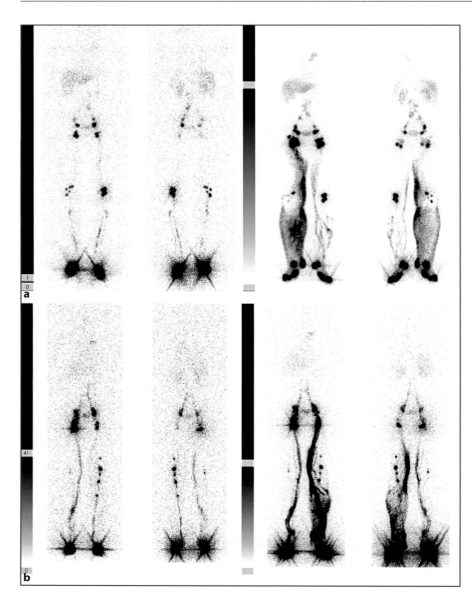

Fig. 17.8. Two cases of unexpected pathological lymphatics of the lower limbs. Both patients demonstrate dysplasia and hypertrophy of the superficial lymphatic system with noticeable dermal diffusion "backflow", and a normal appearance of the deep system. **a** The first patient shows also a star-shaped "lymphatic lake" on the anterior side of the right calf. **b** The second patient has a manifest failure of the deep circulation, compensated by the superficial one. A persistent faint drainage of the para-aortic lymphonodal chain coexists

multiple whole body scans are recommended after centripetal stimulation, obtained by prolonged walking or with an isometric exercise (hand grip), which acts by "squeezing" the deep tissues. It is also possible in some cases to perform a manual draining massage of the area of interest.

With this methodology it is possible to observe the behaviour of a lymphatic flow altered by obstructive phenomena, by the presence of ectasic trunks, by the development of anomalous escape courses, by the presence of dermal diffusion ("backflow"), cross-over with retrograde tracer backflow (reflux) or delayed tracer transport due to inversion of the flow direction. After this first phase of study a multiple subcutaneous injection between the fingers or toes is carried out, followed by an early scan followed by later ones, which are able to highlight with sufficient precision the superficial down flow course [11].

Also in this case it is the direct study of lymphoscintigraphic pattern that guides the clinician in deciding the timing of the subsequent observations. These can be prolonged until the following day if the presence of low speed spare alterations is suspected (Fig. 17.10).

The final diagnostic option is the injection of radiotracer near cystic lesions that have been demonstrated with other methods in order to identify the tributary territories of the lesions themselves or, al-

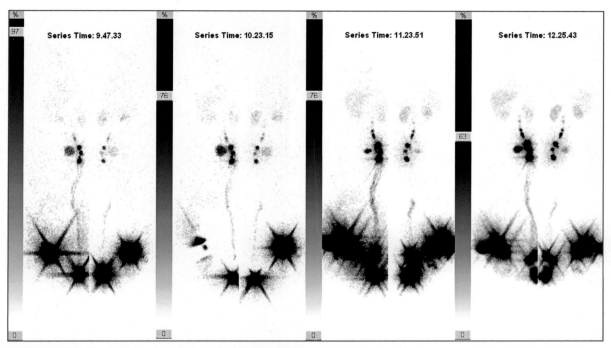

Fig. 17.9. In this patient, the same as in Figure 17.2, a clear deficit of the lymphatic system of the right leg, both deep and superficial, is observed. On the left side, progression of the tracer is prevalently superficial but with an optimal compensation. No oedema or swelling is visible. On the right side there is no evidence of dermal back-flow or venous commission: the examination excluded the presence of lympho-venous shunt and gave evidence of monolateral lymphatic agenesia

ternatively, the direct injection of radio colloid inside the lesion itself, to identify any escape course (Fig. 17.11).

Transarterial Lung Perfusion Scintigraphy (TLPS) (or "Microspheres" Study)

The study of AV shunts by nuclear medicine techniques has long been abandoned because other methods (duplex scan, angiography) are considered far more effective and precise [12–14]. However, in complex congenital vascular malformations (CVM), shunts may be multiple, differently located and of the microshunt variety, detectable with difficulty. To recognize those fistulas, a time consuming duplex scan examination or an invasive catheter angiography with multiple contrast injection is necessary. In this situation a simple and effective nuclear medicine technique is able to give a quick response about existence or not of a shunt, and, if the response is negative, avoid an unnecessary angiography. The method is also capable of evaluating in semi-quantitative terms both the functional impact of the fis-

tula in the malformation system and the arterial and capillary outflow.

The method is based on the same principle used in pulmonary perfusional scintigraphy and consists of intra-arterial injection of micro aggregations (more commonly called microspheres) of purified human albumin radio-labelled with 99m-tecnetium [13]. The examination is possible in the upper and lower limbs. The injection is made in the most easily accessible artery afferent to the malformative area to be examined (femoral artery for the lower limb, axillary, brachial or, in some cases, the ulnar artery if the superior limb is to be studied). The tracer, owing to the size of particles (<100 microns), is normally kept at the capillary circle of the limb (first filter); it is estimated that about one capillary in every 1000 temporarily becomes embolized, a sufficient quantity to recognize and evaluate the blood flow. If fistulas exist, microspheres bypass the capillary circle of the limb (first filter), enter the venous circulation and get trapped at pulmonary capillaries (second filter) (Fig. 17.12) [3, 15, 16].

To confirm or rule out the existence of a shunt, a comparative analysis of the perfusion curves is performed. It is also possible to quantify in percentage

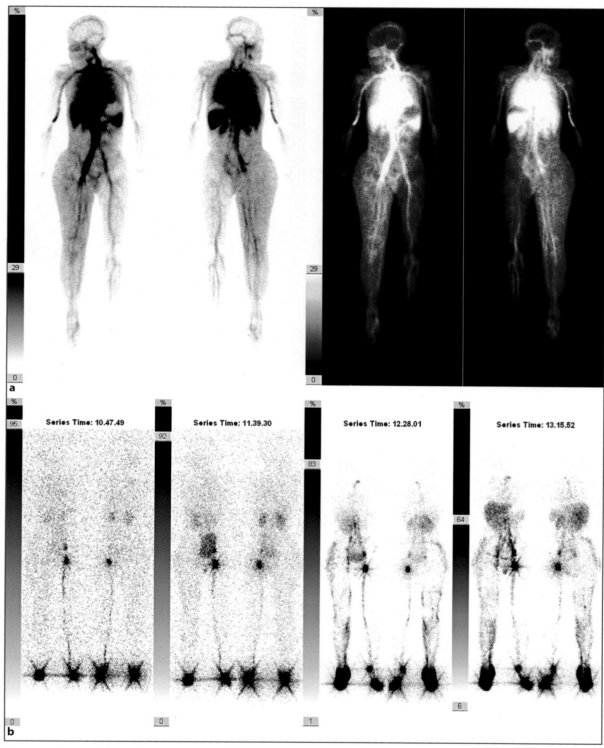

Series Time: 10.47.49   Series Time: 11.39.30   Series Time: 12.28.01   Series Time: 13.15.52

Fig. 17.10. A case of mixed lymphovenous malformation in a female patient. **a** The angioscintigraphy study demonstrates a volumetric asymmetry of the limbs, with an essentially preserved vascular tree and no evidence of AVM. Noticeable is the increased calibre of the iliac vessels. **b** In the lymphoscintigraphic study, lack of right main lymphatic manifolds, in particular the deep one, is observed. The centripetal progression of colloidal tracer is evident with slender superficial vessels, in part in marginal position. Notice the presence of dermal diffusion ("backflow") in the calf and gluteal region. On the left side too, the lymphatic flow is mainly superficial. This agrees with the RBC study

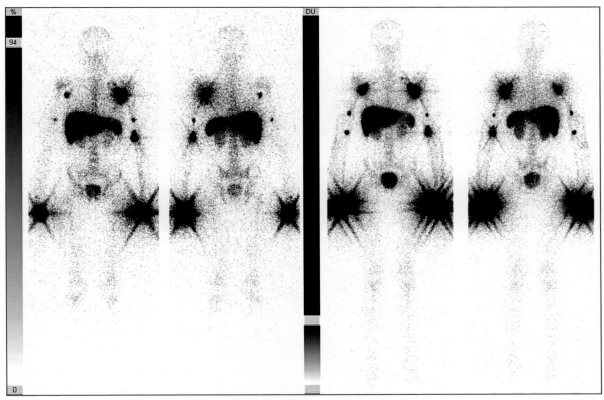

Fig. 17.11. Post-traumatic lymphovenous shunt of the right arm, persistent after repeated surgical treatments. Notice the quick, intense visualisation of liver and reticuloendothelium of the bone marrow (not due to erroneous intra-vein injection!), patent proof of mixing. Consequent lymphatic theft and faint drainage into axillary nodes. The whole lymphatic circulation of both arms is normal

terms the amount of blood diverted by the anomalous circuit: application of a simple mathematical formula indicates the shunted microspheres' quote at the pulmonary level. Moreover, a "morphologically" significant aspect also exists: with optimal arterial injection, whole body spot scans, and with high speed tomographic acquisition, it is possible to notice the capillary flow distribution "visually", demonstrating poor or preferential perfusion areas.

The quantification of the shunt can be estimated as more precise as more tracer is injected near the shunt site; the faster the injection, the greater the bolus dispersion in the capillary circle and therefore the shunted quote will be more of an underestimate. Theoretically, an injection through a catheter placed on the afferent artery would give the most precise data, but in this way the method becomes invasive, like angiography.

The three-dimensional rebuilding of the vascular district improves clinical and instrumental information about the physiopathological effect on the tissues by the "haemal theft" due to the shunt.

TLPS is effective also as a control of treatment in terms of shunting volume reduction, and also as a long term follow-up of the spontaneous evolution of an AV malformation.

It should be considered that arterial puncture is normally not included in the technical skills of the nuclear physician and this may explain the tendency to ignore this procedure. Training by an angiography specialist or by a vascular surgeon is recommended.

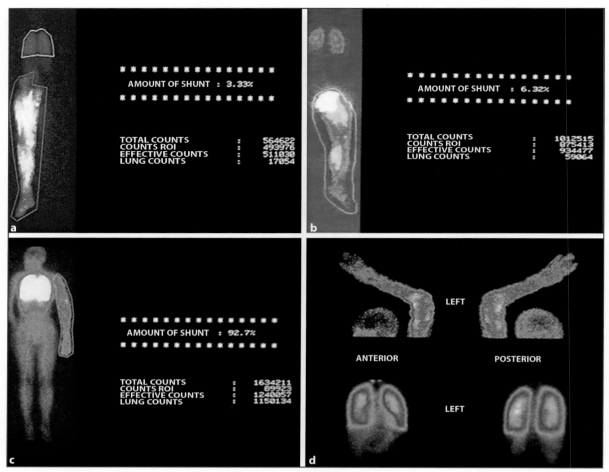

Fig. 17.12. Three cases of a transarterial lung perfusion scintigraphy (TLPS). **a** Normal picture with shunted quote < 4%. **b** A slight positive picture, with shunted quote ≅ 7%. **c** A frank positive picture with clear blood theft and shunted quote of 92%. **d** Spot images of the last case with evident ischemia of the forearm and hand. Fig. 17.12a is reproduced from [3]

References

1. Barton DJ, Miller JH, Allwright SJ, Sloan GM (1992) Distinguishing soft-tissue hemangiomas from vascular malformations using technetium-labeled red blood cell scintigraphy. Plast Reconstr Surg 89:46–52; discussion 53–55
2. Dubois J, Garel L, Grignon A et al (1998) Imaging of hemangiomas and vascular malformations in children. Acad Radiol 5:390–400
3. Dentici R, Mattassi R, Vaghi M (2002) La diagnostica per immagini in medicina nucleare. In: Mattassi R, Belov S, Loose DA, Vaghi M (eds) Malformazioni vascolari ed emangiomi. Testo-atlante di diagnostica e terapia. Springer-Verlag Milano, pp 32-39
4. Witte CL, Witte MH (2000) An imaging evaluation of angiodysplasia syndromes. Lymphology 33:158–166
5. Dubois J, Garel L (1999) Imaging and therapeutic approach of hemangiomas and vascular malforma-

tions in the pediatric age group. Pediatr Radiol 29:879–893
6. Williams WH, Witte CL, Witte MH, McNeill GC (2000) Radionuclide lymphangioscintigraphy in the evaluation of peripheral lymphedema. Clin Nucl Med 25:451–464
7. Sloan GM, Bolton LL, Miller JH et al (1988) Radionuclide-labeled red blood cell imaging of vascular malformations in children. Ann Plast Surg 21:236–241
8. Lee BB, Mattassi R, Kim BT et al (2004) Contemporary diagnosis and management of venous and arteriovenous shunting malformation by whole body blood pool scintigraphy. Int Angiol 23:355–367
9. Solti F, Iskum M, Banos C, Salamon F (1985) Arteriovenous shunts in peripheral lymphedema: hemodynamic features and isotopic visualization. Lymphology 18:187-191

10. Liu N, Wang C, Ding Y (1999) MRI features of lymphedema of the lower extremity: comparison with lymphangioscintigraphy. Zhonghua Zheng Xing Shao Shang Wai Ke Za Zhi 15:447–449

11. Inoue Y, Ohtake T, Wakita S et al (1997) Flow characteristics of soft-tissue vascular anomalies evaluated by direct puncture scintigraphy. Eur J Nucl Med 24:505–510

12. Inoue Y, Wakita S, Yoshikawa K et al (1999) Evaluation of flow characteristics of soft-tissue vascular malformations using technetium-99m labelled red blood cells. Eur J Nucl Med 26:367–372

13. Ennis JT, Dowsett DJ (1983) Radionuclide angiography: intraarterial studies. In: Vascular radionuclide imaging: a clinical atlas. John Wiley, London, pp 122–123

14. Solti F, Iskum M, Banos C, Salamon F (1986) Arteriovenous shunt-circulation in lymphoedematous limbs. Acta Chir Hung 27:223-231

15. Lee MJ, Dowsett DJ, Ennis JT (1990) Peripheral arteriovenous malformation: diagnosis and localization by intraarterial injection of technetium-99m-MAA. J Nucl Med 31:1557-1559

16. Lee BB, Mattassi R, Kim YW et al (2005) Advanced management of arteriovenous shunting malformation with transarterial lung perfusion scintigraphy for follow-up assessment. Int Angiol 24:173-184

Invasive Diagnostics of Congenital Vascular Malformations

18

Jürgen H. Weber

Abstract

Invasive angiographic diagnostics of veins and arteries in congenital vascular malformations (CVM), and especially in arterial congenital malformations (AVM), depend on the character of the lesion, the need for an exact classification and the therapeutic consequences that are indicated by imaging modalities. A "decision tree" quoting the quality of methods for each individual case is recommended. High quality angiography (arteriography and phlebography) should be carried out.

Introduction

It is a fact that clinical pictures of congenital vascular malformations (CVM) vary considerably, which has meant that until now, classification has been difficult [1–4]. The approach chosen to assess a CVM should give detailed data about the clinical appearance, the site and extension of the lesion and all its vascular components by showing all relevant details, including the involvement of adjacent tissues, using the "Hamburg Classification" of the malformation [5, 6].

Compared with new imaging modalities – such as duplex ultrasound, computed tomography (CT) and magnetic resonance imaging (MRI) – the most accurate diagnostic data that can be obtained to date is through angiography (phlebography and arteriography), which directly demonstrates the vessels involved [7–9].

Primary involvement of lymphatic vessels is rarely noticed in CVMs [11].

Clinical Signs

The clinical examination generally opens the "window" to diagnosis by showing remarkable changes compared to the norm; for example, port-wine stains and nevi (Fig. 18.1 a, b, e). The pattern of an abnormally situated subcutaneous truncular vein may directly lead to diagnosis of a persisting marginal vein (MV) (Fig. 18.2 a, b).

However, in other cases there may be only a slight difference in length and circumference to be seen at the site of one extremity (Fig. 18.3 a, b). Gigantism associated with atrophy of the skin and subcutaneous soft tissue gives information about ischemic consequences of an arteriovenous (AV) shunting lesion (Fig 18.4 a). However, many of the clinical signs are ambiguous, and they do not show the full extent of the malformative lesion.

Plain Film

A non-invasive plain film, documented separately or as part of angiographic imaging, enables the exact measurement of differences in length (Figs. 18.3 c, d, 18.4 c) and can demonstrate the extent of a soft tissue mass (Figs. 18.3 c, 18.5 b). The presence of phleboliths may be due to the recurrence of thrombophlebitis and sometimes to a low-flow AV shunting AVM (Fig. 18.5 b).

Morphologic and Functional Aspects

Clinical examination and non invasive functional tests generally help the physician to define the actual appearance of morphologic and hemodynamic

R. Mattassi, D.A. Loose, M. Vaghi (eds.), *Hemangiomas and Vascular Malformations.*
© Springer-Verlag Italia 2009

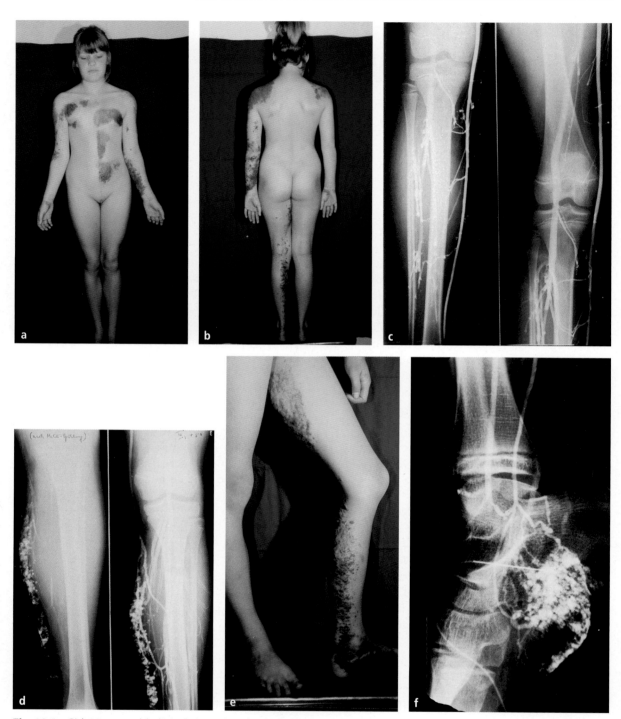

Fig. 18.1. Girl, 11 years old, clinical signs since birth. Strongly separated proliferative and disseminated nevus along the anterior trunk (**a**), on both arms and shoulders (**b**) and the inner side of left foot and leg (**e**). Ascending leg phlebography demonstrates a normal deep venous system of the limb (**c**). Varicography of the lower leg and foot shows phlebectasias connected with a slightly enlarged, valvulated anterior saphenous vein (**d**, **f**). Therapy: partial surgical resection and partial schlerotherapy protecting the intact anterior saphenous vein. No therapy on trunk and upper extremities. Reproduced from [10]

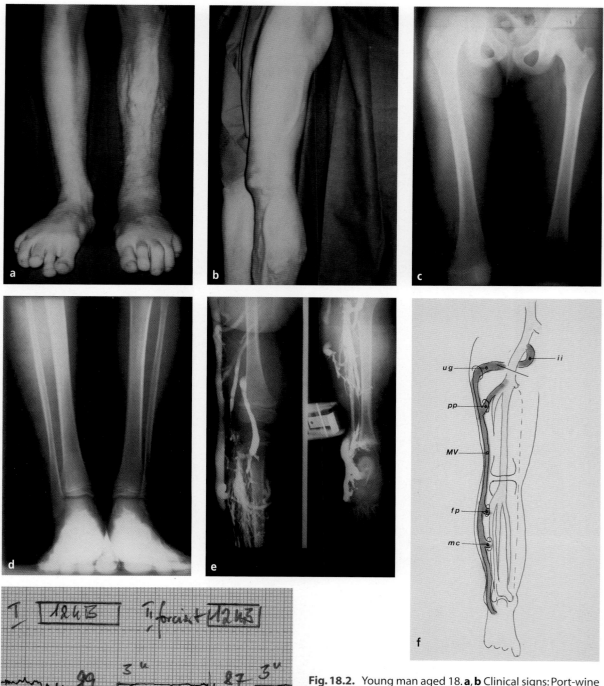

Fig. 18.2. Young man aged 18. **a, b** Clinical signs: Port-wine stain, enlarged lower limb and uncommon subcutaneous venous trunk along the anterolateral side of the limb, typically of a persistent marginal vein. **c, d** Plain film: under orthostatic conditions no difference in length along the lower leg whereas the right upper leg is extended over 3.5 cm with lop-sided hip. **e** Ascending phlebography: dysplastic and enlarged, valveless deep collecting veins. **e** Persistence of a marginal vein, type III (see also Figure 18.4). **f** Sketch of the venous situation, showing the in- and outflow of the persisting marginal vein. **g** Phlebodynamometry: combined with phlebography: reduced pump function under exercise at the right side, e.g. chronic venous insufficiency. Diagnosis: persisting marginal vein in presence of a countinous dysplastic deep venous system of the leg. Therapy: surgical resection of the marginal vein is recommended; partial functional recompensation can be expected. Elastic stockings are mandatory. Reproduced from [10]

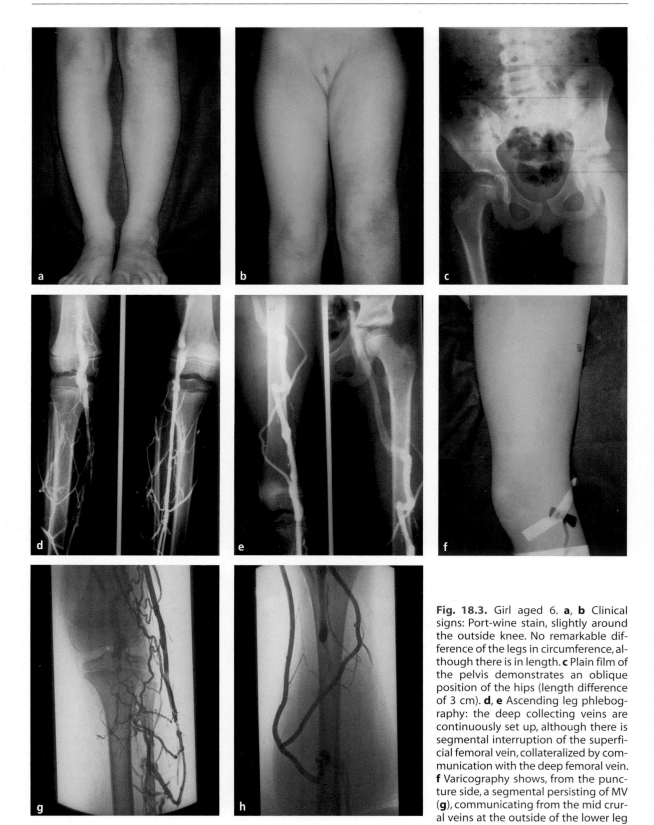

Fig. 18.3. Girl aged 6. **a**, **b** Clinical signs: Port-wine stain, slightly around the outside knee. No remarkable difference of the legs in circumference, although there is in length. **c** Plain film of the pelvis demonstrates an oblique position of the hips (length difference of 3 cm). **d**, **e** Ascending leg phlebography: the deep collecting veins are continuously set up, although there is segmental interruption of the superficial femoral vein, collateralized by communication with the deep femoral vein. **f** Varicography shows, from the puncture side, a segmental persisting of MV (**g**), communicating from the mid crural veins at the outside of the lower leg to (**h**) the upper part of the anterior saphenous vein. Therapeutic consequences: the persisting MV is considered to be the cause of the overgrowth of the leg on this side. Its surgical resection was indicated and performed 1 year later. Follow-up studies showed a complete re-balance in length at puberty, 7 years later. Reproduced from [10]

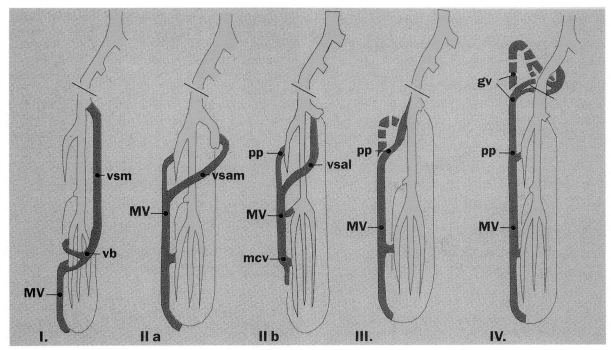

Fig. 18.4. Classification of MV according to Weber. *gv*, gluteal vein; *mcv*, medial crural veins; *mV*, marginal vein; *pp*, deep perforants; *vb*, anterior arched vein; *vsam*, medial accessory saphenous vein; *vsal*, lateral accessory saphenous vein; *vsm*, main saphenous vein. Reproduced from [10]

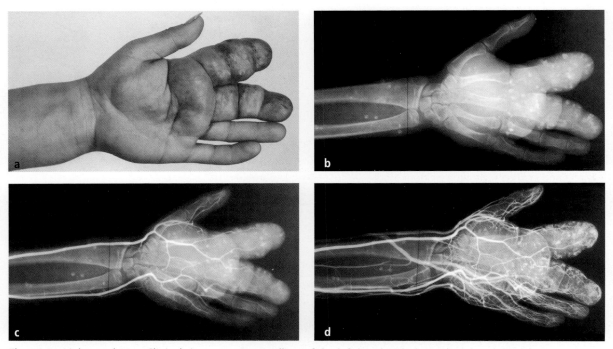

Fig. 18.5. Male aged 30. **a** Clinical signs: massive swelling of the left hand including second and third finger. Ischemic changes along the involved fingers and forehand. Recurrent pain and bleeding starting at 15 years of age. **b** Plain film of the hand: gigantism of second and third finger; multiple phleboliths along hand and forearm. **c** Arteriography: normal anatomy of the vessels, however slight tortuosity is seen in the early arterial phase. At the late arterial phase AV shunting and "pooling" of contrast medium on the venous side (**d**). No signs of increased speed of AV circulation. Diagnosis: low-flow AVM, showing signs of vascular and soft tissue degeneration. No indication for embolotherapy. Conservative treatment using elastic stockings. Reproduced from [10]

characteristics of the malformative lesion. Progressive venous and AV CVM cause – more or less – relevant functional disorders (Fig. 18.3 g), which demand adequate and rapid access to therapy.

A "decision tree" for non-invasive and invasive, morphologically orientated and functional diagnostic procedures is a necessity in our eyes in order to find the earliest and best approach to the diagnosis and classification of the individual lesion (Table 18.1).

The specific value of the main diagnostic procedures dealing with CVM may be worked out by combining different methods (Table 18.2). In any case, functional tests and angiographic methods will be able to calculate the advantages and disadvantages of therapy [8, 12].

The most common CVMs are seen on the venous side, involving venous decompensation in primarily AV lesions [4, 9, 13]. Because of this, phlebography plays a dominant role by showing as well morphologic and functional disorders with excellent overview.

Arteriography should be limited to the patients showing clearly hemodynamic signs of active AV shunting in hyperdynamic AVM [2, 12, 14–16].

Table 18.1. Imaging modalities and functional tests for diagnosis and classification of CVM

I. Functional tests	*II. Non-invasive imaging*
– Doppler/duplex ultrasound	– Duplex scan
– Pressure measurements	– Ultrasound (B-mode)
– Plethysmography	– Computed tomography (CT)
	– Magnetic resonance imaging (MRI)
Localisation of arteriovenous fistulas, definition of low-flow and high-flow arteriovenous malformations, venous reflux, chronic venous insufficiency	Flow direction of arteries and veins, infiltrative forms, subfascial and epifascial manifestations, muscular involvement, cystic degeneration, calcification
III. Phlebography	*IV. Arteriography*
– Ascending leg phlebography	– Arterial overview
– Varicography	– Selective arteriography
– Serial venography	– Subselective arteriography
	– Balloon occlusion arteriography
Pathoanathomy of deep and subfascial veins, venous valves, reflux, phlebectasias, persistent embryonal or marginal veins	Axial arterial anatomy, identification and localization of arteriovenous fistulas, exact definition of low-flow and high-flow lesions, collaterals, cartography of feeding vessels for vaso-occlusive therapy (transcatheter embolization) ↓
V. Lymphography	*Invasive therapy*
– Direct and indirect technique (seldom used)	– Surgery
	– Interventional vasoocclusion

Table 18.2. Imaging modalities and functional tests for diagnosis and classification of CVM

Clinical symptoms	Plain film	Functional tests	Phlebography	Arteriography	MRI
Extremity differences in length	+++				
Predominantly venous defect	(+)	Doppler, duplex, pressure, measurements, plethysmography	+++	(+)	(+)
Low-flow arteriovenous malformations	++	Doppler, duplex	(+)	+++	(+)
High-flow arteriovenous malformations	++	Doppler, duplex	(+)	+++	(+)
Infiltrative forms (arterial and venous)					+++

(+): indicated in special cases; +: indicated; ++: highly indicated; +++: mandatory

Phlebography

Mainly on the level of the lower extremities, ascending leg phlebography using Valsalva's manoeuvre is considered the method of choice. In a good overview it is able to demonstrate the deep (subfascial) veins, muscular and collecting veins and, by reflux, the epifascial veins which are primarily or secondarily involved with the congenital lesion by its progressive functional disorders (Figs. 18.1 c, 18.2 e, 18.3 d, e).

Varicography is an additional very helpful method to complete the sketch of veins, including those not demonstrated with other methods and those not demonstrated clearly enough (Figs. 18.1 d, f, 18.3 f–h). For instance, the persisting embryonal vein – its inflow and outflow as well as its collaterals – can be completely demonstrated (Fig. 18.2 f) [15, 17, 18].

By combining ascending leg phlebography with direct venous pressure measurements (phlebodynamometry in the periphery and central transfemoral measurements), optimal morphologic and functional information can be gained (Fig. 18.2 g).

Our classification of the persisting marginal and embryonal vein depends on their phlebographic overall picture, reducing a wide variety of additional venous components to some characteristic types (Fig. 18.4):

Type I:　The marginal vein (MV) runs from the lateral border of the foot to the anterior arcuate vein, using the anterior saphenous vein as a main drainage.

Type IIa:　The MV drains to the anterior saphenous vein through the medial saphenous accessory vein.

Type IIb:　The MV drains mainly to the lateral saphenous accessory vein.

Type III:　The drainage of the MV is obtained through deep femoral perforator veins and to the lateral circumflex vein.

Type IV:　Drainage of the MV is obtained by the inferior and superior gluteal veins to the internal iliac vein (Figs. 18.2, 18.3).

Supplementary associated truncular dysplasias of the posterior saphenous vein can be identified in some of the cases (Fig. 18.3 d). In those individuals showing a persistent embryonal vein (e.g., persisting MV associated with local or extended segmental aplasia of the deep venous system), phlebography combined with varicography and phlebodynamometry again enables classification and calculation of the degree of hemodynamic disorders. Avalvulia and the secondary loss of venous valves is very common in predominantly venous CVM; however, this is also the case in progressive AVM

due to extended shunting blood volume draining to the venous side (Figs. 18.5, 20.3, 20.4 g) [5–8, 18].

Arteriography

The demonstration of arteries involved in an AVM (and very seldom in huge hemangiomas, see Figure 20.3) should be planned soon after the decision to start therapy [16, 20]. The advantage of arteriography over other non invasive methods is the direct and clear opacification of all afferent ("feeding") vessels (Fig. 18.5 c), demonstrating the "nidus" of the AV shunting malformation and its venous outflow (Figs. 18.5 d, 18.6 f, 20.4 g).

Digital arteriography (DSA) has improved the quality of opacification, including the application of hypo-osmolalic contrast media. However, in AVM a high quality arteriogram depends on some additional factors.

An overview-arteriography may helpful for local orientation and for rating by evaluation of the speed of the run-off of contrast medium, for instance from the abdominal aorta, comparing both extremities being opacified (Fig. 20.2 c-f):

Stationary sequences of films and sub-selected series, realized by sub-selected catheterization, will be needed for demonstrating all relevant details (Fig. 18.6 d-f), at least when planning vaso-occlusion by means of embolization (Fig. 20.4 g) [12, 14, 20].

Reviewing the arteriograms for hemodynamic reasons, normal AV circulation can be differentiated from a low-flow AV shunting malformations by means of the venous backflow (Fig. 18.5 c, d). In so-called high-flow lesions a rapid sequence of pictures (2–4/sec) documents the early venous recirculation of the contrast medium and approximates the "nidus" of the hyperdynamic AV shunting AVM, its extension and – above all – the number of afferent "feeding" arteries (Fig. 18.6 d–f).

The diagnostic arteriography ought to be separated from therapeutic catheterization and opacification in order to permit an interdisciplinary decision: the type of therapy which should be used with the best outcome for the individual patient; embolization versus a surgical approach, or choice of a "combined therapy" (Fig. 18.6) [16, 20].

Lymphography

The application of oily contrast media has been given up completely because of inflammatory lymph node reactions and subsequent worsening of the

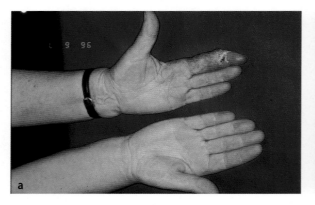
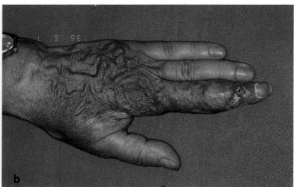
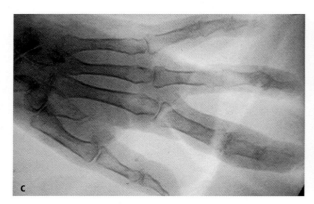
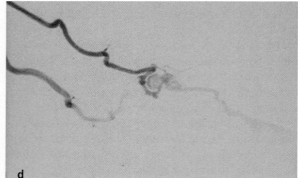
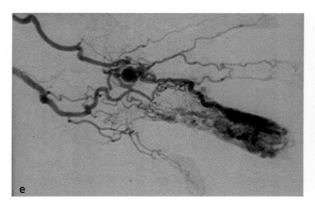
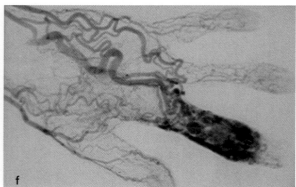

Fig. 18.6. Female, aged 35. **a** Clinical signs: disproportional minus-variant of the left hand showing atrophia of the skin and ischemic ulcerations along the third finger. **b** Condition 18 years after resection of the forefinger because of ulceration and severe recurrent bleeding. **c** Plain film of the forehand: slight decalcification, no destruction of bone. **d** Arteriography, early arterial phase: tortuous main vessels (radial and ulnarian arteries) and beginning of the filling of an arterial aneurysm of the digital artery III. **e** Arteriography, one second later: massive early AV shunting along finger III at the acral space and **f** the aneurysm surrounded by efferent veins. Diagnosis: high-flow AVM showing progressive functional decompensation and steal-phenomenon along the surroundings (including the primarily non-involved finger IV). Therapeutic consequences: subselective transcatheter embolization may be suitable to occlude parts of the shunting lesion. However, at the level of the acral space of the third finger, there is a high risk of over-embolization causing ischemic necrosis (respectively increased steal-effect in case of under-embolization). Surgery will be not effective except in case of the amputation of the finger. Because of recurrent pain and bleeding, embolization should be carried out only by a skilled interventionalist (and in agreement with patient and surgeon) before amputation will be indicated. Reproduced from [10]

lymphatic drainage. Water-soluble contrast medium however, may be used in special cases, getting a rather good orientation at the level of the extremities. On the other hand, most of questions can be analyzed nowadays by means of ultrasound, CT and MRI. Sometimes a direct puncture of lymphocystic malformations may be worthwhile for diagnostic purposes and for sclerotherapy.

All considerations dealing with indication and performance of angiographic techniques that are mentioned above are valid elsewhere also; e.g., at the level of the upper extremities, along the trunk, neck and shoulder space (see Chapter 20).

In conclusion, invasive angiographic diagnostics are imperative when planning interventional therapeutic procedures. They are also needed if non-invasive diagnostic tests are considered to be insufficient for a successful surgical approach. The quality of phlebography and arteriography ought to be superior to other imaging modalities, mainly to MRI and angio-MRI. The indication should follow a "decision tree" from non-invasive to invasive modalities. However, many of the patients nowadays are indicated and treated too late, undergoing multiple sequences of non-invasive studies with unbalanced diagnostic value and cost-efficiency.

References

1. Klippel M, Trenaunay P (1900) Du naevus variqueux osterhypertrophique. Arch Gén Méd 3:641
2. Weber FP (1907) Angioma formation in connection with hypertrophy of limbs and hemihypertrophy. Br J Dermatol 19:231
3. Weber FP (1907) Der umschriebene Riesenwuchs, Typ Parkes Weber. Fortschr Röntgenstr 113:734
4. Belov St, Loose DA, Weber J (1989) Vascular malformations. Einhorn Presse-Verlag, Reinbek
5. Lea Thomas M, Macfie GB (1974) Phlebography in the Klippel-Trenaunay syndrome. Acta Radiol 15:43
6. May R, Nissl R (1970) Beitrag zur Klassifizierung der "Gemischten congenitalen Angiodysplasien". Fonschr Röntgenstr 113:170–189
7. Rau G (1980) Missbildungen des Venensystems. In: Hach W (ed) Die Röntgenuntersuchung des Venensystems (Ergebnisse der Angiologie, Bd 22). Schattauer, Stuttgart
8. Weber J, Ritter H (1989) Diagnostic management of the venous and lymphatic components of av-malformations. In: Belov St, Loose DA, Weber J (eds) Vascular malformations. Einhorn Presse-Verlag, Reinbek, pp 77–84
9. Belov S, Loose DA, Muller E (1985) Angeborene Gefäßfehler. Einhorn Presse-Verlag, Reinbek
10. Weber J (2003) La diagnostica invasiva. In: Mattassi R, Belov S, Loose DA, Vaghi M (eds) Malformazioni vascolari ed emangiomi. Testo-atlante di diagnostica e terapia, pp 40–49
11. Weber J, May R (1990) Funktionelle Phlebologie. Thieme, Stuttgart
12. Weber J, Ritter H (1989) Strategy for the radiological angiotherapy of hyperdynamic av-malformations. In: Belov S, Loose DA, Weber J (eds) Vascular malformations. Einhorn Presse-Verlag, Reinbek, pp 270–274
13. Malan E (1974) Vascular malformations (angiodysplasias). Carlo Erba Foundation, Milano
14. Van Dongen RJ, Barwegen MG, Kormhout JG et al (1985) Congenital arteriovenous dysplasia: Treatment, indications, angiographic documentation, combined percutaneous and operative treatment. Chirurg 56:65–72
15. Weber J (1990) Invasive radiological diagnostic of congenital vascular malformations. Int Angiol 9:175–182
16. Weber J (1998) Invasive Diagnostic angeborener Gefäßfehler. In: Loose DA, Weber J (eds) Angeborene Gefäßfehler. Nordlanddruck, Lüneburg, pp 127–163
17. Weber J (1999) Achnenanomalien im Bereich des Bein-Beckenvenensystems und der unteren Hohlvene. In: Marshall M, Breu FX (eds) Handbuch der Angiologie. Ecomed, Landsberg
18. Weber J, Daffinger N (2008) Congenital vascular malformations: the persistence of marginal and embryonal veins. VASA 35:67–77
19. Vollmar JF, Nobbe FP (1976) Arteriovenöse Fisteln. Dilatierende Arteriopathien (Aneurysmen). Thieme, Stuttgart, p 176
20. Weber J (1987) Embolisationstherapie arteriovenöser Missbildungen. Radiol Diagn 28:513–516

Principles of Treatment of Vascular Malformations

19

Raul Mattassi, Dirk A. Loose, Massimo Vaghi

Abstract

Precise knowledge of the haemodynamic and pathological characteristics of vascular malformations allows individualised treatments to be planned. The therapeutic approach should be flexible and should be addressed to maximise the benefits and to reduce the risks of the treatment. Haemodynamic treatments are beneficial in cases of truncular malformations and AV shunts. Devascularization procedures are useful in cases of infiltrating extratruncular malformations. Each congenital vascular malformation (CVM) should be investigated according to its type, localization and symptoms in order to find the best treatment option [1].

Pediatric patients affected by CVM and vascular bone syndromes should be treated by vascular intervention in order to achieve a normalization of limb length. Orthopedic interventions should be undertaken only in older patients and in children who present a huge limb length discrepancy [2].

Sometimes it may be difficult for a single specialist to successfully treat a complex CVM. This is due to the difficulty in managing a multi-vessel disease which can infiltrate any kind of tissue. The advice of different specialists, according to the location of the malformation, may offer the best option for safely and successfully treating some types of extended and infiltrating CVM.

For each patient, the following issues should be addressed:
1. Therapy should be chosen in order to remove the vascular malformation or the hemodynamic disturbances caused by the vascular malformation.

2. The removal of the vascular malformation may or may not be radical; a strategy based on multiple interventions may often be indicated.
3. Multiple interventions strategy needs a treatment plan and a goal for each single step of treatment.
4. As different strategies may be available, the least invasive and simplest should be selected.

Truncular CVM

For truncular CVM, there are a number of treatment options (Table 19.1).

Revascularization procedures are surgical interventions which are useful in cases of aplasia or hypoplasia of the arteries. Graft interposition is indicated in cases of congenital aneurysm. In venous aneurysm the technique of tangential resection is often the best option. Graft interposition in venous vessels is indicated only if there is the possibility of implanting venous grafts. In cases of segmental vessel stenosis, a patch suture is often possible [3, 4].

Devascularization procedures (Figs. 19.1, 19.2) are based on surgery, radiological and technology-related techniques (laser, radiofreque C). The classical surgical interventions for cases of truncular defects are removal of dilated superficial vessels (almost veins) by normal or hypoplastic deep venous systems. In the latter, step-by-step management should be advised in order to reroute the venous flow from the superficial enlarged vessels to the deep veins.

Surgical resection of dilated vessels is possible also in arteriovenous (AV) shunts. Outflow veins together with the AV shunts can be removed in case of superficial AV shunt [5] (Fig. 19.3).

R. Mattassi, D.A. Loose, M. Vaghi (eds.), *Hemangiomas and Vascular Malformations*.
© Springer-Verlag Italia 2009

Table 19.1. Treatment guidelines in truncular vascular malformations

Aim of the therapy	Operational technique	Indications
Vascular reconstruction	1. Vascular malformation resection and direct reconstruction of vessel patency 2. Vascular malformation resection and graft interposition 3. Endograft placement 4. By-pass graft 5. Patch plasty 6. Membranotomy 7. Percutaneous dilatation of venous webs	Central and peripheral malformations consisting of aneurysmatic dilatation or hypoplasia or congenital stenosis of veins and arteries
	8. Implantation of Denver shunt	Chylous reflux in lower limbs
Devascularization	1. Resection of pathologic veins 2. Resection of deeply located AV shunts	Superficial vein incompetence
	3. Resection of superficially located AV malformations together with efferent veins 4. Trans catheter embolization	AV shunts
	5. Ligation of leaking lymphatic vessels	Lymphatic reflux
Non conventional interventions	1. Resection of all collaterals of the embryonal vein (Belov I) 2. Rerouting of the blood flow from the superficial to the deeply veins (Belov II) 3. Resection of the marginal vein with the aim of Fogarty catheter placement (Loose I)	Marginal vein associated with aplasia of the deep venous system Superficial venous ectasias associate with hypoplasia of the deep venous system Marginal associated with a normal deep venous system
Multidisciplinary treatment	1. Vascular, orthopedic, plastic interventions	Interventions according to the localization and complications of the pathology
Combined approach	1. Embolotherapy + vascular interventions + conservative treatment	AV shunts which can cause difficulties in the surgical approach because of size or anatomical localization

Hemodynamic procedures are typical in AV shunting CVMs (Figs. 19.4–19.6). This group includes some obsolete surgical interventions, such as ligatures of the collaterals of the efferent vein, and of the afferent artery.

Modern interventions for AV CVM are catheter or direct puncture-guided embolization or occlusion by mechanical devices or fluid of the AV communication; this may be followed by surgical resection [6, 7].

A marginal vein (Figs. 19.7, 19.8) with concomitant absence of the deep venous system (rare) and micro AV shunts are treatable by ligation of collateral vessels and skeletonization of the vein in order to ameliorate the venous hemodynamic and the related bone overgrowth [1].

In case of lymphatic disease, characterized by a severe dermal back flow and lymphatic cysts, an in-

ternal shunt from the cysts or cavities to the great deep veins can be implanted.

Enlarged leaking lymphathics with chylous reflux in cavities can be ligated.

Extratrucular CVM

There are a number of treatments for extratrucular CVM (Table 19.2).

Revascularization procedures are indicated to restore arterial patency after a previous surgical ligation or a coil embolization in order to allow an endovascular approach to the nidus of an AV malformation [5].

Devascularization procedures involve removal of the vascular malformation surgically or by percuta-

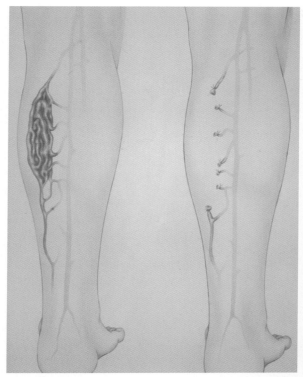

Fig. 19.1. Resection of truncular vein ectasias. Reproduced with permission from [3]

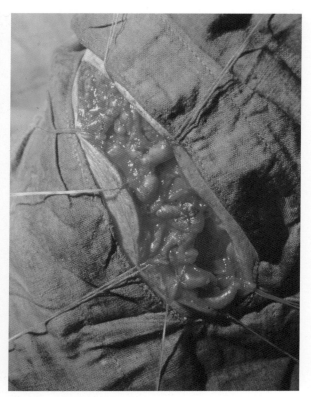

Fig. 19.2. Atypical incision for vein surgery [4]

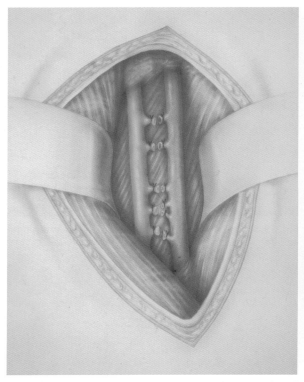

Fig. 19.3. Resection of deep located AV shunts. Reproduced with permission from [3]

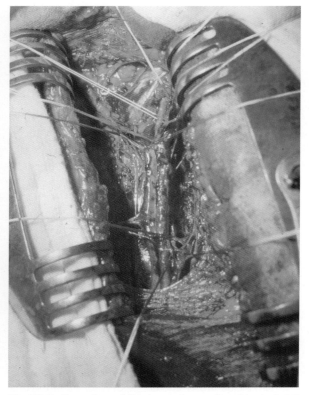

Fig. 19.4. Resection of AV shunts in canalis adductoris [4]

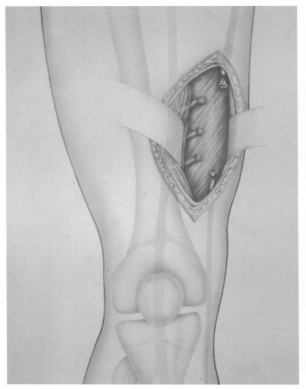

Fig. 19.5. Resection of superficially located AV shunts. Reproduced with permission from [3]

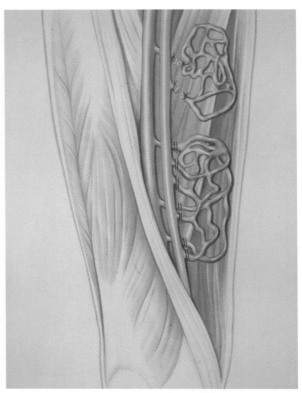

Fig. 19.6. Resection of collateral vessels of principal artery and vein [1]

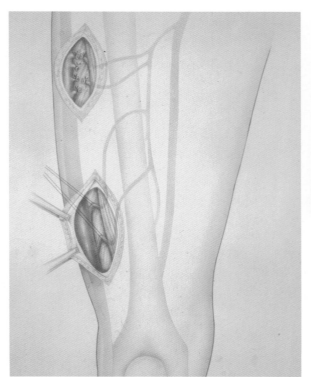

Fig. 19.7. Ligature of afferent vessels to the embryonal vein. Reproduced with permission from [3]

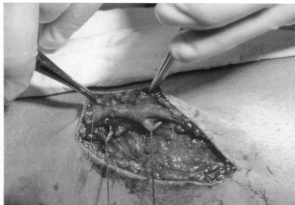

Fig. 19.8. Resection of afferent vessels to the embryonal vein [4]

Table 19.2. Treatment guidelines in extratruncular vascular malformations

Aim of the therapy	Operational technique	Indications
Resection of the malformation	1. Radical resection of the malformation 2. Radical resection of the malformation together with the surrounding tissues	Limited malformations with no infiltration of the surrounding tissues Small size malformations infiltrating surrounding tissues
Reduction of shunt flow	1. Transcatheter embolization 2. Percutaneous embolotherapy 3. Ligation of the afferent artery 4. Ligation of all collaterals of principal artery and vein 5. Ligation in two steps of two vessels in the leg or forearm followed by distal embolization	Extratruncular AV malformations which are not resectable because of dimension or localization Surgical treatment in these cases is replaced by endovascular treatment
Non conventional interventions	1. Tangential resection of involved tissues after positioning of a running suture over clamps	Partial resection of soft tissue infiltrating vascular malformations Indicated according to the size and localization of the malformation
Multidisciplinary treatment	1. Vascular, orthopedic, plastic interventions	Interventions according to the localization and complications of the pathology
Combined approach	1. Embolotherapy + vascular interventions + conservative treatment	AV shunts which can cause difficulties in the surgical approach because of size or anatomical localization

neous injections of sclerosing agents: this is indicated in limited diseases. A radical extirpation of the pathology is then possible.

In cases of infiltrating diseases, radical removal of the defect is only possible by ablating the malformation together along with the surrounding tissues (Figs. 19.9, 19.10). This is seldom possible and other strategies are available. These include surgery: where infiltrated tissues are clamped, a running suture is performed and a partial resection of the underlying tissues may significantly reduce the defect [5] (Figs. 19.11–19.13).

This technique is useful also in case of infiltrating AV shunts detected in the operating room by a hand-held Doppler velocimeter. Endovascular techniques may also be used to remove the defect: percutaneous injection of sclerosing agents causes thrombosis and major damage to the involved vessels. Vessels can also be damaged by thermic injury caused by the use of interstitial or endovascular laser devices.

Hemodynamic procedures are useful in case of AV CVMs and are based on catheter embolization of the nidus of a malformation (Fig. 19.14). If catheter techniques are not feasible, percutaneous direct puncture of the CVM may be the best alternative [8].

Catheter embolization may also be the first step of a so-called combined treatment. This consists of embolization of the afferent arteries, followed by the surgical extirpation of the malformation some days later.

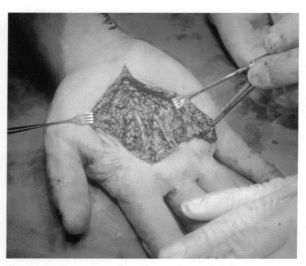

Fig. 19.9. Resection of malformed vessels [4]

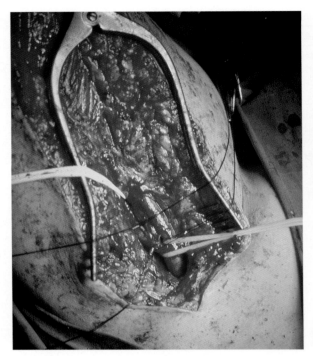

Fig. 19.10. Surgical resection of collaterals in extratruncular AV shunts [4]

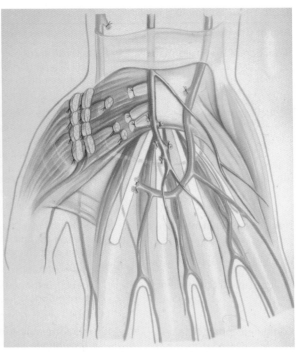

Fig. 19.11. Resection of AV shunts in the hand. Reproduced with permission from [3]

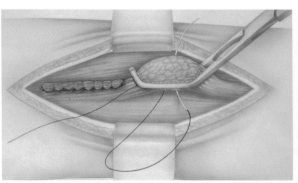

Fig. 19.12. Suture of infiltrating malformed vessels with the aid of Satinsky clamp [4]

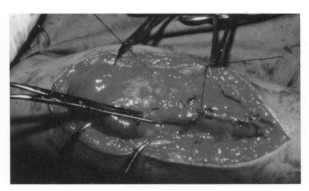

Fig. 19.13. Blalock suture [4]

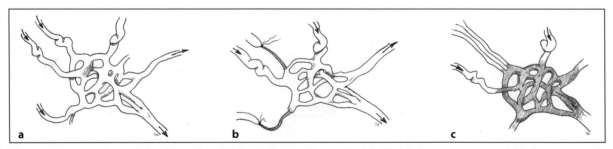

Fig. 19.14. a Drawings of the nidus of an AV shunt. Arrows directed inside (/left/) demonstrate arterial inflow; arrows directed outside show outflow. **b** Effect of ligature of two arterial inflow vessels: collaterals increase in size and maintain inflow to the "nidus" of the fistula. **c** Effect of injection of fluid substances into the "nidus" through a catheter: occlusion of the fistula has been achieved

The aim of the combined treatment is to prevent excessive blood losses and to allow a more radical surgical treatment [5].

Support Therapy

Pain Therapy

Analgesics are important after catheter embolization. The worst problem in these patients is represented by chronic neuritic pain, which responds to antiepileptic drugs. In some cases, when nerves have infiltrated the VM, pain can be controlled only through implantation of a spinal cord stimulator.

Edema Therapy

Elastic stockings are useful in the treatment of venous and lymphatic CVMs. In case of lymphatic defects, manual drainage combined with bandages is the key therapy of lymphedema secondary to lymphatic hypoplasia and dilatation.

Deep Venous Thrombosis Prevention

The use of low weight heparin in prophylactic dosages is indicated in cases of superficial vein ablation. Anticoagulation should be reserved for the patients who undergo vein valve surgery and or the presence of thrombophilia.

References

1. Belov S (1994) Surgical treatment of congenital vascular defects. In: Chang (ed) Modern vascular surgery. Springer-Verlag New York Berlin Heidelberg, pp 383–397
2. Belov S (1993) Correction of lower limb length discrepancy in congenital vascular bone diseases by vascular surgery performed during childhood. Sem Vasc Surg 6:245-251
3. Belov S, Loose DA, Weber J (eds) (1989) Vascular malformations. Einhorn-Presse Verlag, Reinbek
4. Mattassi R, Belov S, Loose DA, Vaghi M (eds) (2002) Malformazioni vascolari ed emangiomi: testo atlante di diagnostica e terapia. Springer-Verlag New York Berlin Heidelberg, pp 83–89
5. Loose DA (1997) Systematik, radiologische Diagnostik, und Therapie vaskulärer Fehlbildungen. In: Hohenleutner U, Landthaler M (eds) Fortschritte der operativen und onkologischen Dermatologie. Blackwell Wissenschafts-Verlag, Berlin Wien, pp 79–94
6. Do YS, Jakes WF, Shin SW et al (2005) Ethanol embolization of arteriovenous malformations: interim results. Radiology 235:674–682
7. Lee BB, Do YS, Yakes WF et al (2004) Management of arteriovenous malformations: a multidisciplinary approach. J Vasc Surg 39:590–600
8. Marshalleck F, Johnson MS (2006) Percutaneous management of haemangiomas and vascular malformations. In Golzarian J, Sun S, Sharafuddin MJ (eds) Vascular embolotherapy. Springer-Verlag Berlin Heidelberg Vol 2, pp 3–30

Interventional Therapy in Arteriovenous Congenital Malformations

20

Jürgen H. Weber

Abstract

Before beginning a session of embolotherapy, all afferent arteries *feeding* the shunt should be clearly demonstrated. To get optimal documentation, large quantities of contrast media injection may be necessary, as selective and superselective angiographies are required. For this reason, and also because of a multidisciplinary discussion necessary to plan the treatment, embolization is best performed in a second session. Materials available for embolization can be divided into fluid, semi-fluid, particulate substances and mechanical devices. Different types of catheter devices are available, including flow-directed Swan-Ganz and Tracker catheters with coaxial combinations, useful for special situations. The strategy and tactic of the treatment should be adapted to the individual case. A step-by-step approach, combination with surgery and other treatments may reduce the risks of complications.

Introduction

For many years surgical therapy was the only generally accepted approach for the treatment of congenital vascular malformations (CVMs), and it still remains very important in predominantly venous CVMs [1]. However, in recent years it has been combined more and more with alternative or additional therapeutic techniques such as percutaneous interstitial laser therapy and sclerotherapy [2, 3].

Percutaneous transcatheter embolization was already in use 1930, when Brooks embolized an arteriovenous fistula in the neuro-cranial space [4]. However, the first sequence of publications (case reports and preliminary communications) did not start before 1975 [5–12].

In order to plan a session of embolotherapy, the arterial and venous structures must be clearly localized and identified, demonstrating the regional morphology [13–17]. Even so, the functional relevance of arteriovenous shunting lesions (*low-flow*, *high-flow*) should be checked by local sequential arteriography and in addition by non-invasive functional tests [18]. All afferent arteries *feeding* the arteriovenous shunting lesion should be demonstrated angiographically, using selective and subselective catheter techniques [6, 19, 20]. Hyperdynamic *high-flow lesions* represent the best indication for transcatheter embolization [21]. In the acral space (e.g., hand, foot) a detailed angiographic diagnostic must also work out the indication for interventional vaso-occlusion versus other therapeutic tactics (surgery, laser therapy), balancing the therapeutic effect against side effects and serious complications (Table 20.1).

Even so, parts of the lesion approached in a selected and safe position may be embolized, whereas smaller vessels and parts of local dysplastic infiltrations may be treated surgically later on. Using combined therapy it will be possible to minimize the disadvantages of both methods and to improve the palliative results [22, 23].

Embolizing Materials

Various materials are available to embolize tissues. A classification of these materials is possible according to their state: we recognize fluid (ethanol and acrylates), semi-fluid substances (Ethibloc®, an alcoholic solution of amino-acids by Ethicon GmbH, Norderstedt, Germany), particulate substances and mechanical devices (such as Gianturco coils and detachable balloons), all of which have been recommended in the current literature (Table 20.2) [5, 9–11, 13, 19, 24–27].

R. Mattassi, D.A. Loose, M. Vaghi (eds.), *Hemangiomas and Vascular Malformations*.
© Springer-Verlag Italia 2009

Table 20.1. Transcatheter embolization of AVMs: indications and contraindications

Localization	Indications	Contraindications
Head and neck	Extracranial space	Intracranial and spinal > neuroradiology
Trunk	All areas, including the parenchymal organs (liver, Spleen, kidney)	Gastrointestinal tract – danger of infarction of terminal arteries without collaterals
Pelvis	All retroperitoneal areas, including the parietal space, gluteal, deep femoral and inguinal collaterals	Step-by-step vaso-occlusion recommended – check collateralization from right and left!
Extremities	All areas, including thoracic and pelvic outflow	Over-embolization must be avoided – above all acral space (hand, foot) terminal vascular structures without collaterals must be respected!

The main indications are for *high flow* AVMs. Combined interventional and surgical therapy must be discussed prior to embolization

Table 20.2. Vaso-occlusive materials, suitable for AVM embolization. Key: 0 - cannot be recommended; (+), (++) - suitable for special cases; +, ++, +++ - suitable for AVMs. * in combination with Ethibloc® only

Materials	Suitability
Particulate materials	
Silicone spheres	(+)
Polivinyl alcohol (Ivalon)	(+)
Dura and fascia lata	0
Mechanical devices	
Steel coils (Gianturco type)	(++ *)
Steel "spiders"	0
Detachable balloons	0
Fluid and semi-fluid materials	
Absolute alcohol (Ethanol)	+
Aethoxysklerol®	(++)
Isobutyl-cyanoacrylate (Bucrylate)	++
Amino-acids (Ethibloc®)	++

However, in view of the special character of hyperdynamic arteriovenous fistulas, particulate and mechanical devices are considered of minor value, causing more or less local blockade of the injected afferent arteries without occluding the "nidus", i.e., the arteriovenous shunting centre of the lesion (Fig. 19.14).

Fluid and semi-fluid solidifying materials, on the other hand, may cause venous shunting with some incidence of pulmonary complications [10]. However, polymerizing acrylates and precipitating amino-acid-Ethibloc® can be fixed at the "nidus" with substantial therapeutic effect [20]. Special handling of these substances is imperative for safe application and for optimal placement [10, 26, 28].

Absolute alcohol (ethanol) remains fluid during the vaso-occlusive procedure. The therapeutic result depends on local damage of the intima of the vessels causing more or less a local arterial thrombosis. In high flow lesions [29, 30] this thrombosis may show a tendency to resolve with recurrence.

Coiling mechanical devices may be useful in combination with Ethibloc® in large arteriovenous shunting fistulas as a "stop cock" at the end of the vaso-occlusive procedure to shorten the placement of the catheter and to avoid reflux of the solidifying material to main local arteries and to the periphery [27]. Coils may be also used prior to the injection of ethanol or Ethibloc® in large arteriovenous shunts in order to reduce the blood velocity and to enhance the contact time with the endothelium.

Catheter Devices

A good knowledge of catheter materials and proper skill in handling the devices is needed for optimal results causing minimal technical complication rate. All catheter devices (including preshaped materials and introducer systems) are now commercially available. Special types may be useful for special situations, such as flow-directed Swan Ganz [31] or Tracker catheters and coaxial combinations (Fig. 20.1a) to achieve superselective positioning in the periphery. Balloon-tipped catheters may also be applied for safety (Fig. 20.1b). All types of catheters should be inserted under heparinization and via a locking catheter sheath introducer system, permitting the exchange of catheters when needed [20, 33]. Acrylates and Ethibloc® must be applied by pre- and post-injection of

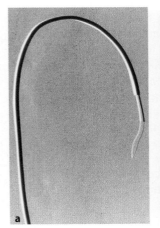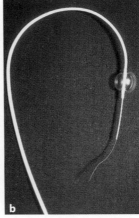

Fig. 20.1. a Vascular catheter with guide. **b** Coaxial catheter with occluding balloon at the tip. Reproduced from [32]

hyperosmolalic 40% glucose for safe delivery and in order to aim the vaso-occlusion just at the level of the "nidus" of the arteriovenous fistula (Fig. 20.2) [10, 26, 28]. Both materials can be added via the oily contrast medium Lipiodol® (iodinated Oleum Pa-

pavery, Guerbet GmbH, Sulzbach, Germany) for better opacification of the substance during embolization and for dilution of the material when working safely with thinner catheters (e.g., co-axial catheters) and in smaller vessels [28].

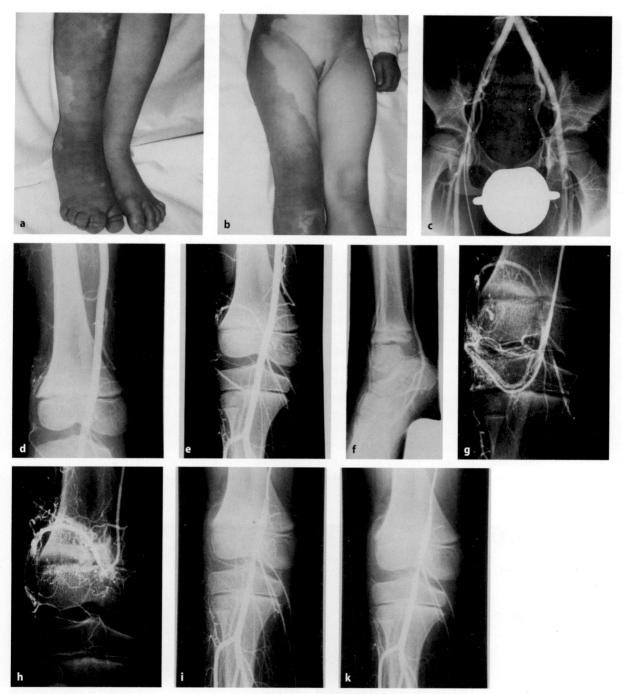

Fig. 20.2. Port wine stain associated with a right lower limb elongation of 3 cm. **a, b** Clinical picture. **c-e** Dilatation of right pelvic arteries, femoral and popliteal artery. **f** Normal vessels in the calf. **g** Selective arteriography of the inferior lateral genicular artery. **h** Selective arteriography of the superior lateral genicular artery. Ethibloc embolization. **i, k** Early and later control of the procedure. Reproduced from [32]

Strategies and Tactics

All maneuvers of catheterization and application of the embolizing materials must be carried out under fluoroscopic control. To get optimal documentation, extensive contrast enhancement is needed. For instance, at the level of the foot, the anterior and posterior tibial arteries and the fibular artery also must be catheterized and injected sub-selectively in order to gain all anatomical and functional information needed, including the collateral distribution of the contrast medium applied. Hyperdynamic arteriovenous shunting lesions generally must be filmed, using multiple series. With good control during embolization, large amounts of contrast medium will be injected repeatedly. For this reason it is important to separate diagnostic arteriography from vaso-occlusive therapy (Fig. 20.3).

Even so, for a serious analysis of the diagnostic output and for interdisciplinary discussion of the therapeutic consequences, embolization should be carried out in a second session.

Ischemic pain reaction, following more or less every successful vaso-occlusion, should be overcome during embolization by working under deep anesthesia. And the subsequent post-embolization syndrome (PES) [34] ought to be balanced by offering pain control by epidural or spinal anesthesia [35, 36].

The accurate documentation and a detailed information on the patient is obligatory and can prevent medico-legal problems in case of complications [17].

Finally, follow-up observations must be emphasized for a critical control of the early and late therapeutic outcome. It is a matter of fact that an angiographic "complete vaso-occlusion" may be the result of an acute arterial spasm rather than a real complete permanent vessel occlusion [11, 20, 21].

Special Interventional Techniques

In slight arteriovenous lesions the indication for transcatheter vaso-occlusion is limited by the small calibers of the feeding arteries. Hunter and Amplatz [37] have demonstrated that local retrograde venous sclerotherapy can be helpful in these patients for palliative improvement of the local clinical symptoms.

By reducing the venous vascular mass, local damage of the skin, compressive pain, etc. can be reduced or may even disappear [30]. In order to optimize the extent of the retrograde venous contamination with the sclerosing agent up to the area of the arteriovenous fistulas, we have used this technique under complete temporary blockage of circulation using short-term Esmarch bandage of the afferent arteries [38].

Belov [39] has pointed out that patients with intraosseous arteriovenous fistulas have poor therapeutic results. Transcatheter embolization also fails in the majority of these cases, as the "nidus" of the arteriovenous fistulas cannot be isolated [39]. Because of this we have carried out an intraosseous vaso-occlusion by direct transosseous puncture [38]. Once again, Ethibloc®, diluted by Lipiodol®, has been injected during temporary blockage of circulation under Esmarch bandage of the involved extremity, in order to control the volume of embolizing agent to be injected and for protection of the "sink" during precipitation of the amino-acids (Fig. 20.4). A direct arteriographic control is possible as long as a separate angiographic catheter has been positioned intra-arterially and adjacent to the lesion.

In a special type of intramuscular predominantly venous low-flow lesion sclerotherapy can be applied with rather good results. By transcutaneous direct puncture of the venous pseudo-aneurysm contrast medium and subsequent sclerosing agent

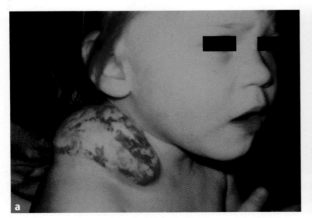
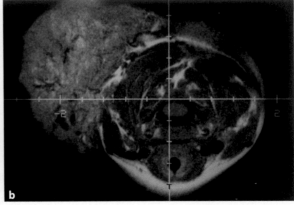

Fig. 20.3. **a** Clinical picture. **b** MRI hypervascular tumor well delineated from muscles   (→ *cont.*)

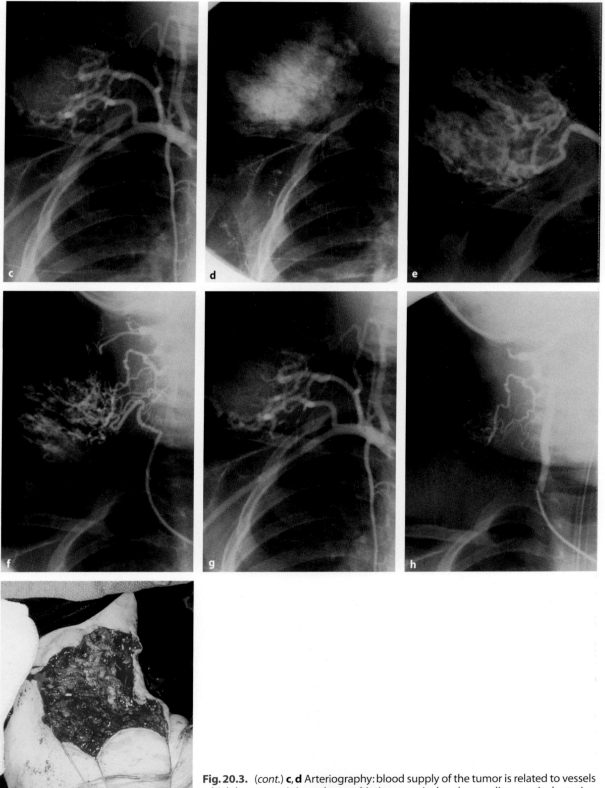

Fig. 20.3. (*cont.*) **c, d** Arteriography: blood supply of the tumor is related to vessels which have an origin at the trunk's tireo-cervical and ascending cervical arteries. **e, f** Embolization with Ethibloc after selective catheterism of the afferent arteries. **g, h** Residual vascularization after the occlusive procedure. **i** Surgical resection. Reproduced from [32]

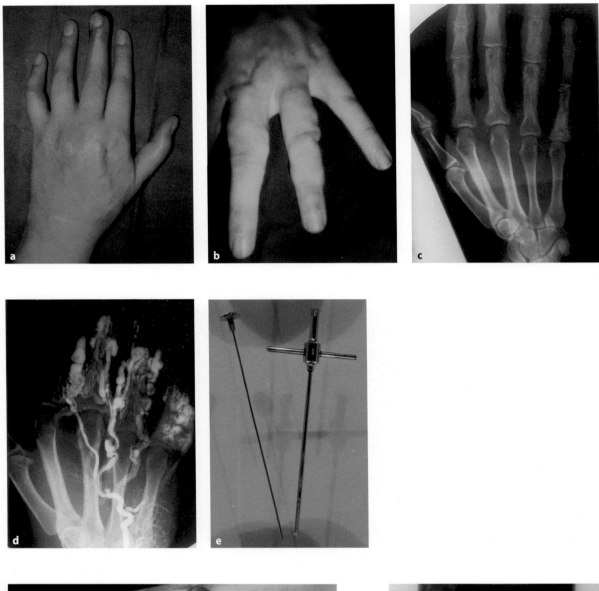

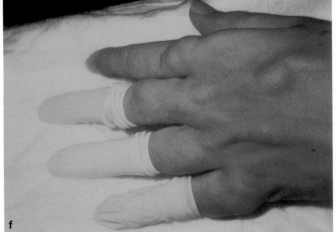

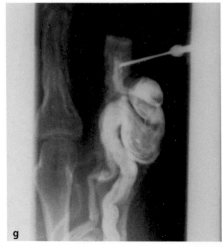

Fig. 20.4 a-l.

($\rightarrow$ *cont.*)

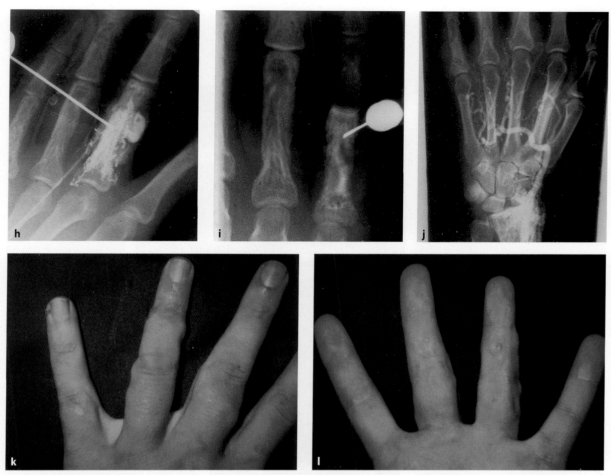

Fig. 20.4. Edema of the fingers and hand. **a, b** Clinical picture. **c** Radiological picture which demonstrates bone alteration in the III, IV and V finger. **d** Arteriography: arteriovenous shunts positioned within and outside the bones. Peripheral steal syndrome. **e** Special needle to perform intraosseous arteriography. **f** Protection of digital finger III to V; equal space to protect embolization. **g-i** Intraosseous arteriography and embolization with Ethibloc. An Esmark bandage was used in order to prevent embolization. **j** Control angiography 6 months after the procedure. **k-l** Clinical picture 2 years after the procedure. Reproduced from [32]

(Aethoxysklerol®) can be applied under fluoroscopy with prolongation of the contact to the venous wall under Esmarch's bandage, blocking the outflow temporarily (Fig. 20.5).

Nowak [40] presents an overview of the current literature dealing with complications resulting from interventional procedures [22]. However, so far there is no special report on statistics of side effects and complications resulting from vaso-occlusive therapy of arteriovenous malformations (AVMs) only. It is misleading to report a "mixture" of common symptoms of the transient PES following vaso-occlusion or of temporary side effects and permanent complications after this treatment [21]. Single case reports, as published so far, are also not representative. However, they may show a risk of skin necrosis in about

2 to 17% of patients [41]. In addition, a certain risk of ischemic neural damage at the site of vaso-occlusion must be considered [21, 23, 39]. Both risks should be discussed with the patient before planning transcatheter vaso-occlusion in AVMs. The PES was first described by Rankin et al. [34] as having typical clinical symptoms, caused by transient local ischemia as a consequence of the therapeutic vaso-occlusion (mild fever, leucocytosis, temporary hypertension, etc.). These are considered more or less common over the first 3–5 days following intervention and should be controlled carefully [36]. Pain depends on the localization of the lesion, the extent of vaso-occlusion, as well as the character of vaso-occlusive agent applied: Ethibloc® for instance is much more painful (but also much more effective)

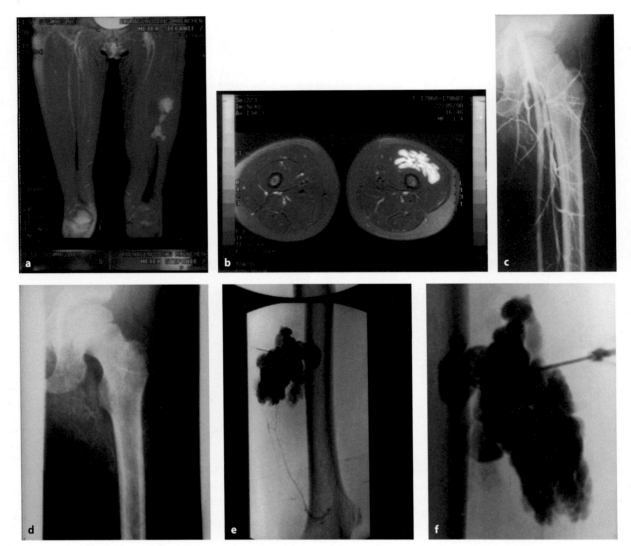

Fig. 20.5. Venous malformations in the quadriceps femoris muscle. **a, b** MR images. **c, d** Arteriography: no sign of an arteriovenous shunt. **e** Direct puncture phlebography. **f** Injection of Atossisclerol 4%. Reproduced from [32]

compared to ethanol [15, 38, 42]. Some of these potential complications can be treated successfully by endovascular procedures, correcting a non optimal position and displacement of Gianturco coils for instance [25].

Combined Therapy

As already mentioned, there are major risks of permanent ischemia and necrosis and/or abscess at the level of the acral AVMs and within the cranio-vertebral space. Side effects and complications can be reduced by skilled procedures and by performing palliation of the lesion with a step-by-step approach

and respecting critical indications (Table 20.1). Combining the advantages of interventional vaso-occlusion, surgical therapy (resection, skeletonization), and other procedures, the range of discomfort and side effects can be reduced dramatically [22]. This goal should be reached with a good interdisciplinary cooperation. Vaso-occlusion should be carried out first, generally to reduce the risks of serious bleeding during vascular surgery. After an interval of about 2–3 months, surgery enables smaller and thinner arteriovenous shunting vessels to be resected, or even to remove the rest of the infiltrative dysplastic vascular mass [22, 43, 44].

Indications (Table 20.1) and therapeutic tactics ought to be worked out critically [22]. Frequently patients have already been treated elsewhere (about 50%). Many of them have been *overdiagnosed* for years, using new imaging modalities (computed tomography [CT], magnetic resonance imaging [MRI]) with a high cost and time commitment, instead of proceeding with the treatment. Many of these patients therefore show typical secondary functional defects such as venous hypertension and ischemic ulceration due to the congenital arteriovenous shunting disease resulting in progressive decompensation. Other patients have been treated only partially by surgeons or by interventionalists without reliable results. Ligation, particularly partial resection of the main feeding arteries (for instance of the internal iliac artery, guiding to an arteriovenous shunting pelvic mass) would be rated as malpractice to our eyes. In some

of these patients we succeeded in convincing the vascular surgeon to reconstruct the interrupted artery, in order to have a direct catheter access again to the lesion [41]. Even so, incomplete results can also be seen after transcatheter embolization, applying particulate materials and/or coils only, while leaving the "nidus" of the fistulas still open, respectively guiding to its collateralization. If possible, a new approach must be offered then, using suitable fluid or semi-fluid materials. However, embolizing collaterals does not make any sense, as it will likely result in undesirable ischemic reactions.

This evidence shows the importance of creating centers for the treatment of CVMs, where interdisciplinary cooperation can be offered and where consultation with specialists will be possible at any time.

References

1. Loose DA, Wang ZG (1990) The surgical treatment of predominantly venous defects. Int Angiol 9(3):183–188
2. Grantzow R, Knorr P (2005) Differentiated therapy of hemangiomas. Przeglad Flebologiczny 13(3):85–90
3. Poetke M, Urban P, Philipp C, Berliner HP (2005) Hemangiomas: classification, diagnostic and laser treatment. Przeglad Flebologiczny 13(3):77–84
4. Brooks B (1930) The treatment of traumatic arteriovenous fistula. Sth Med J 23:100–102
5. Anderson JH, Gianturco G, Wallace S (1975) Mechanical devices for arterial occlusion. Am J Roentgenol 124(3):428–430
6. Berenstein A, Kricheff II (1979) Catheter and material selection for transarterial embolization: technical considerations. I Catheters. Radiology 3(132):619–630
7. Berenstein A, Kricheff II (1979) Catheter and material selection for transarterial embolization: technical considerations. II Materials. Radiology 132(3):631–639
8. Cromwell LD, Kerber CW (1979) Modification of cyanoacrylate for therapeutic embolization: preliminary experience. Am J Roentgenol 132(5):799–803
9. Grace DM, Pitt DF, Gold RE (1976) Vascular embolization and occlusion by angiographic technique as an aid or alternative to operation. Surg Gynecol Obstet 142:469–484
10. Kauffmann G, Wimmer B, Bischoff W et al (1977) Experimentelle Grundlagen für therapeutische Gefäßverschlüsse mit Angiographiekathetern. Radiologie 17:489–495
11. Natali J, Merland JJ (1976) Superselective arteriography and therapeutic embolization for vascular malformations (angiodysplasias). J Cardiovasc Surg 17(6):465–471
12. Stanley RJ, Cubillo E (1975) Nonsurgical treatment of arteriovenous malformations of the trunk and limbs by transcatheter embolization. Radiology 115(3):609–612
13. Weber J (1990) Invasive radiological diagnostic of congenital vascular malformations (CVM). Int Angiol 9(3):168–174
14. Weber J (1997) Invasive Diagnostik angeborener Gefäßfehler. In: Loose DA, Weber J (eds): Angeborene Gefäßmißbildungen. Nordlanddruck, Lüneburg, pp 127–163
15. Weber J (1999) Angeborene Gefäßfehler in Diagnostik und Therapie. In: Marshall M, Breu FX (eds) Handbuch der Angiologie. Ecomed, Landsberg, Vol 2, pp 45–60
16. Weber J (2005) Invasive diagnostic of peripheral congenital vascular malformations. Przeglad Flebologiczny 13(3):111–121
17. Wojtowycz M (1995) Handbook of interventional radiology and angiography. Mosby Year Book, St. Louis, Baltimore, Boston, pp 123–124
18. Vaghi M (2005) Functional diagnostic of peripheral congenital vascular malformations. Przeglad Flebologiczny 13(3):105–109
19. Greenfield AJ (1981) Transcatheter vessel occlusion: methods and materials. In: Athanasoulis CA, Pfister RC, Greene RE, Roberson GH (eds) Interventional radiology. WB Saunders, Philadelphia, pp 40–53
20. Weber J (1990) Technique and results of therapeutic catheter embolization of congenital vascular defects. Int Angiol 9(3):214–223
21. Allison DJ, Kennedy A (1989) Embolization technique in arterio-venous malformations. In: Belov S, Loose DA, Weber J (eds) Vascular malformations. Periodica Angiologica, Einhorn-Presse Verlag, Reinbek, Vol 16, pp 261–269
22. Loose DA, Weber J (1991) Indications and tactics for combined treatment of congenital vascular defects.

Progress in angiology. Minerva Medica, Torino, pp 373–378

23. Triponis V, Vaisnyte B (2005) Diagnostic and prognostic value of birthmarks, symptoms and signs in patients with CVMs of extremities. Przeglad Flebologiczny 13(3):99–104

24. van Dongen RJ (1993) Therapie der angeborenen arteriovenosen Angiodysplasien unter besonderer Berücksichtigung der operativen Embolisation. Angiology 5:169–175

25. Weber J (1980) A complication with the Gianturco coil and its non-surgical management. Cardiovasc Intervent Radiol 3:156–158

26. Weber J (1982) Experimental renal embolization using contrast-labeled Ethibloc® and follow-up observations by computed tomography. In: Oliva L, Veiga Pires JH (eds) Intervention radiology. Excerpta Medica, Amsterdam, pp 23–30

27. Weber J (1989) Embolizing materials and catheter techniques for angiotherapeutic management of the AVM. In: Belov S, Loose DA, Weber J (eds) Vascular malformations. Periodica Angiologic. Einhorn-Presse Verlag, Reinbek, Vol 16, pp 252–260

28. Novak D, Weber J, Wieners H, Zabel G (1984) New liquid and semi-liquid embolizing substances for tumour embolization. Ann Radiol 24:428–431

29. Yakes WF, Haas, DK, Parker SH et al (1994) Symptomatic vascular malformations: ethanol embolotherapy. Radiology 170:1059–1071

30. Yakes WF (1994) Extremity venous malformations. Diagnosis and management. Semin Intervent Radiol 11:332–336

31. Swan JH, Ganz W, Forrester J et al (1977) Catheterization of the heart in men with the use of flow-directed balloon-tipped catheter. N Engl J Med 283:447–454

32. Weber J (2002) Radiologia interventistica. In: Mattassi R, Belov S, Loose DA (eds) Malformazioni vascolari ed emangiomi. Testo atlante di diagnostica e terapia. Springer-Verlag Italia, pp 50–59

33. Weber J, Ritter H (1989) Strategies for the radiological angiotherapy of hyperdynamic av-malformations. In: Belov S, Loose DA, Weber J (eds) Vascular mal-formations. Periodica Angiologica. Einhorn-Presse Verlag, Reinbek, Vol 16, pp 294–298

34. Rankin RN, McKenzie FN, Ahmad D (1983) Embolization of arteriovenous fistulas and aneurysms with detachable balloons. Cand J Surg 26(4):317–322

35. Schilke PM (1989) Special methods of anaesthesia for vascular surgery and interventional radiology. In: Belov S, Loose DA, Weber J (eds) Vascular malformations. Periodica Angiologica. Einhorn-Presse Verlag, Reinbek, Vol 16, pp 299–302

36. Weber J (1989) The post-infarction and pain syndrome following catheter embolization and its treatment. In: Belov S, Loose DA, Weber J (eds) Vascular malformations. Periodica Angiologica. Einhorn-Presse Verlag, Reinbek, Vol 16, pp 294–298

37. Hunter DW, Amplatz K (1989) Sclerotherapy of peripheral AVMs and hemangiomas through a retrograde transvenous approach. In: Belov S, Loose DA, Weber J (eds) Vascular malformations. Periodica Angiologica. Einhorn-Presse Verlag, Reinbek, Vol 16, p 279

38. Weber J (1997) Embolisation von arterio-venosen Malformationen. In: Loose DA, Weber J (eds) Angeborene Gefaßmißbildungen. Nordlanddruck, Lüneburg, pp 245–277

39. Belov S (1990) Hemodynamic pathogenesis of vascular-bone syndromes in congenital vascular defects. Int Angiol 9:155–161

40. Novak D (1990) Complications of arterial embolization. In: Dondelinger RF, Rossi P, Kurdziel JC, Wallace S (eds) Interventional radiology. Thieme, New York, pp 314–324

41. Riche MC, Reizine D, Melni JP, Merland JJ (1984) Les complications et les pieges de l'embolisation des membres. Ann Radiol 27(4):287–291

42. Weber J (1993) Vaso-occlusive angiotherapy in congenital vascular malformations. Semin Vasc Surg 4(6):279–295

43. Belov S, Loose DA (1990) Surgical treatment of congenital vascular defects. Int Angiol 9:175–182

44. Malan E (1965) Surgical problems in the treatment of congenital arteriovenous fistulae. J Cardiovasc Surg 6 [suppl]:251–255

Diagnosis and Management of Soft Tissue Vascular Malformations with Ethanol

21

Wayne F. Yakes

Abstract

Embolization procedures have evolved as one of the cornerstones of modern interventional radiology.

The choice of embolization material is very important in order to achieve long lasting treatment results. The choice of ethanol as an embolizing agent is related to its capacity to destroy the endothelial layer of the vessels. Ethanol may be used in the treatment of both venous, arteriovenous and lymphatic malformations.

Introduction

Vascular malformations constitute some of the most difficult diagnostic and therapeutic dilemmas that can be encountered in the practice of medicine. The clinical presentations are extremely protean, ranging from an asymptomatic birthmark to fulminant life-threatening congestive heart failure. Attributing these varied symptoms to a vascular malformation can be challenging even for the most experienced clinician. Compounding this problem is the extreme rarity of these vascular lesions. If a clinician sees only one affected patient every few years, it is extremely difficult to gain enough experience in order to be able to diagnose and provide optimal treatment. Typically, affected patients bounce from clinician to clinician experiencing disappointing outcomes, complications, and recurrence or worsening of their presenting symptoms.

Vascular malformations were initially treated by surgeons alone. The early rationale of proximal arterial ligation of arteriovenous malformations (AVMs) proved futile, as the phenomenon of neovascular recruitment reconstituted arterial inflow to the AVM nidus. Microfistulous connections became macrofistulous feeders. Complete extirpation of a vascular malformation can be very difficult and, at times, even hazardous, necessitating suboptimal partial resections. Partial resections can result in a good initial clinical response that may last for some time. However, very often the patient's presenting symptoms recur or worsen at follow-up [1–3]. Due to the significant blood loss that frequently accompanied surgery, the skills of interventional radiologists were eventually employed in order to embolize these vascular lesions preoperatively. This not only allowed more complete resections, it also resulted in reduced blood loss. However, complete extirpation of a vascular malformation is difficult and may not always be possible. It has been reported that only approximately 20% of malformations may be amenable to complete extirpation with surgery [2, 4, 5].

D. Emerick Szilagyi, M.D., former editor for the Journal of Vascular Surgery, (USA) said of vascular anomalies: "…with few exceptions, their cure by surgical means is impossible. We intuitively thought that the only answer of a surgeon to the problem of disfiguring, often noisome, and occasionally disabling blemishes and masses, prone to cause bleeding, pain, or other unpleasantness, was to attack them with vigor and with the determination of eradicating them. The results of this attempt of radical treatment were disappointing" [2]. Indeed, of the 82 patients seen in his patient series, only 18 patients were deemed operable and of the 18 operated upon, at follow-up the condition of ten patients was improved, two patients were unchanged and six were worse.

This patient series points to the enormity of the problem posed by vascular malformations. They are best treated in medical centers where this type of patient is seen regularly. The interventional radiologist

R. Mattassi, D.A. Loose, M. Vaghi (eds.), *Hemangiomas and Vascular Malformations*.

or surgeon who evaluates a patient every year or so will never have enough experience to manage these challenging lesions. All too frequently the patient ultimately pays for the physician's initial enthusiasm, inexperience, folly, and lack of necessary clinical back-up. For optimal treatment, a vascular malformation team is needed. On such a team, the various surgical, medical and interventional specialties function together much like a tumor board of specialists. The presentation and regular treatment of patients allows experience to be gained and rational decisions to be made, optimizing patient care. It cannot be emphasized enough that diagnosis and treatment of vascular malformations poses one of the most difficult challenges in the practice of medicine. A cavalier approach to their management will inevitably lead to significant complications and unsatisfactory patient outcomes.

Concepts in Patient Management

Vascular malformations are congenital lesions that are present at birth, even if they are not clinically evident, and grow commensurately with the child. The collective term vascular malformation encompasses any malformed blood vessel of any vascular element, including arteries, capillaries, veins, and lymphatics. Post-traumatic arteriovenous fistulae are different because they are acquired, even though they may be radiographically similar [6, 7]. A thorough clinical exam and history can usually establish the diagnosis of hemangioma or vascular malformation.

Color Doppler Imaging (CDI) is an essential tool in the diagnostic work-up of vascular malformations, allowing accurate diagnosis of both high-flow lesions (AVM, arteriovenous fistula [AVF]) and low-flow lesions (venous malformation, lymphatic malformation). Furthermore, CDI is an important non-invasive method for following patients who have undergone therapy. Documentation of increased arterial flow-rates prior to therapy and decreased arterial flow-rates after therapy is important physiological information. Persistent documentation of thrombosis in low-flow malformations leads to imaging and allows accurate assessment [8].

Computed tomography (CT), although helpful in the diagnostic work-up, is less useful than magnetic resonance imaging (MRI). Unlike CT, MRI easily distinguishes between high-flow and low-flow vascular malformations. Furthermore, the anatomic relationships of the vascular malformation to adjacent nerves, muscles, tendons, organs, bone and subcutaneous fat allow a total assessment. MRI is also an excellent non-invasive method for determining the efficacy of therapy, often obviating repetitive arteriography and venography [9]. The main role of CT is in intraosseous vascular malformations and determination of the cortical margins and their involvement.

After diagnosis is established, the next major hurdle is to determine whether therapy is warranted. Usually the presenting symptoms of the patient are treated. Rarely, the patient may have a serendipitously discovered high-flow AVM and be asymptomatic. However, closer inspection may reveal that this is due to a high output cardiac state, which is due to the patient's youth. This high output cardiac state may be the sole criterion determining therapy. Consultation with multiple medical and surgical specialists may be required to ultimately determine if treatment is warranted.

With the use of ethanol as an embolic agent to treat vascular malformations in all anatomic locations, our patients require general anesthesia. A Swan-Ganz line and arterial line monitoring may be necessary when treating larger lesions. Pulmonary artery pressures can then be constantly monitored to determine if abnormal elevation of pulmonary pressures occurs during the procedure. The embolization procedure can be stopped at this point to allow pulmonary pressures to normalize. If the pressures are high enough, an infusion of nitroglycerine through the Swan-Ganz catheter can help lower the pulmonary artery pressures to normal. General anesthesia is a requirement because intravascular ethanol is extremely painful and constant movement of the patient could compromise an embolization. Post-procedure, the patients are revived from anesthesia and sent to the recovery room for temporary observation. After they are deemed stable, they are usually sent to the routine hospital ward. Medical management consists of decadron therapy to manage the swelling that occurs with the acute thrombosis of embolization. Patients are observed overnight and discharged the following morning unless a complication that requires management occurs.

Patients usually exhibit focal swelling in the area of the malformation after the procedure. In most patients the majority of the swelling resolves within 1–2 weeks. In those patients with lower extremity and foot malformations, swelling may last longer because the leg and foot are not only dependent, but also weight-bearing structures. After 4 weeks all swelling is usually resolved and the patient, at his new baseline, is ready for follow-up therapy as necessary.

MR and CDI can be used to document the efficacy of serial therapy. In those patients who present with pain, serial devascularization of the malformation will usually completely resolve or at least dramatically reduce the amount of pain. At my institution, patients with residual pain undergo neurostimulation therapy with Synaptic 2000, a neurostimulator pain control device (Synaptic Corp., RFP Inc., Aurora, Colorado) [10]. This unique, noninvasive device has proven very helpful in controlling residual pain in selective patients. It has also been useful in reducing the need for oral narcotic medications in patients presenting with pain. Additional applications for this device have been noted in nerve injury recovery, microvascular stimulation in ischemic tissues, decreased swelling, and tissue healing post-injury.

Endovascular Therapy of Vascular Malformations

Embolization procedures have evolved as one of the cornerstones of modern interventional radiology. The extensive array of catheters, guidewires, endovascular embolic materials, and imaging systems used are a tribute to the hard work, insight, and imagination of the many dedicated investigators in this area. The judicious use of embolization is common in modern clinical practice because of significant laboratory research, clinical research, and extensive clinical experience. Now that it is firmly established as an essential therapeutic tool, its role will continue to grow.

There are many embolic agents that are used in various clinical scenarios. The choice of agent depends on several factors: the vascular territory to be treated, the type of abnormality being treated, the possibility of superselective delivery of an occlusive agent, the goal of the procedure, and the permanence of the occlusion required. With regards to vascular malformations, permanence is a significant issue. It has already been documented in the literature that embolization with materials such as polyvinyl alcohol (PVA), tissue adhesives and coils is rarely curative but provides excellent palliation [11–13]. With the advent of the use of ethanol, cures at long-term follow-up have been documented by multiple authors [10, 14–25]. The judicious use of ethanol as an embolic agent has revolutionized our ability to permanently cure these lesions in soft tissues, organs, bone and brain [10, 14–25].

Arteriovenous Malformations

Arteriovenous malformations of soft tissues and organs pose a significantly difficult dilemma (Fig. 21.1). They are typified by hypertrophied in-flow arteries shunting through a primitive vascular nidus into tor-

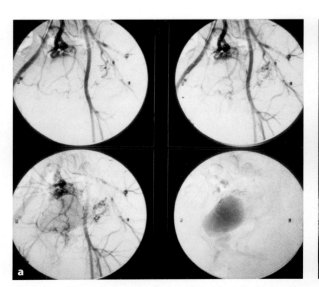
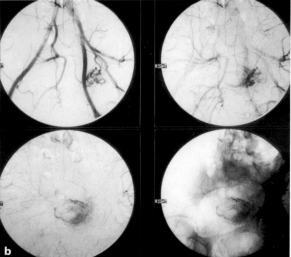

Fig. 21.1. Thirty-four year-old female with pain during intercourse diagnosed with a right pelvic AVM. **a** Right posterior oblique (RPO) pelvic arteriogram demonstrating right pelvic AVM with giant venous aneurysm. **b** RPO pelvic arteriogram 9 months later demonstrating cure of AVM after ethanol endovascular therapy. The patient's painful symptoms during intercourse completely ablated. Reproduced from [26]

tuous dilated out-flow veins. No intervening capillary bed is present. Symptoms are usually referable to the anatomic location of the AVM. The larger and more anatomically central an AVM is, the greater likelihood of high output cardiac. Other presenting symptoms can include pain, progressive nerve deterioration or palsy, disfiguring mass, tissue ulceration, hemorrhage, impairment of limb function and limiting claudication.

When treating AVMs with ethanol, it is essential to be superselective when positioning within the nidus. Being a fluid agent, ethanol will flow into capillary beds if inadvertent embolization occurs. This can lead to extensive tissue devitalization and nerve injury. When catheter placement is not possible due to surgical arterial ligation, coil embolization or vascular tortuosity, then direct percutaneous puncture techniques can be used to circumvent catheterization obstacles. If superselective placement of ethanol in the nidus is not possible, then the use of ethanol must be avoided. Frequently, in-flow vascular occlusion may be required to induce vascular stasis in order to maximize the thrombogenic properties of ethanol. This can be achieved through the use of occlusion balloon catheters, blood pressure cuffs, tourniquets, etc. I empirically use occlusive techniques for approximately 10 minutes. The amount of ethanol used in each embolization procedure is tailored to the flow-volume characteristics of the individual lesion. No pre-determined volume of ethanol is ever considered.

Endovascular therapy of AVMs with ethanol has ushered in a new era in the therapy of these problematic congenital anomalies. Cures and permanent partial oblations have been documented in our patient series, resulting in dramatic symptomatic improvement [10, 14–25]. Neovascular recruitment and recanalizations have not been observed, but permanent partial ablations have also led to long-term symptomatic improvement, obviating the need for further treatment. Despite the success that is possible with ethanol, it must be remembered that ethanol is an extremely dangerous intravascular sclerosant that can cause total tissue devitalization and neuropathy.

Complications are part and parcel of treating vascular malformations, whether surgically or endovascularly. It is crucial for a vascular malformation team to be in place so that complications, if they occur, result in dramatically reduced morbidity.

Arteriovenous Fistulae

Congenital and post-traumatic AVF are similar to AVMs in that they are high-flow vascular malformations. AVF are characterized by an artery connected to a draining vein without an intervening capillary bed. Post-traumatic AVF are usually secondary to blunt or penetrating trauma resulting in injury to an artery and an adjacent vein. Fistulization between the artery and vein is stimulated by preferential vascular shunting through the fistula from the high-pressure arterial system into the low-pressure venous system. Chronic AVF may be confused with AVMs at arteriography because multiple enlarged in-flow arteries can simulate an AVM nidus near the AV connection [6, 7].

The natural history of AVF can be extremely varied. AVF can remain clinically silent and well tolerated by the patient, as seen in iatrogenic dialysis fistula patients or in asymptomatic renal AVF incidentally found at arteriography. If the shunt through an AVF is large, hemodynamic consequences such as cardiomegaly, increased cardiac output, and intermittent bouts of congestive heart failure can occur. Pain and swelling may also be a presenting complaint. Vascular steal alone may cause ischemic symptoms in the tissues and organs adjacent to the AVF. Skin and tissue may demonstrate venous hypertensive (venous stasis) changes with engorged arterialized veins.

Treatment of the AVF requires complete occlusion at the AV connection. As seen in the treatment of AVMs, proximal arterial ligations and distal venous ligations usually fail. Surgical ligations are not only futile, they also remove possible vascular access routes for embolization. Vascular occlusive devices that are successful in curing these difficult lesions in our hands include the use of ethanol or the use of ethanol with coils.

Venous Malformations

Venous malformations of the soft tissues can occur anywhere in the body (Fig. 21.2). They are congenital vascular malformations arising from abnormal vein morphogenesis and incomplete resorption of primitive vascular elements. On plain x-ray films, calcified phleboliths may be present. In-flow arteries are of normal size because there is a normal intervening capillary bed. In the late arterial phase, contrast pooling of the post-capillary dilated venous structures occurs because of slow stagnant flow within the vascular malformation itself. Vein malformations are usually poorly opacified by arteriography. Closed-system venography or direct puncture venography better demonstrate the extent of the abnormal post-capillary vascular spaces.

The work-up of vein malformations includes CDI and MRI as well as closed-system venography and arteriography [8, 9]. MR easily distinguishes vein mal-

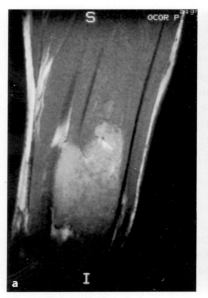
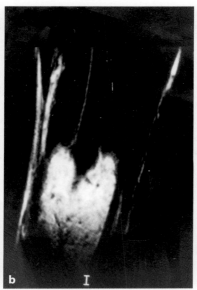
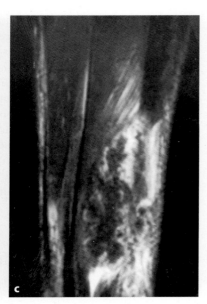

Fig. 21.2. Twenty-two year-old male with painful muscle mass in the right forearm. **a** T-1 weighted MR demonstrating high signal within the pronator quadratus muscle. **b** T-2 weighted right forearm MR demonstrating increased signal in the area of vein malformation infiltrating the quadratus pronator muscle. **c** MR 1 year after therapy. There is markedly decreased signal in the pronator quadratus muscle after treatment. The patient's muscle mass is absent. The patient is functionally normal and is no longer in pain. Reproduced from [26]

formations from AVMs and AVFs, particularly on the T-2 weighted, fat suppressed imaging sequences. Further, MR post-therapy can be compared to initial baseline studies to determine the efficacy of therapy in that the increased signal noted pre-therapy decreases after therapy. This obviates the need for repetitive venography. Venography and arteriography are required only when therapy is warranted, as the imaging sophistication of MRI is normally sufficient for the non-invasive diagnosis of vein malformations and for distinguishing them from other types of malformations.

Vein malformations may be asymptomatic, cosmetically deforming, painful, induce neuropathy, ulcerate, hemorrhage, induce abnormal bone growth, cause pathologic fractures, induce thrombocytopenia, and be a source of rectal hemorrhage and anemia. The anemia can even be life threatening.

I have treated patients with vein malformations in all anatomic locations. Patients are treated by percutaneous puncture to directly access the abnormal vascular vein elements. Transarterial embolization is a possibility, but only in those lesions that are capillary-venous malformations with a dominance in the vein malformation. Direct puncture techniques directly attack the vein malformations, thus the in-flow arterial system and capillary bed are not affected and tissue loss by necrosis is minimized.

A subgroup of vein malformations is the so-called intramuscular hemangioma, which is better termed the intramuscular vein malformation [27–29]. These malformations are largely contained within muscle and may extend from the affected muscle into surrounding tissues. Although histologically identical to vein malformations, they have a different clinical presentation than the non-intramuscular vein malformation subtype. Presentation is in the second or third decade of life, although intramuscular hemangioma may occasionally present earlier or later. All patients present with a growing palpable muscle mass, with or without pain. This subgroup may well be a capillary-venous malformation type in which, on arteriography, hypertrophied arterial in-flow will be seen. In intramuscular vein malformations in which the muscle cannot be totally resected without functional loss, direct puncture ethanol embolization can permanently treat the lesion.

Lymphatic Malformations

Soft tissue lymphatic malformations arise from vein buds. Lymphatic malformations are histologically identical to vein malformations, except that lymphatic fluid rather than red blood cells is present within the vascular spaces. Lymphatic malformations can have large cystic spaces or very small luminal spaces. Lymphatic malformations have the same imaging characteristics as vein malformations on MR in that they demonstrate increased signal on T-2 sequences [9]. As in MR vein malformations, lymphatic malformations are best imaged in T-2 sequences with fat suppression. The inaccurate term "cystic hygroma" should be replaced by the more appropriate term "lymphatic malformation". Lymphatic malformations respond dramatically to percutaneous ethanol therapy in a similar fashion to vein malformations.

Intralipomatous Vascular Malformations

Vascular malformations may occur within fat, although this lesion has not yet been described in the literature. These are complex lesions that involve subcutaneous fat and may or may not have a skin port-wine stain overlying them and they present as a growing fatty mass that may or may not cause pain. These are unusual lesions and require a team approach for effective management. Endovascular occlusion techniques can diminish the vascularity of the malformation. However, it is difficult to determine whether the abnormal fat is being stimulated, or if the abnormal fat is itself stimulating the abnormal malformed blood vessels. However, the fat itself is very dark rather than the usual yellowish color, again indicative of a tissue dysplasia involving fat and blood vessels. To completely treat this lesion, surgery is required to remove the abnormal fat with the abnormal vascular elements.

Conclusion

Vascular malformations pose some of the most significant challenges in medical practice. Peripheral soft tissue malformations and neural axis malformations cause unique clinical problems due to their anatomic location. Clinical manifestations of these lesions are extremely protean. The lesions are rare, meaning that the experience of most clinicians in diagnosis and management is limited, augmenting the problem and often leading to misdiagnosis and poor patient outcome. Vascular malformations are best treated in medical centers where patients with these lesions are seen regularly and a team approach is used. In this fashion, significant experience in the management of these lesions can help to develop definitive statements for their treatment.

References

1. Decker DG, Fish CR, Juergens JL (1968) Arteriovenous fistulas of the female pelvis: A diagnostic problem. Obstet Gynecol Surg 31:799–805
2. Szilagyi DE, Smith RF, Ellliott JP, Hageman JH (1976) Congenital arteriovenous anomalies of the limbs. Arch Surg 111:423–429
3. Flye MW, Jordan BP, Schwartz MZ (1983) Management of congenital arteriovenous malformations. Surgery 94:740–747
4. Halliday AW, Smith EJ, Jackson J et al (1992) Indications for surgery for arteriovenous malformations. Br J Surg 79:361–362
5. Halliday AW, Mansfield AO (1989) Arteriovenous malformations: Current management approaches. Br J Hosp Med 42:196–202
6. Trout HH, Tievsky AL, Rieth KG et al (1987) Arteriovenous fistulas simulating arteriovenous malformation. Otolaryngol Head Neck Surg 97:322–325
7. Lawdahl RB, Routh WD, Vietek JJ et al (1989) Chronic arteriovenous fistulas masquerading as arteriovenous malformations: diagnostic considerations and therapeutic implications. Radiology 170:1011–1015
8. Yakes WF, Stavros AT, Parker SH et al (1990) Color doppler imaging of peripheral high-flow vascular malformations before and after ethanol embolotherapy. Presented at the 76th Scientific Assembly and Annual Meeting of the Radiologic Society of North America, Chicago, November 25–30
9. Rak KM, Yakes WF, Ray RL et al (1992) MR imaging of symptomatic peripheral vascular malformations. AJR Am J Roentgenol 159:107–112
10. Yakes WF (1994) Extremity venous malformations: diagnosis and management. Semin Intervent Radiol 11:332–339
11. Widlus DM, Murray RR, White RI Jr et al (1988) Congenital arteriovenous malformations: Tailored embolotherapy. Radiology 169:511–516
12. Rao VR, Mandalam KR, Gupta AK et al (1989) Dissolution of isobutyl 2-cyanoacrylate on long-term follow-up. AJNR 10:135–141
13. Hashimoto Y, Matsuhiro K, Nagaki M, Tanioka H (1988) Therapeutic embolization for vascular lesions of the head and neck. Int J Oral Maxillofac Surg 18:47–49

14. Yakes WF, Pevsner PH, Reed MD et al (1986) Serial embolizations of an extremity arteriovenous malformation with alcohol via direct percutaneous puncture. AJR Am J Roentgenol 146:1038–1040

15. Takebayaski S, Hosaka M, Ishizuka E et al (1988) Arteriovenous malformations of the kidneys: Ablation with alcohol. AJR 150:587–590

16. Vinson AM, Rohrer DB, Willcox CW et al (1988) Absolute ethanol embolization for peripheral AVMs: Report of two cures. South Med J 1:1052–1055

17. Yakes WF, Haas DK, Parker SH et al (1989) Alcohol embolotherapy of vascular malformations. Semin Intervent Radiol 6:146–161

18. Yakes WF, Luethke JM, Parker SH et al (1990) Ethanol embolization of vascular malformations. RadioGraphics 10:787–796

19. Yakes WF, Luethke JM, Merland JJ et al (1990) Ethanol embolization of arteriovenous fistulas: A primary mode of therapy. J Vasc Intervent Radiol 1:89–96

20. Mourao GS, Hodes JE, Gobin YP et al (1991) Curative treatment of scalp arteriovenous fistulas by direct puncture and embolization with absolute alcohol. J Neurosurg 75:634–637

21. Yakes WF, Rossi P, Odink H (1996) How I do it: Arteriovenous malformation management. Cardiovasc Intervent Radiol 19:65–71

22. Keljo DJ, Yakes WF, Andersen JM, Timmons CF (1996) Recognition and treatment of venous malformations of the rectum. J Pediatr Gastroenterol Nutr 23:442–446

23. Yakes WF, Krauth L, Ecklund J et al (1997) Ethanol endovascular management of brain arteriovenous malformations: Initial results. Neurosurgery 40:1145–1154

24. Yakes WF (1996) Diagnosis and management of vascular anomalies. In: Castaneda-Zuniga WR, Tadavarthy SM (eds) Interventional radiology. Williams and Wilkins, Baltimore, pp 103–138

25. Yakes WF (1996) Diagnosis and management of venous malformations. In: Savader SJ, Trerotola SO (eds) Venous interventional radiology with clinical perspectives. Thieme Medical Publishers, New York, pp 139–150

26. Yakes WF (2002) Diagnosi e terapia delle malformazioni vascolari dei tessuti molli. In: Mattassi R, Belov S, Loose DA, Vaghi M (eds) Malformazioni vascolari ed emangiomi. Testo-atlante di diagnostica e terapia. Springer-Verlag, pp 66–70

26. Jones KG (1953) Cavernous hemangioma of striated muscle: a review of the literature of 44 cases. J Bone Joint Surg 35:717–728

27. Connors JJ, Khan G (1977) Hemangioma of striated muscle. South Med J 70:1423–1424

28. Welsh D, Henger AS (1980) The diagnosis and treatment of intramuscular hemangiomas of the masseter muscle. Am J Otolaryng 1:186–190

Sclerotherapy in Vascular Malformations

22

Juan Carlos Cabrera, Dirk A. Loose

Abstract

Sclerotherapy is performed mainly in venous and lymphatic malformations using different substances. Sclerosis in arteriovenous (AV) forms is contraindicated because an erroneous intra-arterial injection may produce extensive necrosis. Classical sclerosis is mainly performed in venous dysplasias with polidocanol, sodium tetradecyl sulphate and ethanol, among others, while in lymphatic malformations, OK-432 is preferred. Sclerotherapy with the microfoam technique significantly improves results.

Introduction

Sclerotherapy is the removal of an anomalous venous area by injection of a sclerosing agent, classically a liquid, which produces a chemical irritation of the endothelial cells that coat the interior of the vessel. A thrombus is then produced and the vein is finally transformed into a fibrous thread that ultimately disappears (Fig. 22.1).

Indications

Vascular malformations associated with arteriovenous lesions are contraindicated for sclerotherapy because an accidental intra-arterial injection can produce extensive necrosis. It must also be taken into account that head and neck veins lack valves and that those in the upper two-thirds of the facial region communicate directly with the cavernous sinus via the superior and inferior ophthalmic veins (Fig. 22.2). Consequently, sclerotherapy is to be avoided at this level.

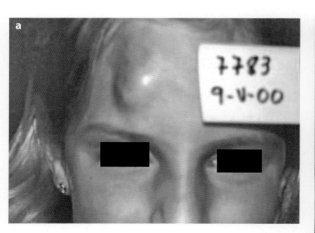
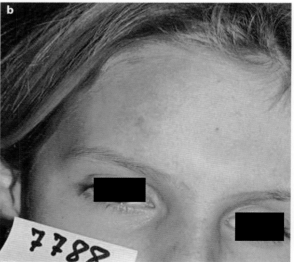

Fig. 22.1. Limited venous malformation of the right forehead. **a** Before and **b** 6 months after sclerotherapy with microfoam

R. Mattassi, D.A. Loose, M. Vaghi (eds.), *Hemangiomas and Vascular Malformations*.
© Springer-Verlag Italia 2009

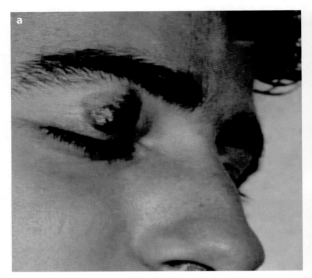
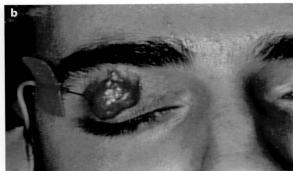
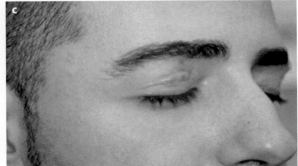

Fig. 22.2. Limited venous malformation of the right upper eyelid. **a** Before, **b** during and **c** 3 months after sclerotherapy with microfoam

Currently, the greatest therapeutic challenges in congenital vascular malformations are posed by venous or low-flow vascular malformations and diffuse lymphatic vascular malformations of a large size or extent or those that show infiltration of muscle masses. Because of their invasion of proximal structures, venous malformations usually have a complex morphology and are often associated with anomalies of the deep venous system of the extremities, therefore limiting the possibilities of complete excision by surgery [1–5].

Sclerosing Agents

The sclerosing agents classically used in the treatment of low-flow venous and of lymphatic malformations include 5% sodium morrhuate, sodium tetradecyl sulphate, polidocanol, ethanolamine oleate, ethanol, ethiblock, hypertonic saline, amidotrizoic acid, bleomycin, dextrose, tetracyclins and OK-432. The selection of the specific agent depends upon the experience and preference of the physician and the morphological appearance and location of the lesion [6–8].

Sclerotherapy with ethanol, the most widely used agent in the treatment of these lesions, is highly aggressive and associated with major complications due to lack of control over the injected liquid. Besides

its general contraindication in children, reported adverse effects include necrosis of skin and mucosa, deep venous thrombosis in extremities, pulmonary embolism, sensory and motor neurologic lesions, superficial cellulitis and cardio-respiratory collapse due to bronchial spasm [6]. Moreover, ethanol treatment is not readily repeatable, and this is essential for sclerotherapy, since partial recanalisation after the intravascular thrombosis is frequent [9].

Technique of Classic Sclerotherapy

The technique of sclerotherapy must ensure that a precise dose is administered and that the agent is homogeneously distributed on the entire endothelial perimeter of the treated venous segment [9]. It must also ensure that the intravascular concentration of the sclerosant is not reduced by dilution in the blood or that this dilution is minimal but always known. Finally, the sclerosant must remain in contact with the endothelium for the necessary time period. In short, the requirements of sclerotherapy must be met:
1. Knowledge of the intravascular concentration of the sclerosant.
2. Homogeneous distribution within the vessel.
3. Control over the duration of contact between agent and endothelia.

4. Sclerotherapy must be selective; i.e., limited to the selected venous area.

These requirements are not met by conventional liquid sclerosants. Using these, the dosage on the endothelia and therefore the sclerosing action is highly difficult to control, and in vessels of a certain volume or flow, the therapeutic effect, besides being unsafe, is generally confined to a short segment.

Ethanol sclerotherapy is indicated before surgery as a preoperative support to reduce the size of the lesion or as a postoperative complement [3, 7]. In contrast, conventional sclerotherapy of large malformations is ineffective because of the intrinsic limitations of the injected liquids, including:

1. Dilution and progressive deactivation of the liquid in a large blood volume.
2. Irregular distribution of the sclerosant on the endothelia of the treated area.
3. Difficulties in manipulating and controlling the injected sclerosant.
4. Imperceptibility within the vessels on duplex ultrasonography.

The general complications of this technique vary according to the agent and the dose used. They include: allergic reactions (especially with sodium tetradecyl sulphate), brain intoxication (especially with ethanol, which must never exceed a maximum volume of 1.2 ml in patients of about 70 kg) [6], haemoglobinuria with possible renal damage, cutaneous necrosis by extravasation or reflux (10%) and neuropraxia due to extravascular injection near a motor or sensory nerve.

Sclerotherapy with Microfoam

The introduction of sclerosants in the specific pharmaceutical form of microfoam has transformed the scenario depicted above, since the microfoam physically displaces the blood contained in the vessels and minimizes dilution, allowing better knowledge of the intravenous concentration. Micronisation of the injected sclerosant exponentially increases its surface area with reductions in the bubble diameter, enhancing its therapeutic action and allowing a major reduction in the total dose injected. Moreover, microfoam facilitates a more homogeneous distribution of sclerosant on the endothelial surface and prolongs sclerosant-endothelium contact time. The echogenicity of the microbubbles makes them indirectly visible and the manipulability of the injected microfoam allows it to be steered to areas distant from the injection site. In this way, microfoam allows the in-

travascular administration of a more precise dose of sclerosant [11–13].

Apart from its safety, a further benefit of sclerosing microfoam is its manageability. The high internal cohesion of microfoam means that it can be aspirated and re-injected after its initial injection. The colour of the aspirated microfoam, visible in the catheter, reveals the degree of dilution or intravascular occupation. It ranges from white, when the occupation is exclusive, to pink or red, when there is moderate or major dilution, respectively. Furthermore, since microfoam can be steered within the vessels, the filling can be intensified or attenuated according to the sensitivity of the venous area under treatment.

Microfoam is made with O_2 and CO_2, which are physiological gases. A priori, injection of a gas into the blood stream raises alarm about the possibility of a gas embolism. However, CO_2 has been intravenously injected at doses of 50–100 cc as a contrast in radiological diagnosis since the 1950s. Among the advantages of CO_2 are its fluidity, allowing the use of fine catheters, the absence of toxicity, even at high doses, and its low costs. Thus, on one hand the high solubility of the gases facilitates metabolism in blood and pulmonary diffusibility, and on the other hand the micronisation increases the surface of the gas in exponential form and facilitates its solubility in the corporal liquids. The sclerosant has a greater active surface area for making contact with the endothelium in comparison with the small surface area available to the liquid form. In this way, the dosage of sclerosant in microfoam is more precise and its action more predictable compared with the liquid form. The microfoam does not mix immediately with the blood but displaces it from within the vessel and fills its lumen, so that the sclerosant contacts the endothelia of the veins homogeneously, without dilution and at a known intravascular concentration. Because the vessel can be kept full of microfoam, the sclerosant-endothelium contact time can also be controlled at will [13, 14].

Technique of Treatment with Microfoam in Vascular Malformations

The technique is based on ultrasound-guided injection of polidocanol microfoam [15]. At each session, 20–100 cc of microfoam is injected, corresponding to 3–6 ml of 2% polidocanol. The concentration of polidocanol injected ranges from 0.25 to 4%, according to the size of the malformation and the haemodynamic characteristics of the area to be treated. Thus, infiltrating malformations (Figs. 22.3–22.6) require higher concentrations (2–4%), whereas malformed lateral veins, e.g., the marginal veins (Fig. 22.7–22.10), are treated with lower concentrations (0.25–0.5%). The procedure is performed without anaesthesia and the number of sessions is variable, ranging from a single to several sessions. The interval between sessions is 2–4 weeks. Clinical and radiological improvement is usually possible in the great majority of patients (over 90%).

The main adverse effects are skin pigmentation (which spontaneously disappears) and small necroses. Deep venous thrombosis, pulmonary embolism and neurologic lesions are extremely rare [15].

These benefits of polidocanol contrast with the aggressive effects of absolute alcohol and/or 5% sodium morrhuate on the malformation and on neighbouring tissues. The injection of these agents is also very painful, and hospitalisation, general anaesthesia and post-sclerosis analgesia are required [6]. Furthermore, sodium morrhuate can produce allergic reactions. These two agents must be administered with great caution.

The therapeutic efficacy of polidocanol microfoam depends on its mechanical action in displacing the blood within the vessel. If the blood flow is elevated, dilution of the injected microfoam can result, reducing its effect.

A precise and extensive phlebographic study must be performed to define the characteristics of a predominantly venous malformation or a combined type.

Thus, the lesions can be divided into four groups:
1. Limited malformations without peripheral drainage.
2. Malformations that drain into normal veins.
3. Malformations that drain into dysplastic veins.
4. Malformations that drain into ectatic veins.

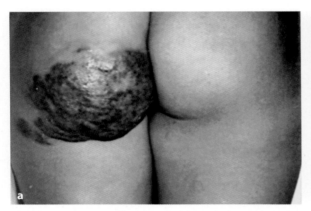 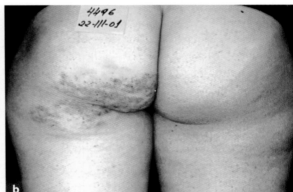

Fig. 22.3. Venous malformation of the right buttock, perineum and genital region, extratruncular, infiltrating form. **a** Before and **b** two years after treatment with ten sessions of sclerotherapy with microfoam

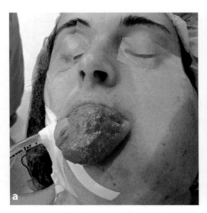 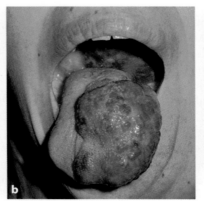 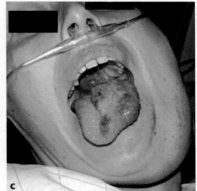

Fig. 22.4. **a** Tongue lesion before treatment. **b** Tongue lesion after two sessions of treatment with microfoam. **c** Tongue lesion and left half of face, after four sessions

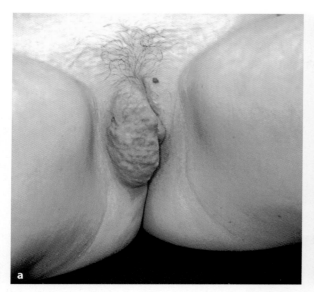
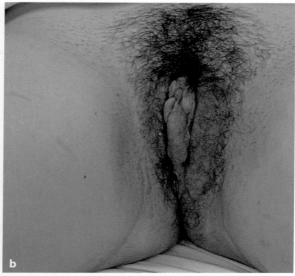

Fig. 22.5. Extratruncular infiltrating venous malformation of the right labium maius with recurrent thrombophlebitis. **a** Before and **b** one year after sclerotherapy with microfoam

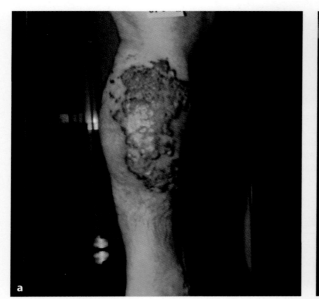
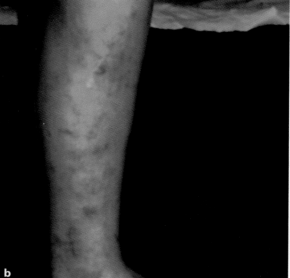

Fig. 22.6. Combined venous malformation of the right lateral shank with extended skin involvement. **a** Before and **b** 2 years after repeated sclerotherapy with microfoam

In routine practice, duplex ultrasonography can often show some areas in venous malformations with abnormal supplies of pulsatile blood delivered by small arteriovenous communications. Therefore, the existence of combined types (see Figs. 22.6–22.11) must be accepted (Table 22.1), or at least the presence of high-flow areas in malformations that are considered low flow. The presence of small arteriovenous fistulas reduces the efficacy of the treatment

and the area initially thromboses after injection, favouring its early partial recanalisation. Attempts can be made to counter this considerable disadvantage by reducing the interval between sclerosis sessions and using a higher concentration of sclerosant. For instance, hand malformations often show a radial artery of increased size and elevated blood flow connected to phlebectasias. In these cases, the high local flow compromises the response to the

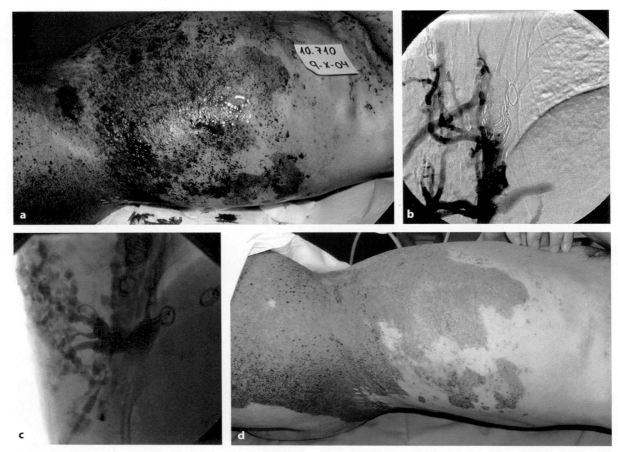

Fig. 22.7. a Combined venous malformation without AV shunt in the skin, extratruncular, with diffuse skin involvement. Important and continued hemorrhage in wall of thorax and abdomen. Severe anemia and progressive general deterioration. **b** Endovascular occlusion of a large vein in the wall of the thorax with coils before treatment with microfoam. **c** After occlusion of the large veins, the wall vessels were treated with large volumes of microfoam over various sessions. **d** Good resolution at the skin level after the end of microfoam treatment

Table 22.1. Classification of vascular malformations (Hamburg, 1988). Data from [1]

Type of defect	Anatomical forms	
	Truncular	Extratruncular
Predominantly arterial	Aplasia or obstruction Dilatation	Infiltrating Limited
Predominantly venous	Aplasia or obstruction Dilatation	Infiltrating Limited
Predominantly lymphatic	Aplasia or obstruction Dilatation	Infiltrating Limited
Predominantly AV shunting	Superficial AV fistulas Deep AV fistulas	Infiltrating Limited
Combined defects	Arterial and venous (without AV shunt)	
	Haemolymphatic (with or without AV shunt)	Infiltrating haemolymphatic Limited haemolymphatic

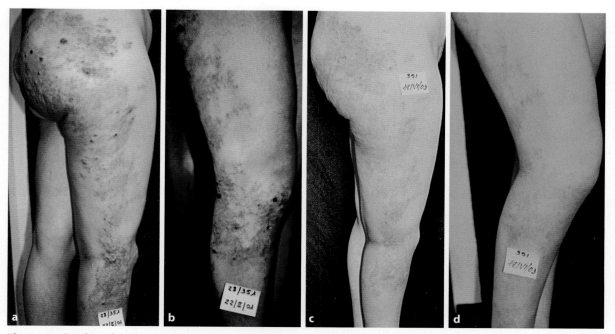

Fig. 22.8. Combined venous malformation without AV shunt, extratruncular, with diffuse skin involvement of the right leg and buttock. **a, b** Before treatment and **c, d** 28 months after several sessions of treatment with sclerosant in microfoam form

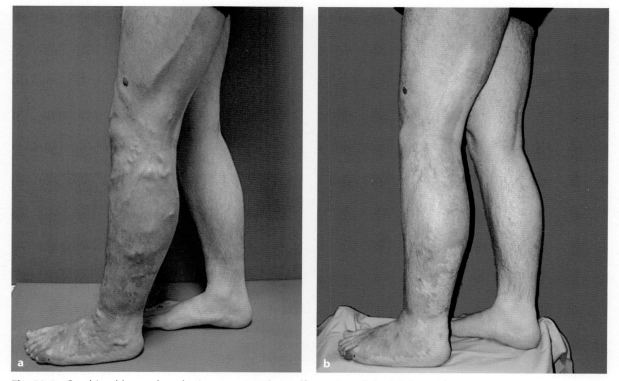

Fig. 22.9. Combined haemolymphatic extratruncular malformation of the left leg with portwine stain and a marginal vein. **a** Before and **b** 6 months after sclerotherapy with microfoam

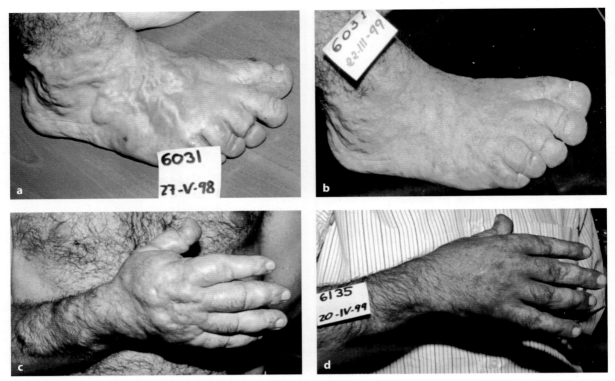

Fig. 22.10. Combined haemolymphatic malformation. The right foot **a** before treatment and **b** 10 months after sclerotherapy and the right hand **c** before treatment and **d** 9 months after sclerotherapy

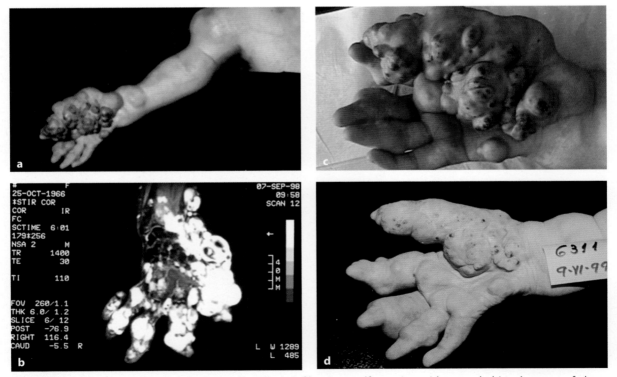

Fig. 22.11. Combined extratruncular haemolymphatic infiltrating malformation with extended involvement of chondrodystrophias and hemangiomatosis of the skin (Mafucci Syndrome). **a**, **b** Before treatment, **c** MRI of the right hand with multiple venectasias, **d** 9 months after several sessions of treatment with sclerosant in microfoam form

sclerosant injection and the technique must be adapted accordingly. For this purpose, we use duplex ultrasonography to identify the most haemodynamically active parts at the start of treatment, compressing the afferent arteries during the injection in order to close up these areas of the malformation. Once the lesion is compartmentalised and haemodynamically "disconnected", it can be more easily closed up in its entirety by successive sessions. Nevertheless, the stability of the vascular occlusion achieved is more precarious than in predominantly venous malformations, and recanalisation is frequent, so that a more rigorous follow-up is required.

We can often only helplessly observe the natural evolution of large venous malformations, unable to provide a definitive effective treatment. Sclerotherapy with microfoam is a therapeutic option that allows the progression of these lesions to be moderated and their size to be reduced in low-flow cases. The simplicity, reproducibility, low cost, safety and strictly out-patient nature of the procedure makes microfoam sclerotherapy the method of choice for the anatomical and

functional elimination of a pathological venous area [15].

With respect to the follow-up, it is evidently essential to differentiate between localized or limited (Figs. 22.1, 22.2) and diffuse or infiltrating vascular malformations (Figs. 22.3–22.5), since the latter require continuous and prolonged treatment, sometimes for years, at best controlling the lesion but never completely eradicating or curing it [4, 10, 16].

Sclerotherapy of Lymphatic Malformations with OK-432

Besides surgery, sclerotherapy with dextrose, tetracyclins and OK-432 has been used to treat lymphatic malformations. The mechanism of action of these substances is diffusion to the stroma and production of irritation and inflammation, favouring the retraction and wound contraction of the lesion. This treatment is extensively explained in the chapter on the treatment of lymphatic malformations.

References

1. Belov S, Loose DA, Weber J (eds) (1989) Vascular malformations. Periodica Angiologica, vol 16. Einhorn Presse Verlag, Reinbek, vol 16, pp 25–27
2. Mulliken JB, Young AE (1988) Vascular birthmarks: hemangiomas and malformations. WB Saunders, Philadelphia
3. Loose DA (2001) Modern tactics and techniques in the treatment of angiodysplasias of the foot. Chir del Piede 25:1–17
4. Lee BB, Mattassi R, Loose DA et al (2005) Consensus on controversial issues in contemporary diagnosis and management of congenital vascular malformation: Seoul communication. Int J Angiol 13:182–192
5. Loose DA (2007) Surgical management of venous malformations. Phlebology 22:276–282
6. Yakes WF, Luethke JM, Parker SH et al (1990) Ethanol embolization of vascular malformations. Radiographics 10:787–796
7. De Lorimier AA (1995) Sclerotherapy for venous malformations. J Pediatr Surg 30:188–194
8. Claesson G, Kuyelenstierna R (2002) OK-432 therapy for lymphatic malformation in 32 patients (28 children). Int J Pediatr Otorhinolaryngol 65:1–6
9. Villavicencio JL (2001) Primum non nocere: Is it always true? The use of absolute ethanol in the management of congenital vascular malformations. J Vasc Surg 33:904–906
10. Belov S (1998) Late results in the treatment of vascular malformations. Int Angiol 7:136–143
11. Cabrera J, Cabrera J Jr, García-Olmedo MA (1997) Elargissement des limites de la sclerotherapie: Nouveaux produits sclerosants. Phlebologie 2:181–188
12. Cabrera J, Cabrera J Jr, García-Olmedo MA (2000) Treatment of varicose long saphenous veins with sclerosant in microfoam form: long-term outcomes. Phebology 15:19–23
13. Cabrera J, Cabrera J Jr (1997) BTG International Limited Assignee. Injectable microfoam containing a sclerosing agent. US patent 5676962
14. Bikerman JJ (1973) Foams. Springer-Verlag, New York
15. Cabrera J, Cabrera J Jr, García-Olmedo MA, Redondo P (2003) Treatment of venous malformations with sclerosant in microfoam form. Arch Dermatol 139:1409–1416
16. Belov S (1990) Classification of congenital vascular defects. Int Angiol 9:141–146

Laser Therapy of Vascular Malformations

23

Hans Peter Berlien

Abstract

In principle the techniques of laser application in congenital vascular tumors and in vascular malformations are similar, but the aim is different. In tumors the aim is to induce regression or fibrosis, in vascular malformations the aim is to destroy the pathologic vascular structure because there is no spontaneous regression. This means that the parameters for treatment of vascular malformations must be more aggressive than for vascular tumors.

Introduction

Due to the potential for regression in congenital vascular tumors, the aim of laser therapy is only to in- duce this regression, while in vascular malformations the pathologic vessels must be destroyed. However, with exception of laser vaporization, all photobiological reactions have a delayed effect. On the other hand, the attitude is that a vascular malformation should be radically excised like a cancer with a high incidence of recurrence, and there is always the danger of massive bleeding and the need for extensive resection which may result in mutilation.

The wide variety of clinical presentations for these anomalies makes it difficult to outline specific management programs. It is important that the appropriate laser and application form be used. Therefore, treatment of these difficult vascular lesions must be carefully individualized. Whereas laser treatments in capillary malformations are the first choice therapy (Fig. 23.1 and Table 23.1), in arteriovenous (AV) mal-

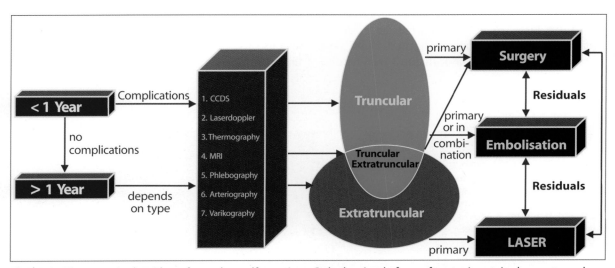

Fig. 23.1. Therapeutic algorithm of vascular malformations. Only the simple form of port wine stain does not need any further diagnostics. In all other cases the visible part of the vascular malformation may be the tip of the iceberg of underlying affections

R. Mattassi, D.A. Loose, M. Vaghi (eds.), *Hemangiomas and Vascular Malformations*.
© Springer-Verlag Italia 2009

Table 23.1. The choice of laser types depends on the depth, the thickness and the kind of malformation. In general more superficial and smaller vessels are an indication for short pulse duration; the deeper and the larger the vessel size and volume, the longer the pulse duration up to CW exposure

Superficial cutaneous

Flat findings	Flash-lamp pumped dye laser
Teleangiectatic findings	Argon laser, KTP
Tuberous findings	Pulsed Nd:YAG laser
Hyperkeratotic findings	CO_2 laser

Intra- and subcutaneous to a depth of 1-15 mm
Impression technique with bare fiber
Transcutaneous Nd:YAG laser with ice-cube cooling

Subcutaneous, voluminous up to a depth of 10 mm
Nd: YAG laser interstitial or intraluminal

Hollow organs, body cavities
Nd: YAG laser endoscopic in air/water

KTP, potassium-tytanyl-phosphate

formations embolization is the first choice therapy. In venous and lymphatic malformations laser therapy is a supplement to surgical excision and sclerotherapy.

Capillary Malformations

Port-Wine Stains (PWS)

Capillary vascular malformations are the most frequent and the oldest indication for laser treatment in both children and adults [1].

With the introduction of the flash lamp pumped pulsed dye laser (FLPDL), PWS can be treated in infancy and early childhood. The high pulse peak power of the pulsed dye laser disrupts the vessels.

The energy fluency ranges from 4 J/cm^2 to 10 J/cm^2 and is varied according to the age of the patient, the anatomic location and the color of the lesion: 5.0 to 5.6 J/cm^2 in children less than 12 months of age, 5.6 to 6.4 J/cm^2 in children 12 months to 4 years of age, and approximately 7 J/cm^2 in children over 4 years of age. Energy is reduced over the eyelids and hands. If blanching or graying of the epidermis occurs during application, energy fluencies should be reduced in order to avoid blistering of the epidermis. Treatments start at the lowest energy density that shows an adequate primary reaction. The lighter the lesion, the higher the energy density for the age range. The darker the lesion, the lower the energy density. Immediately after treatment the area characteristically becomes blue-gray and turns purpuric in a few hours with surrounding erythematous flare: this takes 7–14 days to resolve. Some edema, especially in the periorbital area, is possible. As the purpura disappears, the area lightens progressively for up to 6 weeks. After treatment, the treated areas are covered with panthenol ointment. In case of blistering, parents are instructed to cleanse the area with polyvidone-iodine solution, even if a crust has formed. To avoid postoperative irritation of the treated areas, we instruct the parents to keep their children's fingernails short or that the children wear gloves to avoid trauma to the treated areas. Treatments are usually repeated at 6 week intervals until the desired degree of lightening is achieved.

Adult and teenage patients can often be treated without anesthesia, although this is dependent upon the size and anatomic location of the lesion. General anesthesia is necessary for children with extensive lesions or in case of central facial PWS, because of the need for eye-protection (Fig. 23.2). A significant

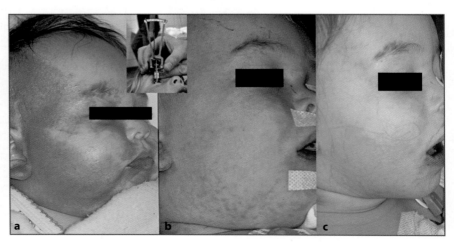

Fig. 23.2. Treatment of Port-Wine stains using the flash-lamp-pumped pulsed dye laser. LPDL-therapy of port wine stain in early childhood. **a** Before treatment. **b**, **c** After 8 and 13 treatments. The earlier the therapy begins, the better the results. Due to intraoperative eye protection in facial lesions general anesthesia is mandatory. In case of Sturge-Weber syndrome anesthesia can be used for further clinical investigations such as instance ophthalmotonometry

reduction of pain as well as skin protection during laser treatment can be achieved using a fluid cooling cuvette or cold air. Some authors use cryogen spray cooling. This can lead to patient discomfort, especially near the nose, eye, mouth or ear.

The incidence of complete clearing is variable. PWS in dermatome V_2 centro-facial regions involving the medial portion of the cheek, upper lip and nose show less lightening than PWS in other locations. Furthermore, lesions on the hand and arm respond less well than lesions on the face, neck, and torso.

Patients younger than 4 years of age require fewer treatments [2]. Treatment of children at the earliest possible age may prevent considerable psychosocial impairment and result in a more complete response. Early treatment of these lesions is expected to prevent the progression of the vessels in the PWS to more ectatic structures that make the lesions dark purple, raised and nodular in many adults. It is hoped that hypertrophy of affected areas, a common complication of extensive PWS, and permanent deformity associated with these lesions can be mitigated. The argon- or potassium-titanyl-phosphate (KTP) laser (power 2 W, pulse duration 0.1 s, interval 0.1 s, spot size 0.05–1 mm) is useful for teleangiectatic PWS and dark purple and nodular PWS of adults, with a good response and a low risk of scarring.

Capillary-Lymphatic Malformation

Capillary-lymphatic malformations may be discriminated from the classical PWS by light staining, and can be bluish-red to black in color. Due to the lower erythrocyte concentration, the basic absorption for the FLPDL is reduced so the results of dye laser therapy are generally worse than for PWS. However, the ectatic venules in the epidermis are a good indication for the KTP, pulsed Nd:YAG or chopped CW Nd:YAG with fluid cooling cuvette (Fig. 23.3). However, in these lesions the birthmark is only the tip of the iceberg. In nearly all cases there is a mixed venous-lymphatic malformation in the underlying organs. Capillary-lymphatic malformations are observed either in association with Klippel-Trenaunay syndrome or alone. So the general anesthesia needed for the laser therapy in childhood may also be used for clinical examinations if necessary.

Hyperkeratotic Capillary Malformation

Angiokeratomas are usually known by their eponyms, matched with the predilection of the lesions: Mibelli for lesions on the hands or feet, Fordyce for lesions on the scrotum, and Fabry for lesions on the trunk or thighs. If only the lymphatic capillaries are affected, this is known as "lymphangioma circumscriptum" [3], but the subcutis may also be affected. Often these lesions bleed easily and weep, either spontaneously or following trauma. Another risk is the high rate of spontaneous erysipelas. The complications provide the indication for laser therapy. KTP laser is mostly not useful due to the high surface absorption. In punctual lesions a pulsed Nd:YAG laser coagulation is helpful but the popcorn-effect due to high energy should be avoided because this can cause bleeding. In disseminated excessive bleeding areas a homogenous CW Nd:YAG laser coagulation through ultrasound

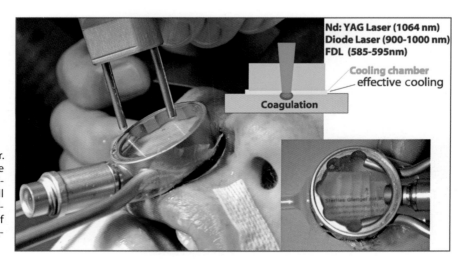

Fig. 23.3. Cooling chamber. The flexible membrane on the patient side of the fluid cooling cuvette can follow all anatomical contours. This allows complete protection of the skin even in difficult regions

jelly is necessary to avoid carbonization. However, this is followed by scarring. In more hyperkeratotic lesions CO_2-laser vaporization is possible, but even this results in scarring (Fig. 23.4).

Port-Wine Stains with Associated Vascular Malformations (Neurocutaneous Syndromes or Phakomatoses)

Capillary or dermal vascular malformations are occasionally associated with deeper vascular anomalies. The key point is that these cutaneous signs permit early diagnosis, thus helping in further recognition of more complex syndromes. Sturge-Weber syndrome is the most well-known vascular malformation complex associated with port-wine staining. The same malformation affects the soft tissue of the face with the risk of subsequent hypertrophy. This can be detected early by color-coded duplex sonography (CCDS) and especially by thermography with hyperthermy. If this is shown despite the FLPDL-therapy, the growing tissue will be treated in cases of dermal hypertrophy with a double pulsed Nd:YAG/pulsed dye laser or in cases of more subcutaneous or soft tissue hypertrophy, with the transcutaneous ice cube-cooled Nd:YAG laser, as for infantile hemangioma but with a higher power of 60 W.

The large PWS of the extremities in Klippel-Trenaunay syndrome sometimes need the same combination of pulsed dye laser, transcutaneous ice cube-cooled Nd:YAG laser or in cases with hyperkeratinization, CO_2 laser. In Proteus syndrome with patchy PWS of the hands or feet the effectiveness of pulsed dye laser therapy is limited, just as it is for other mixed capillary lymphatic malformations. However, even here the treatment of ectatic vessels with pulsed Nd:YAG or KTP laser is possible.

In Wyburn-Mason syndrome/Bonnet-Decaume-Blanc syndrome the facial PWS may be the sign of unilateral arteriovenous malformation of the retina and the intracranial optic pathway (Fig. 23.5). This means that before FLPD laser starts, embolization of the feeding artery is helpful [4].

Nonfading Telangiectasias

Nonfading telangiectasias have been subcategorized under capillary malformations. These present in a spectrum, from the classical spider nevus to the maculopapular punctate anomalies of Osler-Rendu-Weber syndrome, to the characteristic reticulated marbling and cutaneous hypoplasia seen in cutis marmorata telangiectatica congenita (CMTC).

Cutis Marmorata Telangiectatica Congenita (Van Lohuizen Syndrome)

The characteristic lesion of CMTC has a distinctive deep purple color and is depressed in a serpiginous reticulated pattern. In some cases of CMTC-associated deep venous anomalies, ulceration of the reticulated purple areas and hypotrophy of the involved limb and subcutaneous tissue have been reported.

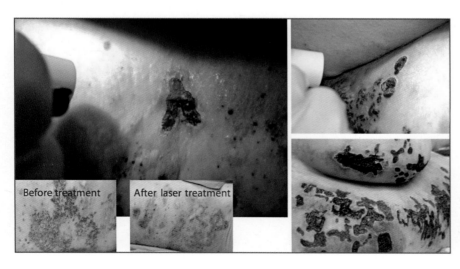

Fig. 23.4. CO_2-laser vaporization. In hyperkeratinization of mixed vascular malformation with the CO_2 laser a bloodless ablation is possible. Due to depth of the disease, scar-free healing is not possible

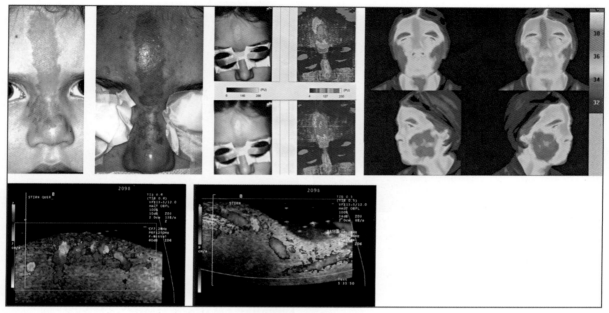

Fig. 23.5. Arteriovenous (AV) malformation. Centro-facial port-wine stains may be only an overlying symptom of a deep vascular malformation. As a screening method thermography is an important investigation. The simple PWS shows normotemperature, whereas a hyperthermia is a sign of an AV malformation. In this case no embolization was possible, so transcutaneous Nd:YAG laser therapy with ice cube-cooling was started to occlude the microfistulas. The result is seen in the CCDS investigation with a decrease in perfusion

The skin atrophy and deep vascular staining can persist into adulthood, along with diffuse ectasia of the veins in the involved extremities. If the steal effect of these pathological vessels causes skin atrophy, coagulation can enhance the microcirculation to avoid further trophic defects. Spider vascular lesions can be obliterated by KTP laser directed at the central artery under compression.

Rendu-Osler-Weber Syndrome (Hereditary Hemorrhagic Telangiectasia)

This disease is classified with the extratruncular capillary malformations and can appear as telangiectasias in the skin and AV malformations widely distributed throughout the body with a predilection for the gums, lips, mucosa of the nose, face and fingers [5].

The major complication is recurrent bleeding, especially of the nasopharyngeal cavity and the gastrointestinal tract with secondary iron deficiency. Beside this manifestation, the most important secondary involvement is the lung [6] and the liver with AV shunts. Cardiac failure, hepatic portosystemic encephalopathy, embolic abscesses, and a variety of neurologic symptoms are complications, resulting in the need for some of these patients to have organ transplantation.

For gastrointestinal bleeding spots, argon beamer electrofulguration is easier to handle endoscopically than side fire laser fiber. However, for all other manifestations Nd:YAG laser therapy is the treatment of choice. For nasal or intraoral spots, including tongue mucous membranes, CW Nd:YAG laser with 600 μ bare fiber in near contact with 12–15 W at 300–400 ms in the repetition mode can be used. Higher power can induce vaporization with opening of the central shunt-artery, and longer exposure times can cause a popcorn effect with massive bleeding. If acute bleeding has occurred one has to remove the blood with continuous saline rinsing during lasering (Fig. 23.6). Here the power must increase to 20–25 W and CW mode. Another option is to compress the bleeding vessel with the Hopf/Jovanovic glass spatula during lasering. Here, even with 20–25 W, the exposure time has to be reduced to prevent carbonization under the glass spatula. For skin lesions including the face, finger or subungual areas, pulsed Nd:YAG laser with intermittent ice cube cooling is the first choice. The parameters vary depending on the laser system, mainly between 50 and 100 J/cm². For micro AV shunts, CCDS-guided interstitial coagulation with 5W and in CW mode is necessary. In larger AV shunts with life threatening bleeding on the face, additional arterial embolization is indicated.

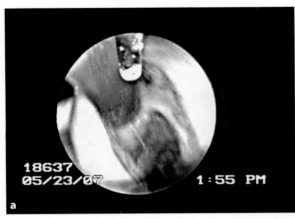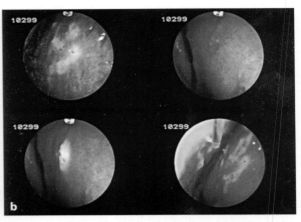

Fig. 23.6. Osler-Weber-Rendu (HHT). The glass spatula compression or rinsing of the blood is necessary during laser therapy of bleeding Osler-spots to prevent vaporization and septum perforation. Nd:YAG-laser, cw; upper septum

Other Telangiectasies

Widespread telangiectasies as a component of other syndromes should also respond to pulsed dye laser treatment [7]. Patients with diffuse telangiectasies as a component of the Rothman-Thompson syndrome or Telangiectasia Macularis Eruptiva Perstans demonstrate dramatic clearing following treatment with pulsed dye laser (Fig. 23.7). Other spider vascular lesions with a central artery show better results with pulsed Nd:YAG laser treatment.

Lymphatic Malformations

Pure lymphatic malformations are only found in the newborn period, but even here the majority of patients show additional venous malformations as mixed malformations [8]. The older the patient, the more the venous part will be important for the complications; e.g., bleeding and overgrowth. The aim of early laser therapy is to reduce this secondary hypertrophy and above all manage these risks.

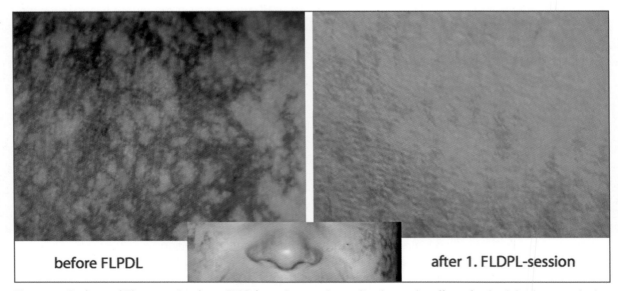

before FLPDL   after 1. FLDPL-session

Fig. 23.7. Rothmund-Thomson-Syndrom. FLPD-laser. One can immediately see the effect of pulsed dye laser on the halo-spaced clearance. A side effect can be long-term persistence of hyperpigmentation due to hemosiderin

Truncular Lymphatic Malformation *Cystic Hygromas*

The isolated single cystic lymphangioma of the neck is a truncular lymphatic malformation and as a rule is better to treat primarily by surgical excision because a previous interstitial Nd:YAG laser coagulation causes fibrosis which affects surgical preparation.

Extratruncular Lymphatic Malformation

If there is an early recurrence after surgery, the lesion was not an isolated truncular lymphatic malformation, but an extratruncular malformation. In extratruncular lymphatic malformations the discrimination between micro- and macrocystic is not precise, but rather like a screen shot. By changing of resorption or production, the size of the cysts can change in short time periods. Furthermore, due to spontaneous rupture of the interseptal pathologic veins massive bleeding can occur. Only a pure microcystic malformation, called solid lymphangioma, is its own entity and is indicated for surgical resection. In all other cases, depending on the actual local situation, different combinations of CW Nd:YAG laser techniques are used.

Intraluminal (Intracystic) Technique

Larger cysts are punctured under CCDS control to prevent a direct puncture of interseptal veins and to string several cysts. If the diameter is more than 2 cm it is helpful to reduce the size by suction of the lymph fluid. In cases of previous hemorrhage, flushing with saline is necessary until the fluid is clear (Fig. 23.8). The kind of puncture cannula depends on the lesion. If possible, 16 or 18 G Teflon vein cannulas are preferred because this material has no heat conduction risk from the heated tip. In larger lymphangiomas or in anatomically difficult regions where the puncture directions must change, a steel cannula is easier to handle but carries the risk of skin burning. As there is a lower basic absorption without erythrocytes, a power of approximately 10 W CW Nd:YAG laser is used [9]. The coagulation is stopped when an extensive color bruit is seen on the CCDS. Near the interseptal veins the power must be reduced to prevent a vein perforation. If there is no risk of communication with vessels or body cavities additional sclerotherapy can be helpful, e.g., with Picibanil [10]. The aim of laser coagulation in this combination is to destroy the lymph cyst's epithelium in order

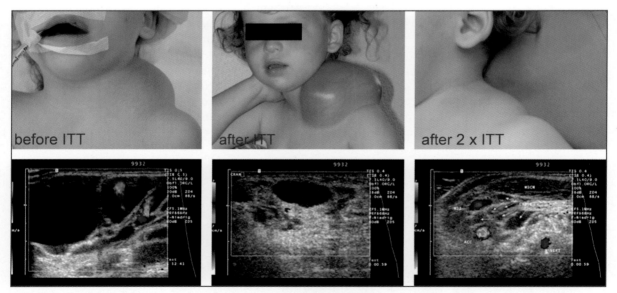

before ITT   after ITT   after 2 x ITT

Fig. 23.8. Interstitial Nd:YAG-lasercoagulation (ITT). The CCDS shows the intraseptal pathological veins which cause recurrent bleeding. During interstitial or intracystic Nd:YAG laser coagulation one has to avoid direct puncture of these veins to reduce the risk of intraoperative bleeding

to enhance the effectiveness of the sclerotherapy. The puncture direction must never cross the nerve direction to avoid direct nerve palsy. However, due to postoperative swelling, an increasing hypesthesia or disesthesia can occur within the next few days. This is transient and heals without any defects within a few weeks.

Microcystic (*Solid*) Lymphatic Malformation "ITT"

If a surgical resection due to the infiltrative growth or other risks is not possible, interstitial laser coagulation is possible. The biophysical basis is that the thin lymph cysts walls are transparent for the Nd:YAG laser near-infrared radiation. This means that not only the direct punctured cyst will be irradiated, but also the surrounding areas. In contrast to the above or to the intraluminal techniques described later in venous malformations, here there exists a direct contact of the 600 µ bare fiber with the adjacent tissue. This means that power of more than 5–7 W leads to a carbonization at the fiber end which absorbs all laser energy. The effect is that vaporization occurs at the fiber but no radiation can transmit to the tissue to perform large volume coagulation. Here additional sclerotherapy makes no sense and is dangerous.

Bare Fiber Contact Vaporization

What was described in the previous section as something to be avoided, must immediately be induced in the treatment of mucous membrane hyperkeratotic cysts, such as intraoral or anogenital cysts, with a high power of 30 W and chopped mode carbonization of the fiber end to prevent uncontrolled deep coagulation and to perform bloodless vaporization. Especially in the mouth there are mixed venous-lymphatic vesicules which have a high risk of recurrent bleeding, superinfection and foetor ex ore (Fig. 23.9). Postoperatively there is no specific treatment necessary, only continuous rinsing with fluid [11].

Endoscopic Coagulation

Palatinal, hypopharyngeal and laryngeal as well urethral, bladder and intravaginal lymphatic cysts are coagulated with the non contact method comparable to the methods described in the chapter on laser therapy of hemangiomas. In the oropharynx, direct coagulation in the near contact procedure is possible with 15–20 W and chopped mode. The more venous the parts with higher basic absorption, the greater the risk of the popcorn effect or direct vaporization. In a frog egg situation on the larynx, the Werner-ice-water-technique gives a good overview of the malformation and prevents carbonization of the surface. The power has to be increased to 20–25 W, depending on the venous component. In the bladder or in the genital tract, endoscopic coagulation is performed under continuous saline rinsing. Even here, the greater the venous component, the greater the risk of popcorn effect. Often the lymphatic malformations are combined with a chylothorax and chylopericardium and a pleural adhesion, and are called Gorham-Stout syndrome (or disappearing bone disease). Here an endoscopic CW Nd:YAG laser coagulation of the ectatic lymph vessels to reduce the chylous extravasation is possible.

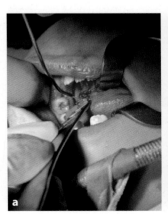 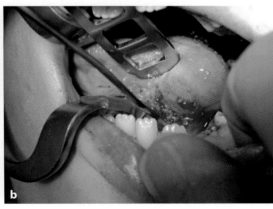

Fig. 23.9. Nd:YAG-laser treatment with direct bare fibre or impression. In contrast to the case described in Figure 23.10, with impression coagulation with a higher power of approximately 30 W and pulse of 0.5 s, contact vaporization of the small lymphatic cysts occurs. For larger cysts with risk of bleeding, a pre-coagulation with lower power and longer pulse duration is helpful

Venous Malformations

Venous malformation of the head and neck region presents in a wide spectrum, from circumscribed venous anomalies in which the venous lacunae are connected to the venous circulation by capillaries, through to localized venous anomalies connected by veins to the venous circulation, and diffuse venous ectasias. Furthermore, multiple venous lesions tend to coexist with venous ectasias and deep vein anomalies [12]. In principle the laser procedures are similar to the lymphatic treatments or the congenital vascular tumor protocols. However, in contrast to lymphatic malformations, here there is a high absorption of the Nd:YAG laser near infrared radiation in the blood, so the parameters have to be adapted to this absorption.

Truncular Venous Malformation

Laser coagulation is, in contrast to sclerotherapy, a local and not a regional procedure. This is not good or bad: it is a fact. This means that no systemic or distant side effects can occur, but it also means that an effect can occur only where the laser hits the tissue. Furthermore, blood is a perfect absorber so the laser radiation does not hit the vessel wall, but cooks the blood. To prevent this effect one has to remove all blood completely by rinsing the fiber. This explains why in simple varicose veins, which can be treated easily with foam or radiofrequency, intraluminal lasertherapy is not used. So laser is an ideal tool for diseases that cannot treated with easier techniques. Large truncular venous malformations, such

as enlarged persistent marginal veins, are a better indication for surgery or sclerotherapy. However, in a difficult anatomical situation such as after previous surgery or in incomplete marginal veins, an intraluminal procedure is indicated. Comparable to the macrocystic lymphatic malformation, under CCDS control the vessel is punctured and a saline rinse is installed to clean up the fiber tip. With an maximum power of 10 W under CCDS the coagulation is performed, while any direct contact of the fiber end with the vessel wall has to be avoided (Fig. 23.10) [13]. This would immediately cause a perforation with bleeding. Another option is the use of diffuse irradiating interstitial applicators, which are used for the therapy of interstitial malignancies, such as liver tumors. The advantage is that vessel wall coagulation is more homogeneous; the disadvantage is that the puncture is larger and more difficult to handle. A string maneuver in kinked vessels is nearly impossible.

Extratruncular Venous Malformation

Similar to extratruncular lymphatic malformations, all tissues can be affected by extratruncular venous malformations and so all the above-described laser techniques are in use. In the following paragraphs only specific parameters that are different from the above will be described.

Soft Tissue Phlebectasias

Because the vessel wall as opposed to the blood is the target, if possible the ectatic vessel will not be punc-

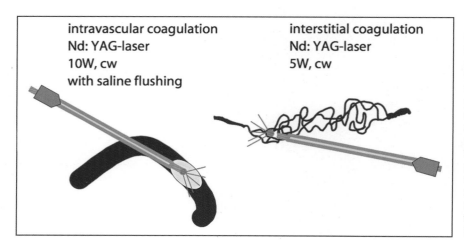

intravascular coagulation
Nd: YAG-laser
10W, cw
with saline flushing

interstitial coagulation
Nd: YAG-laser
5W, cw

Fig. 23.10. Interstitial coagulation. In principle the technique of intraluminal and interstitial Nd:YAG laser coagulation is the same, only the parameters have to be changed. In endovascular laser application the blood has to removed completely from the fiber end with rinsing, so the power has to be increased up to 10 W. In all other cases of interstitial laser application the maximum power for coagulation is 5 W, otherwise vaporization starts immediately

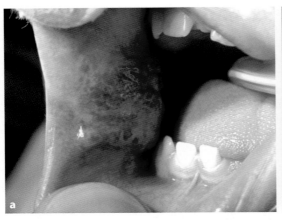
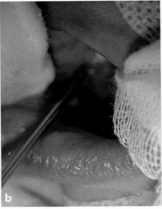
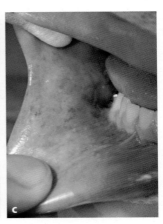

Fig. 23.11 a-c. In smaller lesions or in endangered regions, besides the ITT technique, the impression technique is another option for under surface coagulation. Only on the contact point of the bare fiber with the mucosa is there a fast healing coagulation point. The power is the same as in ITT, the coagulation volume underneath depends on the exposure time

tured, but irradiated paravasally, as with perforator vein laser coagulation (Fig. 23.11). In cases where a paravasal application is not possible, but only an intraluminal application similar to the truncular procedure, the fiber tip has to be rinsed with saline solution to prevent carbonization followed by perforation. If there is no direct drainage over larger veins an additional sclerotherapy can be performed. Postoperatively a compression bandage is obligatory for 24 hours. Localized intravascular coagulopathy (LIC) is not a contraindication for this technique because a thrombus formation can be avoided with this procedure.

Cutaneous/Subcutaneous Malformation

The combination of cutaneous and subcutaneous malformation, also known as the blue rubber bleb nevus syndrome, can be treated like a congenital vascular tumor, with the transcutaneous ice cube-cooled Nd:YAG laser technique (Fig. 23.12). However, here a higher power of at least 50–60 W is needed because induction of regression and also direct coagulation is necessary. In cases of intracutaneous lesions a scar formation in the affected region is not always avoidable.

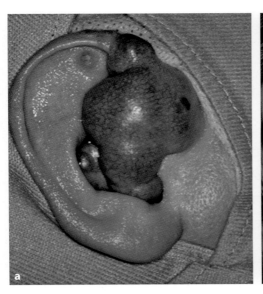
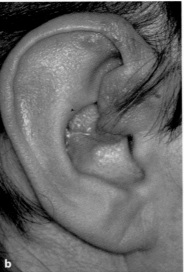

Fig. 23.12. Transcutaneous Nd: YAG-laser treatment with ice cube cooling. **a** Before treatment. **b** After 6 treatments. Comparable to the technique in vascular tumors, the transcutaneous ice cube-cooling Nd:YAG laser irradiation is even used in vascular malformations. In case of enlarged vessels one must take care to prevent a popcorn effect

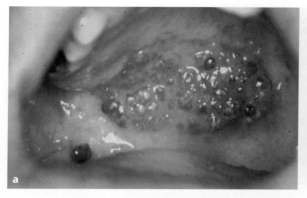

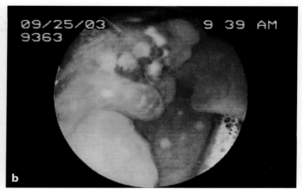

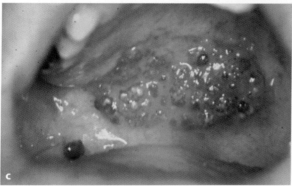

Fig. 23.13. Transmucosal Nd:YAG-laser treatment under ice water protection. In mucous membrane lesions in the oropharynx, Nd:YAG laser irradiation through ice water can prevent vaporization with subsequent bleeding. These small coagulation points on the mucosa will heal without any scars

Mucous Membrane Affection

The main localization for a mucous membrane affection is the oropharynx, followed by the vagina and the rectum. In case of hypopharyngeal or laryngeal lesions the Werner procedure is obligatory in order to avoid any popcorn effect with massive bleeding (Fig. 23.13). In case of laryngeal localization, it is important to coagulate step-by-step over several sessions to lessen the risk of an airway obstruction necessitating a postoperative intubation. In tracheal lesions the procedure is similar to tracheal infantile hemangioma. Vaginal lesions are coagulated endoscopically under water, intrarectal lesion treatment depends on the extent of the lesion.

Glomuvenous Malformation ("Glomangioma")

Cases of large raised, soft, and compressible glomangiomas have been mistakenly diagnosed as blue rubber bleb nevus syndrome [14]. Glomangiomas are less likely to be painful than solitary glomus tumors. An effective therapy for multiple glomangiomas (glomangiomatosis) is treatment with Nd:YAG laser with continuous surface cooling. In solitary lesions the interstitial puncture technique is used as for microcystic lymphangioma.

Arterial Malformations

At present, the first choice therapy for the management of troublesome AV malformations is embolization, either alone or following laser therapy. The therapeutic principle in embolization is to deliver the embolic material into the center of the vascular anomaly (the nidus) in an attempt to block the smallest vessels first, from the inside out. For extensive lesions, interstitial Nd:YAG laser coagulation may help by obliterating all microfistulas in order to collapse the AV malformation permanently, or collateral vessels can develop very slowly.

Truncular Arterio-Venous Fistula

In general the pure truncular AV malformation is successfully treated with embolization. However, in some cases the peripheral smaller vessels remain and are an indication for laser therapy. Depending on the size and origin, the pulsed dye laser, the KTP laser, the pulsed Nd:YAG laser or the CW Nd:YAG laser chopped with the fluid cooling chamber are used. For fistulas which are not treated by embolization, a paravasal or intraluminal Nd:YAG laser coagulation is performed (Fig. 23.14) [15]. The surrounding pathological vessels are treated in the same session with

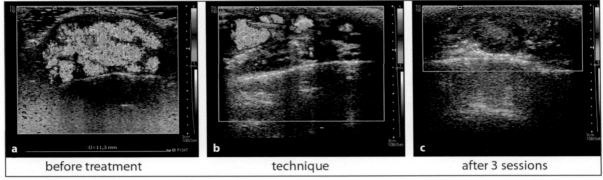

before treatment   technique   after 3 sessions

Fig. 23.14. Scalp-AV-fistula Nd: YAG-laser-ITT-technique. **a** Arteriovenous fistula on the scalp. Due to different feeding arteries, even from the ophthalmic artery, there was no possibility for previous embolization. After three sessions of paravasal interstitial coagulation of the nidus the perfusion decreased (**b, c**)

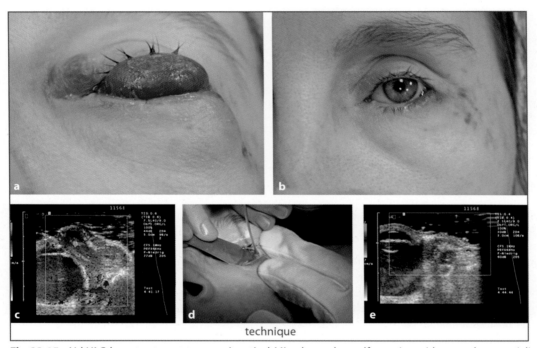

technique

Fig. 23.15. Nd: YAG-laser treatment transconjunctival. Mixed vascular malformation with secondary arterialization (**a** before treatment; **b** after 3 sessions). Due to risk of uncontrolled emboli in the ophthalmic artery, the impression technique allows a precise application of laser energy to subcutaneous volumes. Even though no scattering can occur, near the eye the bulb and the cornea must be protected by a metal spatula (**d**)

high power transcutaneous ice cube-cooled Nd:YAG laser. Depending on the size of the lesion, multiple punctures with the afterloading technique and several sessions are necessary.

Combined Truncular/Extratruncular Arterio-Venous Malformation

Beside the case of the capillary malformations described earlier, the most important malformation for laser therapy is the hamartous AV malformation (*angioma racemosum*). Even in AV fistulas the first choice is embolization. However, this is not always possible and even after successful embolization in the periphery, small fistulas remain. Here an interstitial laser therapy or a transcutaneous ice cube-cooled Nd:YAG laser therapy is needed (Fig. 23.15). Mucous membrane bleeding is directly coagulated because here scar formation is not a concern.

References

1. Noe JM, Barsky SH, Geer DE, Rosen S (1980) Port wine stains and the response to argon laser therapy: successful treatment and the predictive role of color, age, and biopsy. Plast Reconstr Surg 65:130–136
2. Poetke M, Philipp C, Urban P, Berlien HP (2001) Interstitial laser treatment of venous malformations. Med.Laser Appl 16:111–119
3. Whimster IW (1976) The pathology of lymphangioma circumscriptum. Brit J Dermatol 94:473
4. Yakes WE (1989) Alcohol embolotherapy of vascular malformation. Sem Intervent Radiol 6:146–161
5. Menefee MG, Flessa HC, Glueck HI, Hogg S (1985) Hereditary hemorrhagic telangiectasia (Osler-Weber-Rendu disease): an electron microscopy study of the vascular lesions before and after therapy with hormones. Arch Otolarygol 101:246–251
6. Wirbelauer J, Thomas W, Darge K, Singer D (2007) Zentrale Zyanose und Verdichtungen im Thoraxröntgenbild bei einem Säugling. Monatsschr Kinderheilkunde 155:789–792
7. Bekov V, Bonsmann G, Kuhn A (2007) Kollagenosen Monatsschr Kinderheilkunde 156:122–133
8. Vogt R, Gillessen-Kaesbach (2007) Das Noonan-Syndrom. Pädiatr Praxis 69:719–726
9. Poetke M, Bültmann O, Urban P, Berlien HP (1998) Vaskuläre Malformationen im Kindes- und Erwachsenenalter. Therapie mit dem Nd: YAG-Laser. Vasomed 10:338–347
10. Helmstaedter V, Quante G, Roth B et al (2007) Behandlung lymphatischer Malformationen mit Lysat attenuierter Streptokokken (Picibanil/OK-432). Monatsschr Kinderheilkunde 155:1077–1082
11. Poetke M (2003) Laser treatment in haemangiomas and vascular malformations. In: Berlien H-P, Müller G. Applied Laser Medicine, Springer
12. Sürücü O, Sure U, Stahl S et al (2007) Neue CCM1-Mutation bei einem 2-jährigen. Monatsschr Kinderheilkunde 155:1161–1165
13. Urban P (2006) Vaskuläre Malformationen. In: Kubale R, Stiegler H. Farbkodierte Duplexsonographie. Thieme, Stuttgart
14. Höger P (2005) Kinderdermatologie, Differenzialdiagnostik und Therapie bei Kindern und Jugendlichen. Schattauer, Stuttgart
15. Poetke M, Philipp C, Großewinkelmann A et al (2001) Die Behandlung von Naevi flammei bei Säuglingen und Kleinkindern mit dem blitzlampengepumpten Farbstofflaser. Monatsschrift Kinderheilkunde 32:405–415

The Combined Treatment of Arteriovenous Malformations

24

Dirk A. Loose

Abstract

In arteriovenous malformations (AVM), the tactics and techniques of combined treatment have been worked out adapting surgical and non-surgical methods. The most common combinations include surgery, catheter embolization and ethanol sclerotherapy. Strict indications should be followed when choosing the appropriate procedures and timing. The best long-term follow-up results are obtained with the combination of presurgery catheter embolization and surgery. Alcohol sclerotherapy has gained an important role in combined treatment. Experience has demonstrated that the indication for catheter embolization in the limbs when distally performed should take into consideration the danger of peripheral necrosis. Correct combination with surgery and/or ethanol sclerotherapy may avoid such a complication.

Introduction

The first documented treatment of cases with length discrepancy and arteriovenous (AV) malformations of the extremities occurred in 1853, but it is only recently that the true connection between these two entities has become obvious. The Hamburg Classification allowed the latest therapeutic concept in the modern era of vascular surgery to be developed: the combined treatment. This consists not only of operative occlusion of the vascular malformation with obstruction by sutures of its feeding arteries and, if possible, excision, but also of further surgical and non-surgical methods.

This treatment is the therapy of choice in predominantly AV congenital vascular defects. It is a logical improvement over the formerly recommended sole approach of skeletonization of the fistula feeding segment of the afferent artery. It makes it possible to treat even the smallest AV shunting vascular defects. This approach became feasible through the development of new catheter technologies and occlusive materials. Skeletonization of the afferent stem artery as sole treatment, or its application after embolization, is no longer recommended, because this removes any further opportunity for embolization of persisting AV fistulas with renewed hemodynamic activity. In fact, in some cases where skeletonization therapy had already been performed, it has been necessary to reattach the larger of the ligated arterial branches in order to allow embolization therapy to be performed.

The therapy consists of non-surgical and surgical treatment and is the therapy of choice in severe predominantly arteriovenous congenital vascular defects. It does not consist of alternative or competitive techniques; rather, the non-surgical and the surgical forms of treatment are complementary.

Non-Surgical Methods of Treatment

Non-surgical methods of treatment include laser-therapy, sclero-therapy and embolization-therapy.

The indications for non-surgical treatment are:
1. Laser-therapy: appropriate for all persisting capillary AV lesions, where no feeder artery for embolization treatment is present.
2. Sclero-therapy: the foam technique is a good alternative and/or adjunctive treatment for superficial malformed vessels; the ethanol technique is also indicated for deep AV malformations.
3. Embolization-therapy: appropriate for all hypervascular lesions with AV shunting (dependent on the morphological form and the site of the lesions).

R. Mattassi, D.A. Loose, M. Vaghi (eds.), *Hemangiomas and Vascular Malformations*.
© Springer-Verlag Italia 2009

Surgical Methods of Treatment

Surgical methods include operations to remove the vascular defect, where feasible; operations to reduce the hemodynamic activity of the vascular defect; and other, non-hemodynamic procedures.

Because the different morphological forms of AV defects most frequently appear in mixed combinations, many cases will require combined treatment, using multidisciplinary skills. In many cases severe enough to require treatment, surgery or embolization alone cannot succeed and may not be appropriate because of an inaccessible location of the defect or the impossibility of reaching the "nidus" by catheter. Thus, surgical treatment and embolization may have to be combined or completed with other non-surgical methods.

Surgery can be combined with embolization, performed preoperatively, intraoperatively or postoperatively.

Preoperative Embolization

Preoperative embolization is extended over several sessions and is the most effective approach. Ideally, it can be combined with surgical occlusion-sutures in persisting very small AV fistulas which cannot be reached by the catheter. This can be performed after the ischemic reactions and inflammatory signs of the embolized tissues have abated (Figs. 24.1–24.8).

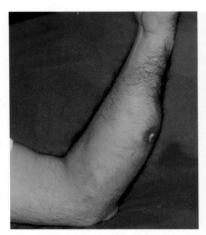

Fig. 24.1. Typical clinical aspect of a left lower arm with ulceration and swelling caused by an AVM. The patient complained of continuous pulsating pain and heat in his left arm

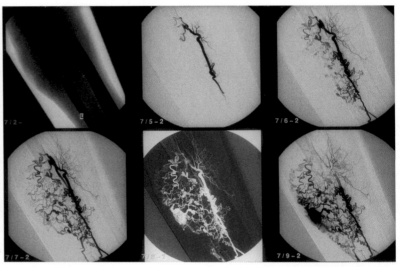

Fig. 24.2. Only a super selective arteriography is able to reveal AV fistulas originating mainly in the interosseal artery and its side branches

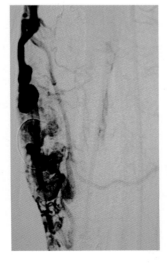

Fig. 24.3. After interventional embolization treatment of the interosseal artery the control arteriography demonstrates residual AV fistulas in the region of the ulnar artery

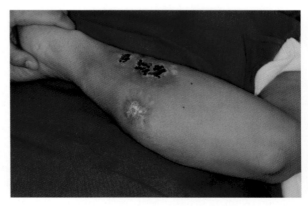

Fig. 24.4. The clinical aspect 2 weeks after embolization demonstrates the reduction of the ischemic ulceration of the lower arm and a superficial skin necrosis resulting from interventional embolization treatment

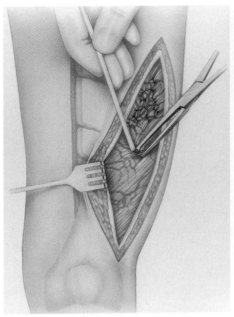

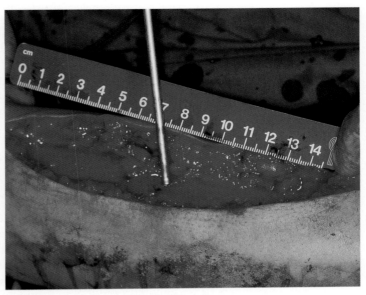

Fig. 24.6. Loose II technique (1997) during surgery

Fig. 24.5. Representation of the Loose II (1997) technique: Doppler identification and mapping of AV fistulas during surgery and subsequent ligation. Control of fistula occlusion by Doppler during surgery

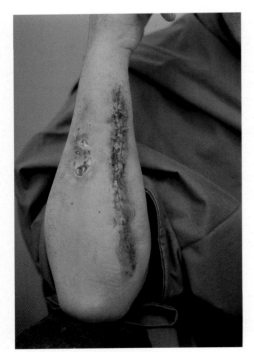

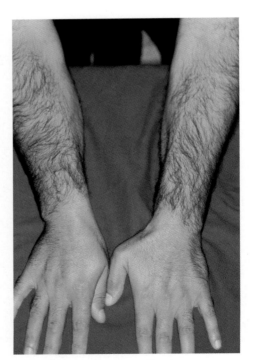

Fig. 24.7. Clinical aspect of the left arm 12 days after surgery. The ischemic necrosis as well as the underlying AV fistulas were resected or occluded. A superficial skin necrosis after interventional embolization treatment is healing up

Fig. 24.8. Clinical aspect of both arms 3 years after surgery of the left arm

Intraoperative Embolization

Intraoperative embolization techniques have several disadvantages:

1. A higher rate of complications because the method of application results in a diffused distribution like an embolic shower, and is not directed into a specific artery and aimed at the nidus, as in the catheter technique.
2. In most cases it is not possible to perform embolization, surgical occlusion of the feeding arteries and excision of the AV defect in one step. The ischemic reaction would potentially be too intense and the extremity could even be lost. That is why multiple operations would be required, each becoming more difficult. In contrast, the catheter embolization performed over several sessions, followed by a well-planned operation, as indicated, gives much better long-term results.
3. The majority of operating rooms do not have the latest imaging devices with specialized technical refinements found in departments for interventional radiology. These are necessary for embolization therapy to be safely and accurately applied.

Postoperative Embolization

Postoperative embolization can be performed if, after preoperative embolization and surgical excision of the AV defect, residual AV fistulas remain or newly appear and have to be occluded.

Ethanol sclerotherapy can be combined with surgery and/or catheter embolization.

Before treatment starts, the precise plan of attack has to be decided upon. Ordinarily it should be coordinated by the vascular surgeon. When working as a multidisciplinary team, the main question is whether treatment should be predominantly surgical or predominantly embolization.

Although the treatment of every patient has to be individualized, there are some major guidelines that can be followed. It is essential to understand that the relative risks and benefits of the combined treatment depend to a great degree on the location of the congenital vascular defect.

For the upper extremity, catheter embolization therapy should generally not be applied distally beyond the wrist. Here, severe peripheral vasospasm and/or digital necrosis can occur.

For the lower extremity, embolization-therapy should generally not be applied distally, beyond the proximal calf level. Should it be necessary to perform treatment distal to the above-mentioned levels, then surgery is clearly the method of choice, although we have had a few patients with diffuse, infiltrating AV lesions in the foot where surgery has been successfully combined with embolization therapy. Thus, for both upper and lower extremities, embolization therapy dominates for the most proximally located lesions (i.e., shoulder and buttock regions). Beyond that level, surgery predominates, combined with embolization therapy mainly around the elbow or knee (Tables 24.1–24.3, Figs. 24.9–24.14).

Our experience has shown that the pathoanatomical form of the congenital defects with predominantly shunting greatly influences the recommended choice of treatment. For truncular forms with deep AV fistulas, surgery predominates as the treatment of choice. For truncular forms with superficial AV fistulas, surgery is mainly indicated where the AV communications must be removed together with segments of dilated afferent veins. The main candidates for the combined treatment are those with extra-truncular forms, either diffusely infiltrating or localized. In both instances, combining surgical and non-surgical treatment is recommended (Table 24.3). The most appropriate course of treatment is determined on the basis of the specific hemodynamic aspects of each individual case (Figs. 24.15–24.33).

Table 24.1. Recommended application of combined treatment relative to location of lesion: upper extremity

Location of Lesion	Type of Combined Treatment	
	Predominantly Surgery	**Embolization**
Shoulder	X	X
Upper arm	X	X
Elbow	X	X
Forearm to wrist	X	(X)
Hand distal to wrist joint	X	(X)

Table 24.2. Recommended application of combined treatment relative to location of lesion: lower extremity

Location of Lesion	Type of Combined Treatment	
	Predominantly Surgery	**Embolization**
Buttocks	X	X
Upper thigh	X	X
Knee	X	X
Proximal calf	X	X
Distal calf	X	(X)
Ankle	X	(X)
Foot	X*	(X)

* Dependent on pathoanatomic form

Table 24.3. Recommended application of combined treatment relative to the pathoanatomic form for predominantly AV shunting defects

Pathoanatomic Form	Type of Treatment	
	Surgery	**Embolization**
Truncular Forms		
Deep AV fistulas	X	
Superficial AV fistulas	X	(X)
Extratruncular Forms		
Diffuse, infiltrating	X	X
Localized	X	X

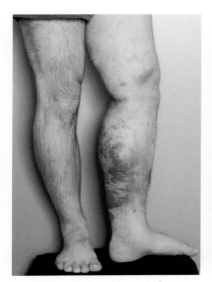 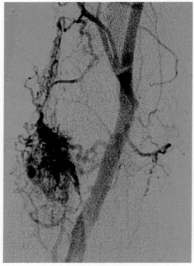 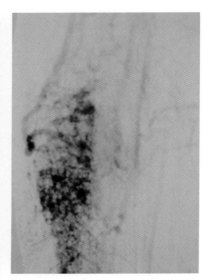

Fig. 24.9. Clinical aspect of an extended AV malformation of the left calf with skin involvement and ischemic pre-ulcerations as a consequence of untreated AV malformation

Fig. 24.10. After interventional embolization treatment, residual infiltrating AV fistulas are obvious in the control arteriography of the popliteal artery

Fig. 24.11. After interventional embolization treatment, residual infiltrating AV fistulas are obvious in the control arteriography also of the posterior tibial artery

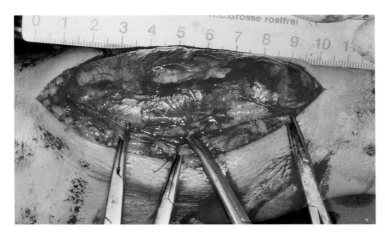

Fig. 24.12. During surgery the gastrocnemius muscle infiltrated by AV fistulas is developed

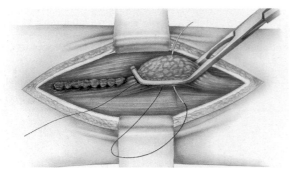

Fig. 24.13. In the technique of Belov IV (1992) the main part of the infiltrated muscle is clamped and the basis is oversewn by an over-and-over Blalock suture

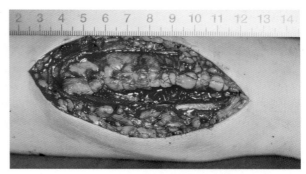

Fig. 24.14. The aspect after a partial excision of the gastrocnemius muscle which was infiltrated by AV fistulas

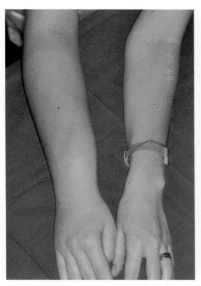

Fig. 24.15. A lower right arm demonstrating a swelling caused by an AV malformation. The patient complained of heat and pain

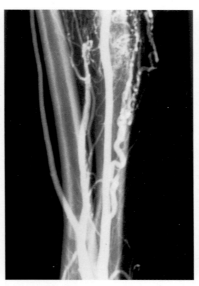

Fig. 24.16. The arteriography of the arteries of the forearm demonstrates AV fistulas nourished by a hyperplastic interosseal artery

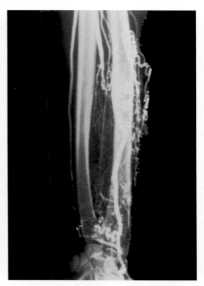

Fig. 24.17. By interventional embolization treatment the interosseal artery was embolized and the arteriography demonstrates a plain circulation of the ulnar artery whereas the radial artery still nourishes some infiltrating AV fistulas

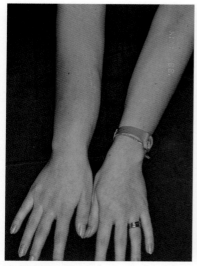

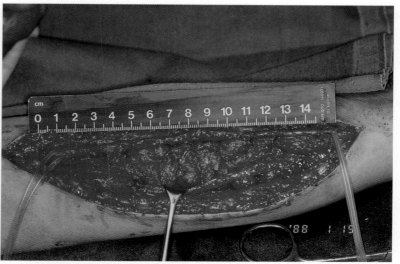

Fig. 24.18. Clinical aspect 4 weeks after embolization treatment: the swelling of the right lower arm is dramatically diminished

Fig. 24.19. In the concept of a combined treatment during surgery, many AV fistulas have to be ligated (skeletonization of the radial artery with the technique of Malan 1974) and occlusion of infiltrating AV fistulas with the technique of Loose II (1997) by means of ultrasonic control. The figure demonstrates the situation during surgery after these techniques had been performed

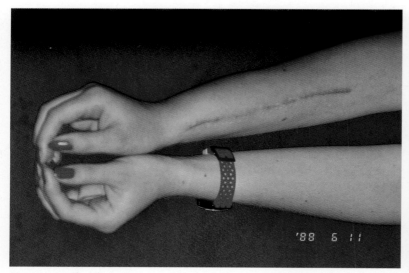

Fig. 24.20. The clinical aspect of both lower arms 4 weeks after surgery (combined treatment) of the right lower arm

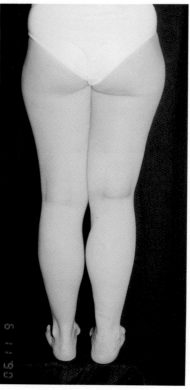

Fig. 24.21. Clinical aspect of legs with a length discrepancy (hypoplasia of the thigh and hyperplasia of the right calf)

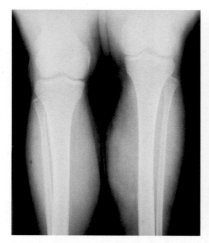

Fig. 24.22. X-ray of both lower legs demonstrating length discrepancy of the right tibial bone

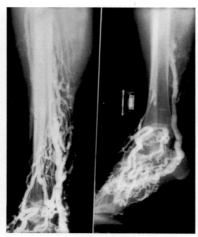

Fig. 24.23. Phlebography of the right leg with many dysplastic veins in the foot and calf region. The venous system is secondarily dilated by AV fistulas

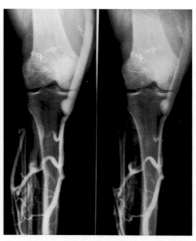

Fig. 24.24. Phlebography of the right leg with many dysplastic veins in the foot and calf region. The venous system is secondarily dilated by AV fistulas

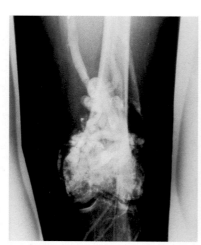

Fig. 24.25. Femoral arteriography of the right leg revealing huge AV fistulas in the knee joint region

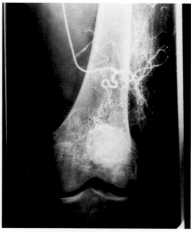

Fig. 24.26. Interventional embolization treatment of AV fistulas in the distal thigh region and in the knee joint as the first step of combined treatment

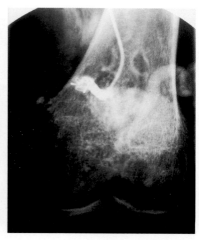

Fig. 24.27. Interventional embolization treatment of AV fistulas in the distal thigh region and in the knee joint as the first step of combined treatment

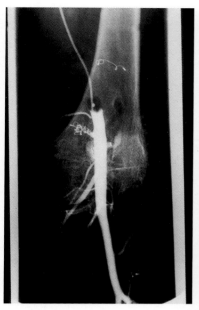

Fig. 24.28. Control arteriography (occlusion balloon technique) of the popliteal artery demonstrating that no hemodynamically important AV fistulas remained

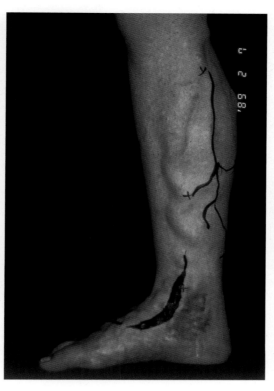

Fig. 24.29. Clinical aspect of the right calf and foot region with extensive dilation of veins as a result of congenital AV fistulas. It is important to realize that in congenital AV malformations not only the AV fistulas, but also the secondarily dilated veins have to be treated, in order to remove peripheral venous insufficiency and prevent venous ulceration

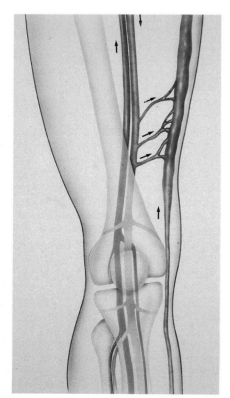

Fig. 24.30. Schematic representation of residual AV fistulas in combined treatment. These fistulas have to be ligated surgically

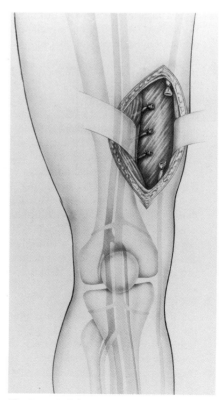

Fig. 24.31. Schematic representation after ligation of residual AV fistulas and after en bloc resection of muscle with superficial veins and with AV fistulas

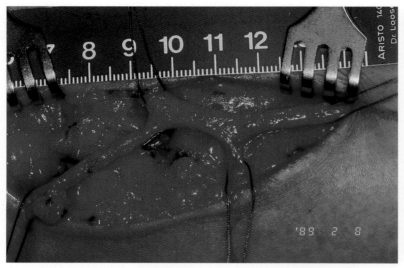

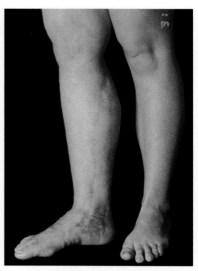

Fig. 24.32. Intraoperative picture demonstrating left-over AV fistulas and dilated veins

Fig. 24.33. Clinical aspect 2 years after combined treatment

References

1. Allison DJ, Kennedy A (1989) Embolization techniques in arteriovenous malformations. In: Belov S, Loose DA, Weber J (eds) Vascular malformations: Periodica Angiologica, Vol 16. Einhorn Presse, Reinbek, pp 261–269
2. Belov S, Loose DA, Müller E (1985) Angeborene Gefäßfehler. Einhorn Presse Verlag, Reinbek, pp 24–25
3. Belov S, Loose DA, Mattassi R et al (1989) Therapeutical strategy, surgical tactics and operative techniques in congenital vascular defects (multicentre study). In: Strano A, Novo S (eds) Advances in vascular pathology, Vol 2. Excerpta Medica, New York, pp 1355–1360
4. Belov S (1989) Surgical treatment of congenital predominantly arteriovenous shunting defects. In: Belov S, Loose DA, Weber J (eds) Vascular malformations: Periodica Angiologica, Vol 16. Einhorn Presse, Reinbek, pp 229–234
5. Belov S (1992) Operative-technical peculiarities in operations of congenital vascular defects. In: Balas P (ed) Progress in angiology. Minerva Medica, Torino, pp 379–382
6. Kromhout JG, van der Horst C, Peeters F et al (1990) The combined treatment of congenital vascular defects. Int Angiol 9:203–207
7. Loose DA (2008) Contemporary treatment of congenital vascular malformations. In: Dieter R (ed) Textbook on peripheral arterial disease. McGraw Hill, New York
8. Loose DA, Weber J (1991) Indications and tactics for a combined treatment of congenital vascular defects. In: Balas P (ed) Progress in angiology. Edizioni Minerva Medica, Torino, pp 373–378
9. Loose DA (1989) The combined surgical therapy in congenital av-shunting malformations. In: Belov S, Loose DA, Weber J (eds) Vascular malformations, Einhorn Presse, Reinbek, pp 213–225
10. Loose DA (1997) Systematik, radiologische Diagnostik und Therapie vaskulärer Fehlbildungen. In: Hohenleutner U, Landthaler M (eds) Operative Dermatologie im Kindes- und Jugendalter. Diagnostik und Therapie von Fehl- und Neubildungen. Blackwell, Berlin, Wien
11. Loose DA (2000) Combined treatment of vascular malformations: Indications, methods and techniques. In: Chang JB (ed) Textbook of angiology. Springer, New York, pp 1278–1283
12. Malan E (1974) Vascular malformations (angiodysplasias). Carlo Erba Foundation, Milan, p 17
13. Mattassi R (1990) Surgical treatment of congenital arteriovenous defects. Int Angiol 9:196–202
14. Rosen RJ, Riles TS, Berenstein A (1995) Congenital vascular malformations. In: Rutherford, RB (ed) Vascular surgery. WB Saunders, Philadelphia, pp 1218–1232
15. Van Dongen RJ (1983) Therapie der angeborenen arteriovenösen Angiodysplasien unter besonderer Berücksichtigung der operativen Embolisation. Angiology 5:169–179
16. Weber J (1990) Techniques and results of therapeutic catheter embolization of congenital vascular defects. Int Angiol 9:214–223
17. Weber J (1989) The post infarction and pain syndrome following catheter embolization and its treatment. In: Belov S, Loose DA, Weber J (eds) Vascular malformations. Reinbek, Einhorn Presse, pp 294–298

Multidisciplinary Surgical Treatment of Vascular Malformations

25

Raul Mattassi

Abstract

The introduction of non surgical techniques for the treatment of congenital vascular malformations (CVMs) has dramatically diminished the frequency of operations. However, in some cases, surgery is still the best option. In some locations that are difficult to approach, surgical expertise in the anatomical area allows a safer and more radical operation to be performed. The main locations in which multidisciplinary surgery may be helpful include muscle, joints, hand, face and skin.

Introduction

CVMs may appear in diverse forms, sizes and sites: from small, limited, superficial defects to diffuse deep infiltrating forms, with all kind of variables possible. In the past, surgery was the only treatment option, but today there are a variety of other techniques available. This has resulted in a dramatic reduction in the number of operations performed for CVM.

However, there are still some cases for which surgery may be the best approach. Unfortunately, when the CVM is in a location that is difficult to access, surgical resection of a CVM may be difficult. The most hazardous CVMs to treat surgically are the diffuse infiltrating forms found in difficult-to-approach areas, such as the orbita, cheek and pelvis. Involvement of non vascular but non resectable structures may create technical difficulties for the vascular surgeon approaching the defects. To perform the best and safest surgical treatment, surgery should be performed together with other specialists who have expertise in approaching the non vascular tissues involved.

Anatomical localizations in which a multidisciplinary approach may be required include muscle, joints, intraosseous locations, hand, skin, head and neck and the pelvis.

Muscle

In these cases two main problems have to be solved: surgical approach and limits to the removal of muscular tissue. The surgical approach may be crucial for the outcome of the operation. According to the site of the malformation, orthopaedic, vascular or atypical approaches may be possible. Discussion with an orthopaedic surgeon will help to select the best option, which may be atypical for both vascular and orthopaedic specialists (Figs. 25.1, 25.2).

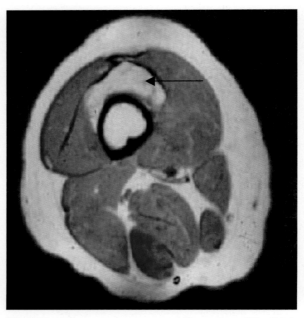

Fig. 25.1. Intramuscular venous malformation of the thigh (*arrow*), visibile on magnetic resonance image

R. Mattassi, D.A. Loose, M. Vaghi (eds.), *Hemangiomas and Vascular Malformations*.
© Springer-Verlag Italia 2009

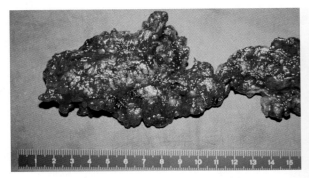

Fig. 25.2. Resected vascular malformations of the same case as in Figure 25.1. The surgical approach was chosen because it was the simplest option, due to extension to the subfascial layer of the malformation and the limited extension. Surgery was performed with an orthopaedic surgeon

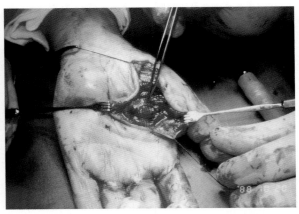

Fig. 25.3. Resection of AV malformations of the hand together with hand surgeon

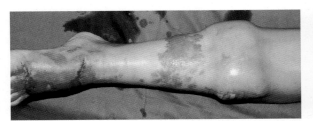

Fig. 25.4. Treatment of a capillary malformation of the calf with plastic surgery, using a skin expander

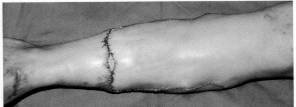

Fig. 25.5. Same case as shown in Figure 25.2, final result

Joints

Intra-articular CVMs, mostly venous, destroy cartilage and should be removed as soon as possible. If surgery is chosen, joint opening and VM removal is best performed with the assistance of an orthopaedic surgeon.

Intraosseous

Surgery of intraosseous malformations has proven to be difficult and dangerous because non controllable bleeding may occur, mainly in arteriovenous (AV) malformations. More effective and less dangerous options are described in another chapter.

Hand

Palmar and wrist malformations should be operated on only with the help of an experienced hand surgeon. Fine hand structures are best approached by a specialist. Sometimes microsurgical techniques and mag-

nification by microscope are required. In our experience, with these techniques, some deep infiltrating AV or venous malformations can be removed radically. The site of fistulas in hand malformations is sometimes difficult to recognise even with microscope magnification. We have observed some cases in which tortuous bundles of veins circumscribed an artery but the fistula was only at a single limited point. Intraoperative Doppler is the decisive technique with which to recognise a fistula (Fig. 25.3). Principles, techniques and results are described in another chapter.

Skin

In cases of infiltration of skin by CVM, plastic surgery of the skin is best performed by a plastic surgeon. Vascular surgeons should participate in the operation in order to treat the subcutaneous CVMs, if necessary. Sometimes in combined superficial and deep CVMs, plastic and vascular surgeons will decide together on the best incisions with which to approach the CVM and skin plastic surgery may be performed in the same session (Figs. 25.4, 25.5).

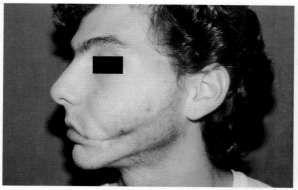

Fig. 25.6. Infiltrating malformation of the cheek. The visible scar is from a former operation

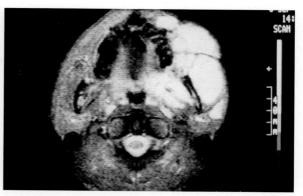

Fig. 25.7. MRI of the same case as in Figure 25.6, demonstrating the extension of the defect

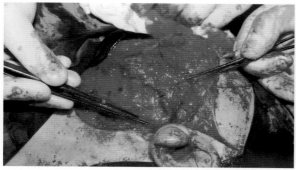

Fig. 25.8. Surgical resection of vascular malformation. First step was the preparation of facial nerve through the malformation

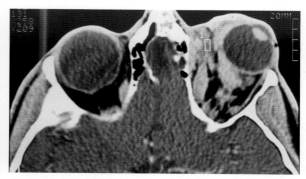

Fig. 25.9. Cranial MR in a retro orbital AV malformation of the right eye; the left eye was blind. Endovascular treatment was refused

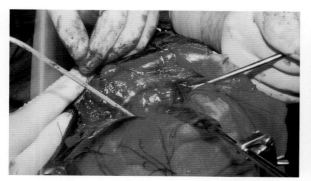

Fig. 25.10. Surgical resection of AV malformation together with a neurosurgeon. Approach via craniotomy

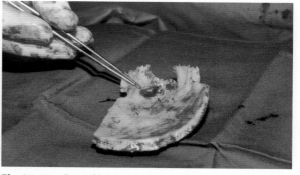

Fig. 25.11. Cranial bone erosion of AV malformation in the same case as Figure 25.6

Head and Neck

Surgical resection of CVMs below and above the mandibula should be performed together with an expert in facial nerve approach, as damage to this structure is a major risk. We prefer to prepare the facial nerve proximally first and to follow it through the malformation. Only after this step is resection of CVM performed (Figs. 25.6–25.8). Collaboration with a plastic surgeon may be also extremely useful in different types of resections. In selected cases, in which an approach to the orbita is required, an oculist or a neurosurgeon may be helpful (Figs. 25.9–25.11). Otorhinolaryngologists may collaborate in cases of external ear or nose CVMs. Malformations sited in the larynx are mainly approached with non surgical techniques.

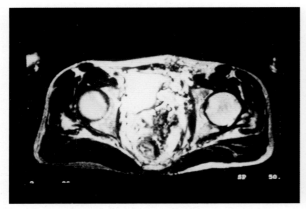

Fig. 25.12. MRI demonstrating large pelvic AV malformation

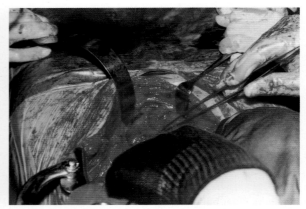

Fig. 25.13. Resection of pelvic AV malformation together with an urologist

Pelvis

CVM on the pelvis floor, sited in connection with bladder and prostate, may be approached safely together with an urologist (Figs. 25.12, 25.13).

Conclusion

Although today surgery is less frequently performed, the concept of involving another specialist in resection of an awkwardly sited CVM should always be considered because it may result in alternative approaches that may lead to more appropriate treatments. In our opinion, a physician who wants to treat CVMs should be able to perform, alone or (often) together with other specialists, all kind of techniques, including surgery. To be open to collaboration widens the possibilities for approaching CVMs.

Suggested Readings

Belov S (1990) Surgical treatment of congenital vascular defects. Int Angiol 9(3):175–182

Belov S (1992) Operative-technical peculiarities in operations of congenital vascular defects. In: Balas P (ed) Progress in angiology 1991. Minerva Medica, Turin, pp 379–382

Belov S, Loose, DA, Müller E (1985) Angeborene Gefäßfehler. Einhorn-Presse Verlag, Reinbek

Mattassi R (1992) Individual indications for surgical and combined treatment in so-called inoperable cases of congenital vascular defects. In: Balas P (ed) Progress in angiology 1991. Minerva Medica, Turin, pp 383–386

Treatment of Arterial Malformations

26

Raul Mattassi, Dirk A. Loose

Abstract

Pure arterial malformations represent only about 8% of all vascular anomalies. They can be divided into aneurysms, hypoplasia (stenosis), aplasia and anomalies of site and course. Many are asymptomatic, but some require treatment because the disease can be severe or may even become life-threatening.

Introduction

Pure arterial malformations are uncommon and represent only about 8% of all vascular malformations. Arterial defects may affect central, visceral and peripheral vessels. The great majority of them are truncular defects and can be dilatations, including aneurysms, stenosis/hypoplasia or aplasia of a main artery. Moreover, anomalies of the site and course of an artery are possible.

Aneurysms

Congenital aneurysms of main arteries are rare; however, there are reports of dilatations of many arteries in the whole body. Intracranial congenital arterial aneurysms with symptoms in infancy are relatively rare. Usually they exist in the internal carotid bifurcation, in the posterior circulation and sometimes within the territory of the distal middle cerebral artery. Beside unspecific symptoms, such as irritability, vomiting, lethargy and coma, the most severe manifestation is subarachnoid hemorrhage. Sometimes, the first symptom can be a peripheral facial paresis [1]. Symptomatic intracranial aneurysms

in the adult are well known and remain a field for neurosurgeons and neuroradiologists.

Congenital aneurysms of the extracranial carotid arteries can be located in the common, external or internal carotid. These aneurysms can be often symptomatic with thromboembolic complications, rupture, bleeding and even stroke. Sometimes, past medical history may reveal a tonsillectomy, although the relationship with the aneurysm is not clear. Surgical treatment with interposition of a vein graft is recommended [2]. The internal carotid may be aneurysmatic also on the skull base and difficult to approach surgically. A lateral skull base approach through the intratemporal fossa may be the best option [3].

Vertebral artery congenital aneurysms are even rarer than carotid ones; mainly single cases are reported. As these defects may be the cause of embolic phenomenon in the posterior circulation, treatment is recommended. Treatment options include surgical ligation, reimplantation on the carotid artery after aneurysm resection or endovascular occlusion [4–6].

The ascending aorta may be aneurysmatic at birth [7]. Rupture of the aneurysm is possible. Treatment is surgical, with replacement of the involved aorta with a synthetic graft [8].

Pulmonary artery aneurysms are rare, although some cases have been reported [9–11]. Controversy remains concerning treatment opportunities.

Abdominal aorta congenital aneurysms are rarely described in the literature. Two cases have been reported in neonates [12]. These aneurysms may be related to a generalized arterial wall defect and aneurysms in other areas may be present or be only a local defect without aneurysms in other vessels. [13]. Congenital aortic aneurysms may be voluminous and not always symptomatic, but rupture is possible [14]. Prosthetic replacement is required.

R. Mattassi, D.A. Loose, M. Vaghi (eds.), *Hemangiomas and Vascular Malformations*.
© Springer-Verlag Italia 2009

Visceral artery aneurysms are very rare in children, but possible in all main vessels. Treatment may be surgery or endovascular occlusion [15].

In the upper limb, congenital subclavian artery aneurysms are described in single cases in the literature [16]. Surgical treatment with resection and direct reimplantation on the carotid artery is possible if the artery is also tortuous [17]. An aberrant left subclavian artery with a retroesophageal course and large aneurysm has been reported. Treatment was surgical, with resection and end-to-side subclavian-carotid anastomosis [18]. Aneurysm of an aberrant right subclavian artery is also treated surgically [19]. The brachial artery may also present with congenital aneurysm; treatment is surgical with resection and end-to-end anastomosis, or graft interposition [20]. Aneurysms of distal arteries of the upper limb are extremely rare; a single case of palmar arch aneurysm has been reported [21].

Congenital aneurysms of the lower limb arteries can be found at any level (Figs. 26.1, 26.2) [22].

A persistent sciatic artery (PSA) may have aneurysms (25% of cases) [24], although it is unclear if these are congenital or represent a late degeneration of the vessel. These aneurysms may cause pain by nerve compression [25, 26] or by ischemia due to thrombosis or embolization [27]. Rupture with life-threatening hemorrhage is possible [28]. Symptomatic cases should be treated by resection and graft replacement.

Multiple congenital aneurysms in different vessels have been also reported [29, 30].

Stenosis, Hypoplasia and Aplasia

Aplasia and hypoplasia of the carotid artery is rare; a recent study reported an incidence of 0.13% in an angiographic screening of 5100 patients [31]. Aplasia of one or both carotid arteries has been reported [32]. These anomalies are mainly asymptomatic, but patients have an increased risk of life-threatening conditions, such as subarachnoid hemorrhage due to increased stress through the collateral circulation [33]. Intracranial aneurysm may coexist and may be treated surgically [34, 35]. Vertebral artery aplasia and hypoplasia has been also reported [36, 37]. Incidence seems to be more frequent than carotid aplasia/hypoplasia: 11.5% of morphological anomalies have been found in a study of 768 cases [38]. This anomaly may be the cause of cerebral hypoperfusion leading to vertigo and dizziness and, after long lasting symptoms, to lacunar brain infarcts [38].

Aortic arch coarctation is widely known and surgical treatment is well established. Recently, endovascular treatment of thoracic aorta coarctation has been described [39]. Long thoracic and abdominal aortic coarctation is a rare condition, reported in about 0.5–2% of aortic coarctations [40]. Symptoms typically occur within the first three decades of life and include hypertension, lower extremity claudication, and mesenteric ischemia [41]. The condition is considered a life-threatening emergency as a result of the complications associated with severe hypertension [42]. Treatment is surgical and based on patch or bypass implant. Infrarenal aortic aplasia is very rare; the anomaly may be asymptomatic and discovered only occasionally [43].

Aplasia of a pulmonary artery is very rare. The patient may complain of respiratory symptoms, such as recurrent hemoptysis, fatigue or pulmonary infections [44].

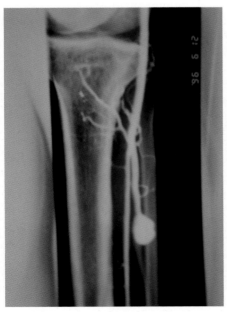

Fig. 26.1. Angiogram of a congenital aneurysm of the interosseous artery in a 20 year old male. Reproduced from [23]

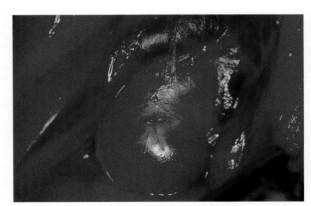

Fig. 26.2. Exposed interosseous artery aneurysm. Treatment performed was a tangential resection without occlusion of the artery. Reproduced from [23]

Anomalies of the visceral arteries are common; the great possibilities of anastomosis explain the lack of symptoms. Treatment is not required, but the anomalies should be known in case other surgery is planned in this area [45–47].

Iliac arteries may be hypoplastic without symptoms [48] or show intermittent claudication [49].

In the lower limb, the most common anomaly is hypoplasia or aplasia of the superficial femoral artery in combination with persistent sciatic artery, which is an embryonal vessel, a continuation of the internal iliac artery which follows the sciatic nerve and connects distally with the popliteal artery. The vessel normally disappears spontaneously during embryogenesis (Figs. 26.3, 26.4) [24]. The incidence of PSA has been estimated at as low as 0.025–0.04% [28]. The anomaly is asymptomatic and does not require treatment. The main complications are aneurysm degeneration or occlusion by thrombosis or emboli, as discussed above. Atherosclerotic occlusion may be treated successfully only by medical therapy [50]. If necessary, bypass implants from the common femoral to popliteal artery are recommended. Failure to recognize the anomaly may lead to inappropriate treatment in ischemic disease of the lower limbs [51, 52].

Arterial Course Anomalies

Many different arterial anomalies of site and course are known. The great majority are asymptomatic and are occasionally discovered: they need no treatment. However, some anomalies may create disturbances and need to be treated; the most frequent is the aberrant right subclavian artery, or *arteria lusoria*.

The *arteria lusoria* is an aberrant right subclavian artery that passes dorsally between the esophagus and spine after branching off from the aortic arch. The first case was described in 1794 by Bayford and was called *lusoria* to indicate a joke of nature (*lusus naturae*). An incidence of 0.36% has been reported [53]. Patients complain of dysphagia due to a compression of the esophagus between the abnormal subclavian artery and spine. Treatment is surgical, directed to the removal of the vascular compression. Transposition of the subclavian artery into the ipsilateral common carotid artery is the preferred technique by most authors [54]. In infants, reimplantation on the aortic arch of the abnormal artery is also possible [55]. Recently, endovascular hybrid techniques with catheter plugging of the anomalous artery to decompression, combined with a carotid-subclavian bypass using right supraclavicular access have been proposed [56].

In conclusion, arterial anomalies are rare defects which may remain asymptomatic throughout life. However, in some cases disturbances may appear that may become severe or even life-threatening. Knowledge of these anomalies is essential to treat the diseases and also to avoid incorrect approaches in common vascular diseases combined with one of these anomalies.

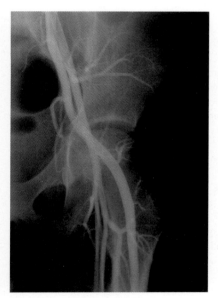

Fig. 26.3. Angiography demonstrating a persistence of sciatic artery. Notice the large hypogastric artery continuing laterally in the sciatic artery. Reproduced from [23]

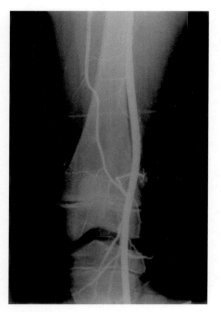

Fig. 26.4. Sciatic artery connecting distally with popliteal artery. Reproduced from [23]

References

1. Iglesias S, Hinojosa J, Esparza J et al (2007) Congenital aneurysm presenting as peripheral facial paresis. Pediatr Neurosurg 43:504–506

2. Pourhassan S, Grotemeyer D, Foukou M et al (2007) Extracranial carotid arteries aneurysms in children: single-center experiences in 4 patients and review of the literature. J Pediat Surg 42:1961–1968

3. Hazarika P, Sahota JS, Nayak DR, George S (1993) Congenital internal carotid aneurysm. In J Pediatr Otorhinolaryngol 28:63–68

4. Ekeström S, Berqdahl L, Huttunen H (1983) Extracranial carotid and vertebral artery aneurysms. Scand J Thorac Cardiovasc Surg 17:135–139

5. Gaskill SJ, Heinz ER, Kandt R, Oakes WJ (1996) Bilateral congenital anomalies of the extracranial vertebral artery: management with balloon therapy. Pediatr Neurosurg 25:147–150

6. Post EM, Owen MP, Cacayorin ED (1985) Vertebral artery aneurysm in a 6 year old child. AJNR 6:977

7. Ramaswamy P, Haberman S, Kleinman C et al (2006) Ascending aortic aneurysm in a fetus due to a benign nodular fibromyoblastic lesion. Cardiovasc Pathol 15:294–296

8. Noordzij MJ, Hanlo-Ploeger AE, Peters JA et al (2001) Rupture of thoracic aneurysm in a 10-year old boy. Ned Tijdschr Geneeskd 145:2388–2891

9. Salhab K, McLarty A (2007) Idiopathic pulmonary artery aneurysm. Thorac Cardiovasc Surg 55:329–331

10. Castañer E, Gallardo X, Rimola J et al (2006) Congenital and acquired pulmonary artery anomalies in the adult: radiologic overview. Radiographics 26:349–371

11. André V, André M, Le Dreff P et al (1999) Congenital aneurysm of the trunk of the pulmonary artery. J Radiol 80:391–393

12. Saad SA, May A (1991) Abdominal aortic aneurysm in a neonate. J Pediatr Surg 26:1423–1424

13. Sterpetti AV, Hunter WJ, Schultz RD (1988) Congenital abdominal aortic aneurysm in the young. Case report and review in the literature. J Vasc Surg 7:763–769

14. Mehall JR, Saltzmann DA, Chandler JC et al (2001) Congenital abdominal aortic aneurysm in the infant: case report and review of the literature. J Pediatr Surg 36:657–658

15. Oechsle S, Vollert K, Buecklein W et al (2006) Percutaneous treatment of a ruptured superior mesenteric artery aneurysm in a child. Pediatr Radiol 36:268–2671

16. Beissert M, Jenett M, Trusen A et al (2000) Asymptomatic aneurysm of the proximal right subclavian artery: a rare ultrasound diagnosis. Eur Radiol 10:459–461

17. Mergan F, Naitmazi D, Dereuma JP (2004) Congenital right subclavian artery aneurysm: a case report. Acta Chir Belg 104:118–119

18. Harrison LH Jr, Batson RC, Hunter DR (1994) Aberrant right subclavian artery aneurysm: an analysis of surgical options. Ann Thorac Surg 57:1012–1014

19. Kokostakis JN, Lazopoulos GL, Lioulias AG et al (2003) Surgical treatment of aneurysm of an aberrant right subclavian artery. Ann Vasc Surg 17:315–319

20. Jones TR, Frusha JD, Stromeyer FW (1988) Brachial artery aneurysm in an infant: case report and review of the literature. J Vasc Surg 7:439–442

21. Lourie GM, Kleinmann WD (1993) Congenital pseudoaneurysm of the superficial palmar arch in a child: a case report. J Hand Surg (Am) 18:151–152

22. Rainio P, Biancari F, Leinonen S, Juvonen T (2003) Aneurysm of the profunda femoris artery manifested as acute groin pain in a child. J Pediatr Surg 38:1699–1700

23. Mattassi R, Belov S, Loose DA, Vaghi M (eds) (2003) Malformazioni vascolari ed emangiomi. Springer-Verlag, Milano

24. Anger P, Seidel K, Kauffmann G, Urbanyi B (1984) Unusual variations of the large arteries of the thigh. Rofo 141:318–326

25. Shinozaki, T, Arita S, Watanabe H, Chiquira M (1998) Aneurysm of a persistent sciatic artery. Arch Orthop Trauma Surg 117:167–169

26. Mazet N, Soulier-Guerin K, Ruivard M et al (2006) Bilateral persistent sciatic artery aneurysm discovered by atypical sciatica: a case report. Cardiovasc Intervent Radiol 29:1107–1110

27. Wu HY, Yang YJ, Lai CH et al (2007) Bilateral persistent sciatic arteries complicated with acute left lower limb ischemia. J Formos Med Assoc 106:1038–1042

28. Sindel T, Yilmaz S, Onur R, Sindel M (2006) Persistent sciatic artery. Radiologic features and patient management. Saudi Med J 27:721–724

29. Bordeaux J, Guys JM, Maqnan PE (1990) Multiple aneurysms in a seven-year-old child. Ann Vasc Surg 4:26–28

30. Pourhassan S, Grotemeyer D, Klar V, Sandmann W (2007) The Klippel-Trenaunay Syndrome with multiple visceral arteries aneurysms. Vasa 36:124–129

31. Tasar M, Yetiser S, Tasar A et al (2004) Congenital absence or hypoplasia of the carotid artery: radioclinical issues. Am J Otolaryngol 25:339–349

32. Gonzales-Cuyar LF, Lam-Himlin D, Tavora F et al (2008) Bilateral internal carotid absence: a case report of a rare congenital anomaly. Cardiovasc Pathol 17:113–116

33. Lee HJ, Oh CW, Lee SH, Han DH (2003) Aplasia of the internal carotid artery. Acta Neurochir (Wien) 145:117–125

34. Zink WE, Komotar RJ, Meyers PM (2007) Internal carotid aplasia/hypoplasia and intracranial saccular aneurysms: series of three new cases and systematic review of the literature. J Neuroimag 17:141–147

35. Funiu H, Kondo R, Sakurada K et al (2006) Aneurysms of the anterior communicating artery and subclavian artery in association with congenital absence of unilateral internal carotid artery. No To Shinkel 58:257–261

36. Altmann S, Fröhner S, Diegeler A, Urbanski PP (2004) Atresia of the right vertebral artery in a patient with acute aortic dissection. Ann Thorac Surg 78:1465–1467

37. Sakellaroupoulos A, Mourgela S, Kyrlesi A, Warnke JP (2008) Hypoplasia of multiple cerebral arteries: report of an unusual case. J Stroke Crebrovasc Dis 17:161–163

38. Paskoy Y, Vatansev H, Seker M et al (2004) Congenital morphological abnormalities of the distal vertebral arteries (CMADVA) and their relationship with vertigo and dizziness. Med Sci Monit 10:316–323

39. Fink-Josephi G, Gutierrez-Vogel S, Hurtado-López LM, Calderón C (2008) Endovascular surgery by means of a Talent endoprosthesis implant in adult patients with thoracic aorta coarctation. J Cardiovasc Surg (Torino) 49:483–487

40. Nomura K, Nakamura Y, Iwanaka T et al (2005) Thoracoabdominal coarctation of the aorta: surgical repair in a 7-year-old boy. Jpn J Thorac Cardiovasc Surg 53:227–229

41. Celik T, Kursaklioglu H, Iyisoy A et al (2006) Hypoplasia of the descending thoracic and abdominal aorta: a case report and review of literature. J Thorac Imaging 21:296–299

42. Terramani TT, Salim A, Hood DB et al (2002) Hypoplasia of the descending thoracic and abdominal aorta: a report of two cases and review of the literature. J Vasc Surg 36:844–848

43. de Albuquerque FJ, Coutinho AC, Castro Netto EC et al (2008) Infra-renal abdominal aorta agenesis: a case report with emphasis on MR angiography findings. Br J Radiol 81:e179–183

44. Simsek PO, Ozcelik U, Celiker A et al (2008) A case of congenital agenesis of the right pulmonary artery presenting with hemoptysis and mimicking pulmonary hemosiderosis. Eur J Pediatr [Epub ahead of print]

45. Losanoff JE, Millis JM, Harland RC, Testa G (2007) Hepato-spleno-mesenteric trunk. J Am Coll Surg 204(3):511

46. Petscavage JM, Maldjian P (2007) Celiomesenteric trunk: two variants of a rare anomaly. Australas Radiol 51:B306–B309

47. Yi SQ, Terayama H, Naito M et al (2008) Absence of the celiac trunk: case report and review of the literature. Clin Anat 21:283–286

48. Kawashima T, Sato K, Sasaki H (2006) A human case of hypoplastic external iliac artery and its collateral pathways. Folia Morphol (Warsz) 65:157–160

49. Loose DA, Wang Z (1990) Surgical treatment in predominantly arterial defects. Int Angiol 9:183–188

50. Kritsch D, Hutter HP, Hirschl M, Katzenschlager R (2006) Persistent sciatic artery: an uncommon cause of intermittent claudication. Int Angiol 25:327–329

51. Brantley SK, Rigdon EE, Raju S (1993) Persistent sciatic artery: embryology, pathology, and treatment. J Vasc Surg 18:242–248

52. Vaghi M, Mattassi R, Tacconi A (1989) Persistence of sciatic artery: case report. In: Belov S, Loose DA, Weber J. Vascular malformations. Einhorn-Presse Verlag, Periodica Angiologica, Reinbek, pp 132–134

53. De Luca L, Bergman JJ, Tytgat GN, Fockens P (2000) EUS imaging of the arteria lusoria: case series and review. Gastrointest Endosc 52:670–673

54. Kieffer E, Bahnini A, Koskas F (1994) Aberrant subclavian artery: surgical treatment in thirty-three adult patients. J Vasc Surg 19:100–109

55. van Son JA, Vincent JG, van Oort A, Lacquet LK (1998) Reimplantation of an aberrant right subclavian artery into the ascending aorta in dysphagia lusoria in childhood. Tijdschr Kindergeneeskd 56:126–129

56. Shennib H, Diethrich EB (2008) Novel approaches for the treatment of the aberrant right subclavian artery and its aneurysms. J Vasc Surg 47:1066–1067

Treatment of Arteriovenous Malformations

27

Dirk A. Loose

Abstract

Arteriovenous malformations (AVM) can be treated by endovascular embolization, surgery, sclerotherapy and laser. Endovascular embolization is today the most frequent treatment, followed by surgery. Sclerotherapy and laser treatments are other possibilities. Treatment strategy depends on the type, symptoms and evolution of the defect. Truncular forms are treated mainly by surgery while the techniques listed may be used alone or in combination when treating extratruncular defects.

Introduction

Clinical pictures of arteriovenous malformations (AVM) may vary greatly; from slight, asymptomatic limited defects to extended life-threatening malformations. Although AVMs are the second most common malformation after venous malformations, some of the cases are difficult to treat. Experience, skill, multidisciplinary approach and the capacity to find original solutions may be required to treat some of the most complex cases of AVM. The general principles of treatment of congenital vascular malformations and different treatment procedures are described in other chapters of this atlas.

Therapeutic Options

Available treatments for AVM include: endovascular embolization; surgery; sclerotherapy and laser treatment.

Endovascular embolization is actually the most frequent treatment for congenital vascular malformations (CVMs). Occlusion of the nidus, not only of feeding vessels, should be the main goal of treatment. Occlusion of feeding vessels by a covered stent is not a successful procedure and should not be used. This topic is discussed in detail in Chapters 20 and 21.

Surgery to remove or to reduce the hemodynamic effect of AVM is the second main option. Stefan Belov developed a simple and useful scheme of the different surgical procedures available [1]. Details are discussed in Chapter 19.

Sclerotherapy with alcohol injections, through a catheter or by direct puncture is another well established technique. For details, see Chapter 22.

Laser treatment is less often used for treatment of AVM; however, in some cases an echo-guided percutaneous treatment may be effective for small and localized defects. This topic is discussed in detail in Chapter 23.

The different techniques, in combined form and performed stepwise or with a multidisciplinary approach (see Chapter 25), are options to be considered and to be adopted to individual cases.

Treatment Strategy

Treatment strategy should be chosen according to the type, symptoms and evolution of the AVM.

Type of AVM

AVMs may be truncular or extratruncular (see Chapter 15).

R. Mattassi, D.A. Loose, M. Vaghi (eds.), *Hemangiomas and Vascular Malformations*.
© Springer-Verlag Italia 2009

Truncular AVMs, i.e., those with a direct connection between main arteries and veins, are rarely congenital. Much more common is an area of extratruncular fistulas situated outside the main vessels. In cases of true truncular AVM, surgery to ligate the fistula should be the first option. Endovascular implant of a covered stent in cases of direct AV fistula is a good alternative to surgery, but only in cases of direct AV connection. If, however, an AV fistulous area exists (which is much more frequent), such an endovascular procedure will only lead to early recurrence.

Extratruncular AVMs are by far more common than truncular AVMs. Limited, superficial AVMs can be treated successfully by surgical resection and even cured if the surgeon succeeds in removing the malformation completely (Figs. 27.1–27.5). Embolization, if the nidus is totally occluded, is a good alternative. Sclerotherapy with ethanol or glue through a direct puncture is also possible. Echo-guided percutaneous laser treatment is possible in limited AVMs. A combined procedure with embolization of the feeding arteries to reduce bleeding, followed by surgical resection is often the best option (Figs. 27.6–27.12).

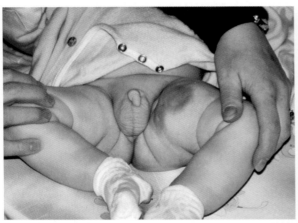

Fig. 27.1. AV malformation of the left thigh in a 5 month old child. The indication for treatment was continuous severe pain and impending perforation

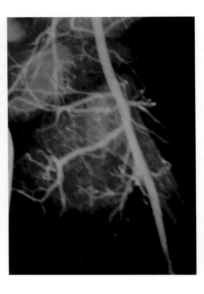

Fig. 27.2. Angiography of the external iliac artery, common femoral artery and superficial femoral artery with pathologic side branches and big AV fistulas

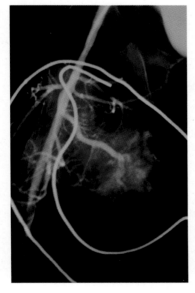

Fig. 27.3. Control angiography, demonstrating the closure of the main feeding vessels of the AV malformation

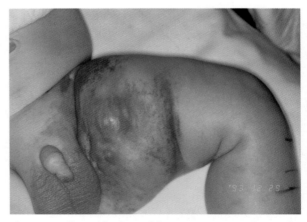

Fig. 27.4. Clinical finding of the tissue reaction during the post-embolization syndrome with local pain, fever and leucocytosis, secondary to local tissue infarction. During surgery, some days later, the remaining AV fistulas were ligated and extirpated together with involved muscle tissue

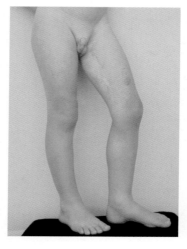

Fig. 27.5. Clinical appearance of the 6 year old boy, 5.5 years after treatment

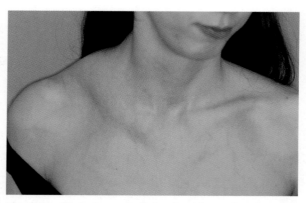

Fig. 27.6. Clinical aspect of the shoulder and neck region of a patient, where a right supraclavicular swelling is obvious, caused by an AV malformation

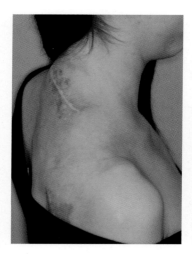

Fig. 27.7. The side aspect of the shoulder/ right cervical region also demonstrates scar tissue after two trials of treatment. The patient complained of a growing mass in the right cervical region in combination with pulsating pain

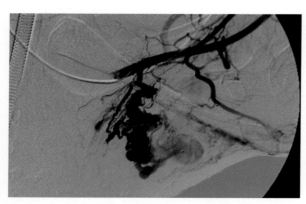

Fig. 27.8. Arteriography of the subclavian artery, demonstrating the AV malformation of the supraclavicular region with a large nidus

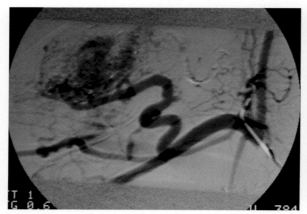

Fig. 27.9. Arteriography of the subclavian artery, demonstrating the AV malformation of the supraclavicular region with a large nidus

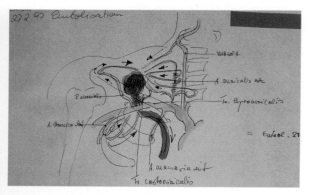

Fig. 27.10. Schematic representation of the circulation of the involved vessels of the AV malformation. Several attempts to abate the malformation by interventional radiological treatment were not successful, which is why, in this case, direct treatment by vascular surgery was indicated

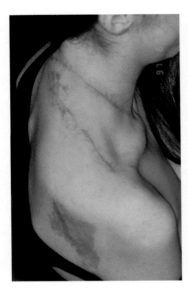

Fig. 27.11. Clinical aspect of the shoulder and right cervical region 3 months after surgery and after subtotal resection of the AV malformation and the involved tissue

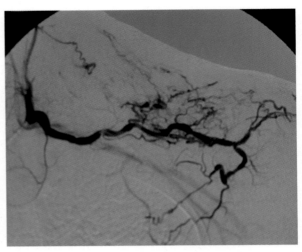

Fig. 27.12. Control arteriography of the right subclavian artery demonstrating a satisfactory treatment result

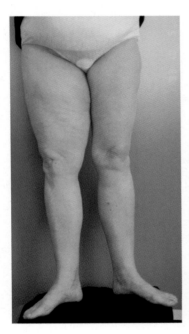

Fig. 27.13. Clinical aspect of the lower extremities of a woman with circumferential overgrowth of the right thigh without severe length disparity. The patient complained of recurrent thrombophlebitis, swelling and heaviness of the thigh with impediment during walking

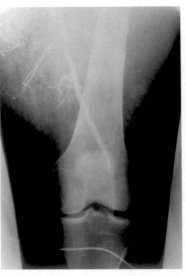

Fig. 27.14. Arteriography of the right thigh, demonstrating numerous AV fistulas of different calibers, some of which are infiltrating the muscles

Extratruncular infiltrating forms may be some of the most difficult cases to treat. The goal of the treatment should be occlusion or removal of the nidus; i.e., the real area where the connections between arterial and venous flow occur. The nidus should be clearly distinguished from inflow and outflow vessels: this may be difficult in extended forms. All available techniques can be applied to treat infiltrating AVMs (Figs. 27.13–27.21).

Symptoms

Asymptomatic AVMs may be simply followed by controls, looking for signs of secondary effects (limb overgrowth and cardiac effects, which are rare). In extended forms with secondary effects, treatment should be performed early in order to avoid progression and worsening.

Symptomatic malformations that create discomfort

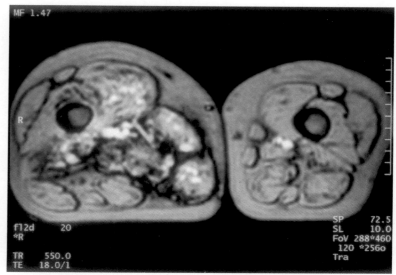

Fig. 27.15. Magnetic resonance image (MRI) in cross-section demonstrating that the AV fistulas have involved many sections of the thigh muscles of the right leg. Distinct circumferential change of the right thigh

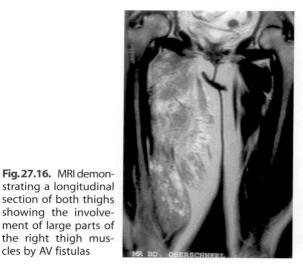

Fig. 27.16. MRI demonstrating a longitudinal section of both thighs showing the involvement of large parts of the right thigh muscles by AV fistulas

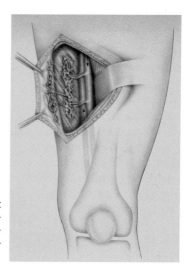

Fig. 27.17. Schematic representation of infiltrating AV malformation in the thigh muscles

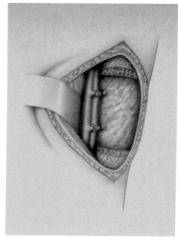

Fig. 27.18. Situation during surgery 4 weeks after embolization treatment of large AV fistulas of the right thigh. During surgery, persisting subcutaneous and subfascial AV fistulas are clamped or are oversewn respectively. The sartorius muscle has been prepared. The ultrasonic Doppler mapping during surgery demonstrates AV fistulas involving the muscle tissue

Fig. 27.19. Schematic representation of surgical technique: Ligation of AV fistulas and partial resection of infiltrated muscles

220   D.A. Loose

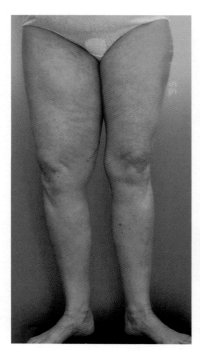

Fig. 27.20. Clinical aspect 6 months after combined treatment of AV fistulas of the right thigh. The volume of the thigh is distinctly diminished. The patient is no longer in pain

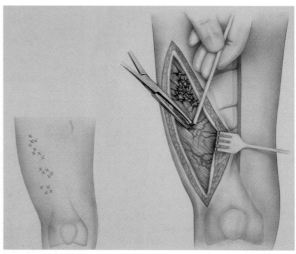

Fig. 27.21. Schematic representation of the Loose II technique: Preoperative identification of AV fistulas by color Doppler imaging and precise marking on the overlying skin. During surgery, ultrasonic Doppler mapping of AV fistulas; clamping and oversewing of the AV fistulas and ultrasonic Doppler control of the complete closure of the AV fistulas

should be treated as early as possible. Sometimes, even in extended forms, a treatment with only a partial success may lead to a cessation of symptoms. The goal of the treatment must, however, not be forgotten: i.e., hemodynamic control of the malformation, where no peripheral ischemia is caused by persisting AV fistulas. Otherwise, the disease behaves as a "vascular cancer".

Evolution

It is not uncommon that asymptomatic AVMs remain stable for a long time without patient disturbance.

AVMs with symptoms and which are complicated by pain or bleeding need prompt treatment. In severe cases with bleeding, embolization of feeding vessels in an attempt to stop bleeding is justified. Further treatment will be necessary to prevent bleeding recurrence. In some cases, a well directed surgical resection preceded by embolization may be more effective than repeated embolizations alone.

Limb length discrepancy developing during childhood should not be left untreated, as late orthopedic correction is not always successful. Early correction or reduction of the hemodynamic effect may stop the pathologic growth and even completely correct length discrepancies. Staples can be implanted to stop growth, but a very precise calculation of the expected growth is required to implant them at the correct age. This concept is unfortunately not widely known and too often children are not treated promptly or they undergo orthopedic surgery with a wrong indication and incorrect treatment concept.

Conclusion

Treatment of AVMs is a difficult and a complex issue. Precise diagnosis and treatment, considering all therapeutic options and stepwise combinations of techniques, are necessary in order to select the best treatment for the individual patient.

References

1. Belov S (2000) Vascular malformations and hemangiomas: Surgical treatment. In: Chang JB (ed) Textbook of angiology. Springer, New York, pp 1284–1293
2. Belov S, Loose DA, Weber J (eds) (1989) Vascular malformations. Einhorn-Presse Verlag, Reinbek/Hamburg, pp 29–30
3. Loose DA (1997) Malformaciones vasculares. Sistemática para el diagnóstico radiológico y la terapéutica. Forum FL 2:101–108
4. Loose DA (1997) Therapie angeborener Gefäßmißbildungen. In: Göroch J, Brambs H-J, Sunder-Plassmann L (eds) Endovaskuläre Chirurgie "State-of-the-Art" Symposium, W Zuckrschwerdt, München, Bern, Wien, New York
5. Loose DA (1999) Modern concepts and combined treatment of congenital vascular malformations. XXIst European Congress of the International College of Surgeons. Prague, Czech Republic, June 2–5. In: Milos Hajek: Abstracts of the Congress, Galéu, Prague
6. Loose DA, Weber J (1997) Angeborene Gefäßmißbildungen. Interdisziplinäre Diagnostik und Therapie von Hämangiomen (Angiodysplasien). Periodica Angiologica, Vol 21, Nordland-Druck, Lüneburg
7. Loose DA, Belov S, Mattassi R et al (2001) Long follow-up results in active causal treatment of vascular malformations. A review of 1378 cases (Multicenter Study). In: Clement D, Rieger H (ed) Proceedings of the 14th Congress of the European Chapter of the International Union of Angiology. Cologne, Germany, Monduzzi Edit, Bologna, pp 431–450
8. Loose DA (2000) Vascular malformations and hemangiomas: clinical features and their basis. In: Chang JB (ed) Textbook of angiology. Springer, New York, pp 1248–1257
9. Loose DA (2008) Contemporary treatment of congenital vascular malformations. In: Dieter R (ed) Textbook: Peripheral arterial disease. Mc Graw Hill, New York
10. Lumley JSP (1986) A colour atlas of vascular surgery. Wolfe Medical Publications, London
11. Mattassi R (1990) Surgical treatment of congenital arteriovenous defects. Int Angiol 9(3):196–202
12. Shoab SS, Scurr JH (2000) Arteriovenous malformations of the upper limb. In: Chang JB (ed) Textbook of angiology. Springer, New York, pp 1270–1277
13. Weber J (2000) Radiological diagnostic strategies and interventional radiology. In: Chang JB (ed) Textbook of angiology. Springer, New York, pp 1261–1269
14. Belov S (1993) Correction of lower limbs length discrepancy in congenital vascular-bone diseases by vascular surgery performed during childhood. Seminars in Vasc Surg 6(4):245–251

Treatment of Venous Malformations

28

Raul Mattassi

Abstract

Treatment of venous malformations (VM) is based on the following concepts: conservative treatment, sclerotherapy, laser treatment and surgery. Conservative treatment with elastic stockings is recommended mainly in minor cases with little discomfort. Sclerotherapy may be performed with classic sclerosis, foam and absolute alcohol. Foam sclerosis, performed with a mixture of sclerosant fluid and gas (such as air or other gases) has been reported to offer good results, although experience in this area is only recently beginning to grow. Alcohol sclerosis, with radioscopic control of the injected area, is one of the preferred treatments for VM. Laser application is possible by percutaneous, superficial and intravascular approaches. Percutaneous puncture with fiber introduction through the needle allows extratruncular limited forms or infiltrating forms to be treated. An intravascular approach may be useful to close superficial dysplastic veins.

Introduction

Surgery still has a central place in treatment, although introduction of other procedures has reduced the need for surgery. Truncular dysplastic vessels are resected, while aneurysms may be replaced or resected tangentially. A persistent marginal vein is resected if the deep veins are normal. Extratruncular limited VM can be resected radically, if accessible; sclerosis by direct puncture is always a good alternative procedure. Infiltrating forms may be resected partially or treated in combination with sclerosis or laser.

Venous malformations (VM) are the most common vascular anomalies. As with other vascular defects, the type, site, extension and tissue involvement is extremely variable. Treatment strategy and the treatment techniques employed depend on a correct evaluation of all these factors.

Treatment options include conservative treatment, sclerotherapy, laser treatment and surgery.

Conservative Treatment

Conservative treatment is based on elastic stockings and is mainly indicated in patients with little or no discomfort. The role of phlebotonic drugs is not cleared, although some patients indicate some improvement with this therapy.

Sclerotherapy

The injection of a solution that acts as an endothelial irritant in the dysplastic vessels causing immediate thrombosis is the easiest and most active treatment for VM. However, early results have not been completely successful and the efficacy of this treatment has not been accepted universally [1–3]. More recently, sclerotherapeutic techniques have been improved and a consensus has been reached; today sclerotherapy is the most frequent treatment for VM.

Three different types of sclerosants and techniques are used: classic sclerosis, foam sclerosis and absolute alcohol sclerosis.

Classic Sclerosis

Classic sclerosis is the same procedure as used for varicose veins treatment; different solutions with variable strengths are available. The most frequently

R. Mattassi, D.A. Loose, M. Vaghi (eds.), *Hemangiomas and Vascular Malformations*.
© Springer-Verlag Italia 2009

used solutions for the treatment of VM are polidocanol and sodium tetradecyl sulphate. Often higher concentrations than for the treatment of varicose veins are required for greater efficacy. The technique of injection is the same as for the treatment of varicose veins. After vein puncture, the leg is elevated to empty the vein and sclerosant injection is performed. If pain or a burning sensation is experienced, injection should be stopped because of extravasation and needle replacement is required. An elastic bandage is placed and maintained for 3–7 days.

The efficacy of classic sclerotherapy for VM treatment is controversial.

Foam Sclerosis

The foam used in sclerosis is the result of an extemporaneous mixture of fluid tension-active sclerosants, such as polidocanol or sodium tetradecyl sulphate, with air or other gases, such as CO_2. A quick and easy method to prepare foam is to mix the sclerosant fluid in one syringe with air from a second syringe through a three way stop-cock connection [4]. Foam has several advantages over liquids: complete filling of the vessels by displacement of blood is obtained; the bubbles have a tendency to remain in the vessel for a longer time, increasing the sclerosing effect; a lower dosage of sclerosant is required; and the bubbles are visible by echography, allowing direct control of vessel filling.

Technically, the procedure is simple. After percutaneous puncture of the vessels, obtaining blood reflux, the foam is prepared and immediately injected. By duplex scan control, the progression of the foam in the vessels can be followed (Figs. 28.1, 28.2). Foam can be displaced into the vessels to be treated by finger pressure under duplex control, if required.

Good results have been reported with foam treatment of VM [5, 6].

Absolute Alcohol Sclerosis

Alcohol denatures endothelial proteins rapidly, with immediate thrombosis. In stagnant channels the effect is increased, as alcohol has a low viscosity and readily passes through vessels. The technique of alcoholization of VM is based on percutaneous direct puncture of the dysplastic vessels [7]. An echo-guided puncture is recommended for deep sited malformations. After getting venous reflux, contrast injection under fluoroscopy is performed. This procedure is useful to recognize venous outflow, to establish the quantity of alcohol to inject (according to the quantity of contrast which fills the malformation) and to exclude arterial injection. If a large outflow vein is demonstrated, a localized finger compression (the efficacy is controlled by a new contrast injection) may stop these quick flows, increasing the alcohol effect. A tourniquet on the limb to completely stop venous flow has been tried; these procedures may be dangerous if large quantities of ethanol are being used because at tourniquet removal a massive emission of ethanol may create heart disturbances. Ethanol can be mixed with lipiodol to directly visualize the injection [8]. It has been recommended that not more than 1 cc/kg or 60 ml per procedure of ethanol be injected [9]. As alcohol injection in vessels is extremely painful, it should be performed under general anesthesia; local anesthesia is not effective for pain prevention (Figs. 28.3, 28.4). A new technique of intravascular local anesthesia is experimented in our department; results will be reported.

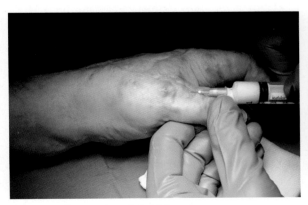

Fig. 28.1. Foam sclerosis in VM

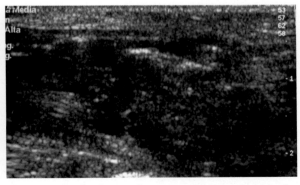

Fig. 28.2. Duplex image demonstrating foam bubbles inside the vein

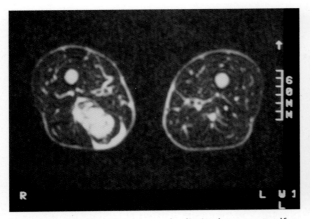

Fig. 28.3. MR of an intramuscular limited venous malformation of the right thigh

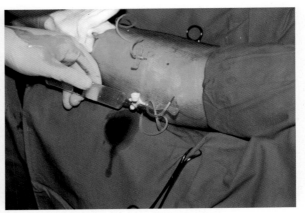

Fig. 28.4. Percutaneous alcohol treatment

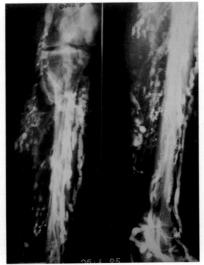

Fig. 28.5. Phlebography of an extensive venous dysplasia of the calf

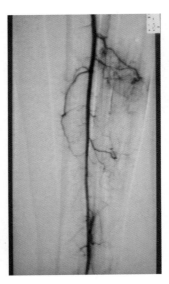

Fig. 28.6. Arteriography of the same case as Figure 28.5, demonstrating slight fistulous areas

A technique that, in our experience, has given good results is the immediate re-aspiration of the injected ethanol after the malformation has been filled. This procedure has the advantage of reducing the introduction of ethanol into the circulation and the effect has been shown to be similar or even better than with the traditional injection without aspiration. Noticeable is that in these cases there is generally not an immediate hardening by thrombosis of the treated mass; however, a few hours later the effect is very intense.

A swelling with relative pain is common after successful alcohol injection of dysplastic vessels; symptoms usually disappear in 2–3 weeks and shrinkage of the treated anomalous venous mass is noticed if the treatment has been successful.

Good results have been reported in large casuistics with ethanol sclerotherapy [10, 11].

Endovascular Catheter Embolization

Arteriography performed in VM, mainly in extratruncular forms, may often show slight arteriovenous (AV) fistulas which coexist with venous dysplasias, although without significant hemodynamic effects [12]. Often these patients are studied by angiography and, if AV fistulas are demonstrated, transcatheter embolization is performed. This procedure is not effective and is mainly the result of an incorrect understanding of venous malformations (Figs. 28.5, 28.6).

Laser Treatment

Extratruncular and truncular VMs can be treated successfully with laser: Nd:Yag (1064 nm) laser is one of the most commonly used lasers, as it offers the best combination of terminal effect and penetration (up to 5 mm). In the past, only cutaneous applications were considered, limiting the treatment to port wine stains and superficial small lesions [13]. Superficial facial VMs, such as of the cheek, lips and tongue, have also been treated successfully. The intravascular and percutaneous approach has enabled laser therapy to be extended to many other VMs [14].

In extratruncular forms, the percutaneous direct approach is the best option. General anesthesia is required. The fiber is introduced into the malformation through a cannula and laser application is performed while slowly retracting the fiber. If correctly regulated, laser provokes a shrinking of the dysplastic area. In deeper malformations, an echo-guided puncture allows even deeply located malformations to be reached. By duplex scan, the laser effect can be constantly controlled. After treatment, a temporary swelling of the treated area is common; this effect normally disappears in 1–2 weeks (Fig. 28.7).

In truncular forms, endovascular closure of dysplastic veins, such as the marginal vein, is possible. The vein is cannulated distally and a catheter containing the laser fiber is introduced until the proximal end of the vein is reached. As in saphenous vein treatment, laser spots are administered while the fiber is slowly retracted. Duplex scan continuous control follows the procedure and the effect (shrinkage) in the vein. These procedures have not been widely used. In our cases, we have noticed that the patient often complains of an uncomfortable painful reaction, as the marginal vein is often very superficial. It is possible that some additional procedures, such as infiltration with saline solution along the vein to increase the distance between the skin and the vein and less laser power may improve the technique. More experience is required.

Surgery

Although the improvement in sclerosing techniques has reduced the frequency of surgical treatment, this is still an important and sometimes irreplaceable option for VM treatment. Different techniques are available, according to the type of malformation.

Truncular Forms

According to the Hamburg Classification, truncular forms of VM are dysplasias of main veins, such as dilatation, hypoplasa or aplasia.

Dysplastic dilatation of superficial veins is best treated by surgical resection. As these veins may have a very unusual distribution, incisions should be planned carefully and may often be atypical. Diffuse superficial dysplastic veins should be treated in multiple steps.

Congenital venous aneurysms may exist in different vessels, in locations such as the neck, face, superior and inferior cava, pelvic veins and limbs. The most common sites are the popliteal and saphenous veins. Surgical resection is the best option for treating aneurysms in some collateral veins, such as the saphenous vein. In aneurysms of main veins, such as the popliteal vein, a tangential resection or a venous graft implant is the best option. Banding technique is also possible, although not commonly performed (Figs. 28.8–28.10).

In hypoplasia of main veins of the limbs, dilated insufficient superficial veins coexist and may create significant venostasis. Segmental stenosis is generally of a short vein segment, often in the popliteal or superficial femoral vein. If the deep vein anomaly is not a complete occlusion, a step-by-step resection of the superficial veins is possible. The increased pressure in the deep veins brings a progressive dilation of the stenosis, often to an almost normal calibre (Fig. 28.11) [15, 16]. Some authors are of the opinion that some stenoses are due to an anomalous fibrous band compression, but others disagree. An instrumental recognition of an external compression (by duplex scan, magnetic resonance (MR), computed tomography (CT) or flebography) is not very accurate. Only surgical exposition of the area of the

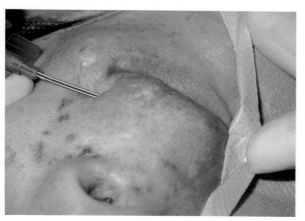

Fig. 28.7. Percutaneous laser treatment of venous malformation of the lip

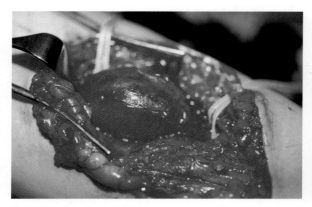

Fig. 28.8. Popliteal vein aneurysm

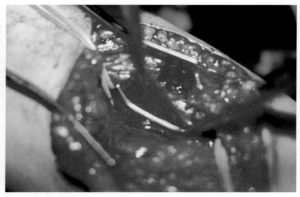

Fig. 28.9. Tangential clamping of the venous aneurysm

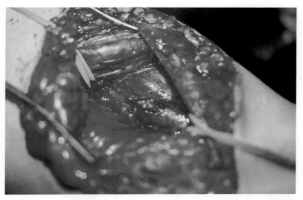

Fig. 28.10. After tangential resection of the aneurysm and suture an almost normal caliber popliteal vein is obtained

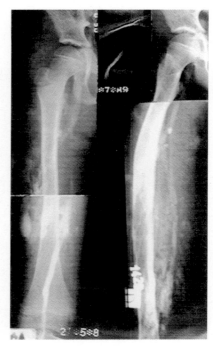

Fig. 28.11. Phlebography of a case with congenital hypoplasia of superficial femoral vein (*left*). After resection of superficial dilated veins, a dilation of the hypoplastic vein is noticed (*right*)

stenosis may resolve the dilemma. There is no agreement as to whether these approaches should be performed every time, in selected cases, or not at all. In our personal experience of 12 cases, we obtained a good dilation of deep veins after superficial vein resection without exploring the stenotic vein, indicating that in these cases there was no compression.

Congenital stenosis of larger veins, such as the iliac veins, can be treated by balloon dilatation. Congenital stenosis of inferior caval veins (Budd-Chiari syndrome) is more common in Asian countries. Treatment options include balloon angioplasty, with or without stent implantation, digital membranotomy, patch application and shunt techniques (caval-atrial, meso-caval or meso-atrial) [17].

Aplasia of deep veins is rare and mainly limited to short segments (poplitea, superficial femoral or iliac veins); aplasia of the whole deep veins of a limb is much rarer (Fig. 28.12). Collateral circulation occurs via dilated superficial veins or through a persistent marginal vein. Surgical removal of these superficial collateral veins should be avoided. Very often in deep vein aplasia, AV fistulas coexist which may stimulate bone growth, creating a limb length difference. If those fistulas are mainly on the marginal vein, skeletonization is possible, reducing the inflow overloading of the vein and the venostasis (Fig. 28.13) [18]. However, this procedure is rare. Aplasia of the infrarenal cava and iliac veins is normally well compensated through collaterals and may not require treatment.

The persistence of a marginal vein, which is a remnant of the primitive veins and is situated on the lateral side of the limb, may create significant discomfort because of venostasis, as this vein is valveless. Before treatment, precise study of the deep veins through duplex scan and/or flebography should rule out hypoplasia of the deep vein. Marginal veins may connect with deep veins by abnormally large insufficient perforators which should be recognized precisely before surgery is planned, in order for direct ligation to be performed. The best treatment is surgical resection by a semi closed technique. Closed stripping, as in varicose veins, may be dangerous because of the risk of getting a large hematoma by rupture of a large perforator or by stripping of multiple small AV fistulas which sometimes connect with the marginal vein (Fig. 28.14) [19].

Treatment of Venous Malformations

Recently, we have noticed that some patients with marginal veins may have also lymphatic dysplasias, such as defects of the deep lymphatic trunks. In some patients we have demonstrated abnormal superficial lymphatics, sited near the marginal vein: we call this a "marginal lymphatic". If deep lymphatic anomalies also coexist, damage to this abnormal lymphatic during surgery may cause lymphedema. Lymphoscintigraphy performed before resection of the marginal vein will rule out this anomaly.

Extratruncular Forms

Subcutaneous limited areas of dysplastic veins may be treated by surgical resection although sclerosis is also possible. In deeper malformations, such as intramuscular forms, surgery is possible by carefully entering the muscle along fibers and resecting the malformation en bloc (Figs. 28.15, 28.16).

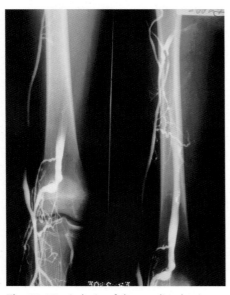

Fig. 28.12. Aplasia of the popliteal vein

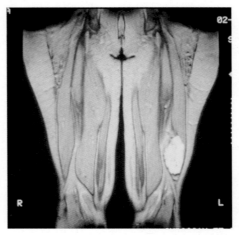

Fig. 28.15. Intramuscular limited venous malformation of the thigh, demonstrated by MR

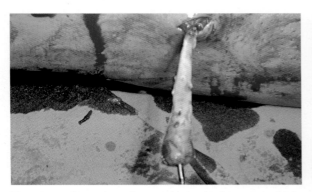

Fig. 28.14. Resection of a marginal vein through multiple incisions

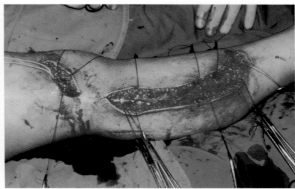

Fig. 28.13. Skeletonization of a marginal vein

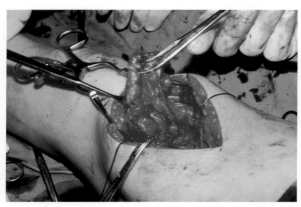

Fig. 28.16. Surgical resection en bloc of the venous malformation

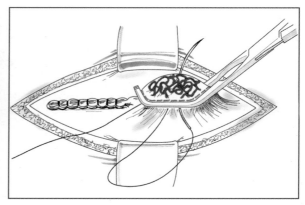

Fig. 28.17. Tangential resection and suture of the venous dysplastic area

Infiltrating venous malformations may often represent a difficult challenge for surgery. Muscles may be deeply infiltrated and very difficult to separate from VM. Sometimes muscular fibers are fibrosed, resulting in a loss of their function. Tendons of the hand and feet may be surrounded by dysplastic, fragile vessels which make surgery difficult because of severe bleeding.

Surgical options include resection together with tissues, if possible; step-by-step resection with stitches; tangential partial resection, using a Satinsky clamp (Fig. 28.17); and en bloc suture of the dysplastic area.

Decision to perform surgery in these cases should be taken only after evaluating feasibility; otherwise other techniques (such as sclerosis or laser) should be considered. In difficult cases with extended tissue involvement, the approach supported by different specialists should be considered.

Gastrointestinal bleeding focal VM should be treated by resection. Multifocal lesions, such as seen in blue rubber bleb nevus syndrome, are treated by multiple resections [20].

References

1. Sigg K (1976) Varizen, Ulcus Crucis und Thrombose. Springer, Berlin, p 157
2. Malan E (1974) Vascular malformations (angiodysplasias). Carlo Erba Foundation, Milan
3. Van der Stricht (1990) The sclerosing therapy in congenital vascular defects. Int Angiol 9:224–227
4. Tessari L (2000) Nouvelle technique d'obtention de la sclero-mousse. Phlebologie 53:129
5. Cabrera J, Cabrera J Jr, Garcia-Olmedo A, Redondo P (2003) Treatment of venous malformations with sclerosants in microfoam form. Arch Dermatol 139:1409–1416
6. Bergan J, Pascarella L, Mekenas L (2006) Venous disorders: treatment with sclerosant foam. J Cardiovasc Surg 47:115–124
7. Yakes W, Prevsner P, Reed M et al (1986) Serial embolization of an extremity VM with alcohol via direct percutaneous puncture. AJR 146:1038–1040
8. Suh JS, Shin KH, Na JB et al (1997) Venous malformations: sclerotherapy with a mixture of ethanol and lipiodol. Cardiovasc Intervent Radiol 20:268–273
9. Hammer FD, Boon LM, Mathurin P, Vanwijck RR (2001) Ethanol sclerotherapy for venous malformations: evaluation of systemic ethanol contamination. J Vasc Interv Radiol 12:595
10. Lee BB, Do YS, Byun HS (2003) Advanced management of venous malformations with ethanol sclerotherapy. Mid-term results. J Vasc Surg 37:533
11. Shireman PK, McCarthy WJ, Yao JS, Vogelzang RL (1997) Treatment of venous malformations by direct injection with ethanol. J Vasc Surg 26:838–844
12. Leu JL (1990) Pathomorphology of vascular malformations. Int Angiol 9:147–154
13. Landthaler M, Hohenleuthner U (1990) Laser treatment of congenital vascular malformations. Int Angiol 9:208–213
14. Berlien HP, Waldschmidt J, Mueller G (1988) Laser treatment of cutaneous and deep vessels anomalies. In: Waidelich W (ed) Laser optoelectronics in medicine. Springer, Berlin, pp 5–25
15. Belov S, Loose DA (1990) Surgical treatment of congenital vascular defects. Int Angiol 9:175–182
16. Mattassi R (1992) Individual indications for surgical and combined treatment in so-called inoperable cases of congenital vascular defects. In: Balas P (ed) Progress in angiology. Minerva Medica, Torino, pp 383–386

17. Wang Z (1989) Congenital defects of the inferior vena cava causing Budd-Chiari syndrome (personal experience in 50 cases). In: Belov S, Loose DA, Weber
J (eds) Vascular malformations. Einhorn Presse,
Reinbek, pp 138–145

18. Belov S (1972) Congenital agenesia of the deep veins
of the lower extremity: surgical treatment. J Cardiovasc Surg 13:594–598

19. Mattassi R (2007) Approach to marginal vein: current
issue. Phlebology 22:283–286

20. Fishman SJ, Burrows PE, Leichtner AM, Mulliken
JB (1998) Gastrointestinal manifestation of vascular anomalies in childhood: varied etiologies require
multiple therapeutic modalities. J Pediatr Surg
33:1163

Treatment of Lymphatic Malformations

29

Byung-Boong Lee, James Laredo, Jeong-Meen Seo, Richard F. Neville

Abstract

The development of the Hamburg Classification, along with a better understanding of vascular malformations, has allowed a more concise description of lymphatic malformation (LM). The management of LM has become clear: "lymphangioma" should no longer be considered a single LM lesion, but rather one of two different LM lesions belonging to an extratruncular lesion, even though the management of lymphangioma is different from its "truncular" LM lesion counterpart that clinically presents as primary lymphedema. Although they often present as discrete clinical entities, the lesions can occur together, making clinical management confusing.

Treatment options for lymphangioma should be approached cautiously with appropriate consideration of its embryologic characteristics, as for any other extratruncular lesion, when options such as sclerotherapy and/or surgical excision are being considered.

Primary lymphedema should be managed as a truncular lesion, where decongestive physiotherapy remains the mainstay of treatment to improve lymph-transporting function. Additional surgical therapy, either reconstructive or ablative, should only be carried out as a supplemental therapy with justifiable indications.

Introduction

Before the development of the Hamburg Classification for congenital vascular malformations (CVM) [1], the lymphatic malformation (LM) had been solely represented by the "extratruncular" form of the lesion, the "cystic/cavernous/capillary lymphangioma"

(Fig. 29.1a) [2, 3]. The "truncular" LM lesion had been neglected since it presents clinically as "primary" lymphedema (Fig. 29.1b). Infrequently, both extratruncular and truncular lesions may occur together; therefore, a precise understanding of the difference between the two lesion types (extratruncular versus truncular lesions) is important for appropriate management (Fig. 29.2) [4, 5].

LM may also occur with other CVMs, further complicating the clinical picture. They often occur with venous malformations (VM) [6, 7] and/or arteriovenous malformations (AVM) [8, 9]. These complex lesions are separately classified as hemolymphatic malformations (HLM) and are also known as Klippel-Trenaunay syndrome and Parkes-Weber syndrome [10, 11]. Knowledge and thorough understanding of these mixed CVMs is required for proper diagnosis and appropriate management of the LM itself (Figs. 29.3, 29.4) [12].

This chapter focuses on the extratruncular LM lesion, the so-called lymphangioma, which remains among the most clinically challenging of the LM lesions. A brief summary of the management of the truncular LM lesion that presents as chronic lymphedema is also included [13–15].

General Principles and Guidelines

The vast majority of extratruncular LMs occur as independent lesions, known as a lymphangioma. This lesion is derived from embryonic lymphatic tissue and maintains its mesenchymal cell characteristics [16, 17]. The treatment decision should follow a complete and appropriate assessment of recurrence risk. Recurrence often follows unnecessary stimulation by ill-planned treatment, especially with incomplete excision [18].

R. Mattassi, D.A. Loose, M. Vaghi (eds.), *Hemangiomas and Vascular Malformations*.
© Springer-Verlag Italia 2009

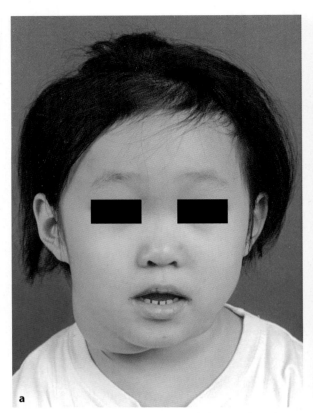
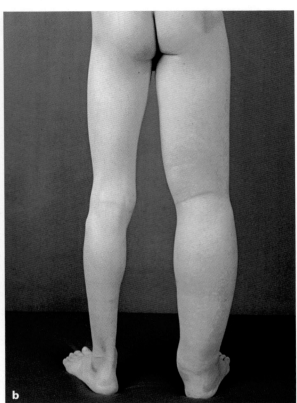

Fig. 29.1. Lymphangioma. **a** A typical shape of lymphangioma presented as a localized swelling along the right neck extended to submandibular region. The extratruncular lymphatic malformation (*LM*) lesion is the second most common vascular malformation after the venous malformation (*VM*); it is a generally localized swelling present as a soft boggy mass, although it also may be the tip of a quite extensive deep-seated lesion in the head and neck region. **b** A common form of primary lymphedema, affecting the right lower extremity of young male patient. This hypoplasia of the lymph-transporting vessel is a clinical outcome of truncular lymphatic malformation. It manifests as a diffuse swelling along the entire area affected by lymphatic obstruction/stasis. However, a localized/limited form of lymphedema seldom mimics lymphangioma until it progresses further

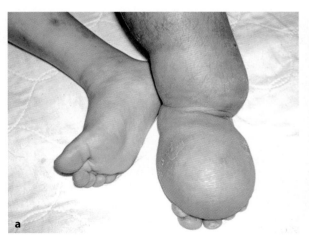
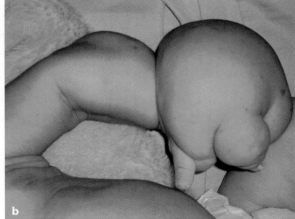

Fig. 29.2. An extreme case of massive swelling on the **a** foot or **b** hand should be investigated in order to determine whether it is a truncular, extratruncular or mixed LM lesion. If there is any doubt of its status, a tissue biopsy is recommended before the treatment decision is taken, although a proper combination of various non-invasive and invasive tests (such as direct puncture percutaneous lymphangiography) is generally sufficient. Both of these cases were shown to have a mixed condition of truncular with an extratruncular LM lesion

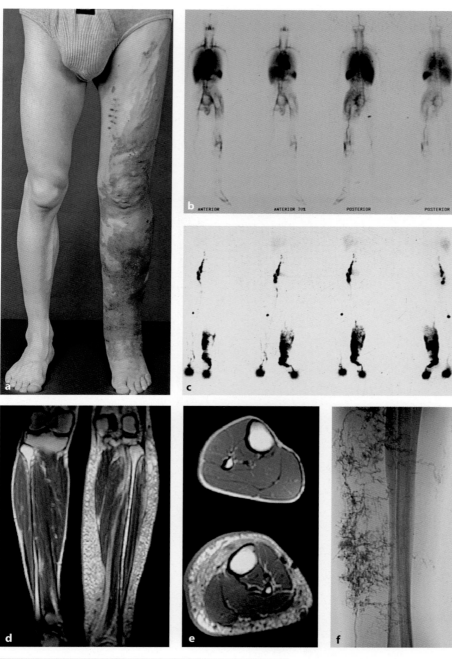

Fig. 29.3. A complex form of vascular malformation. **a** A clinical condition of the swollen left lower extremity is often called Klippel-Trenaunay Syndrome (*KTS*). However, the condition is a lot more complicated than a simple name, with many different combinations of various vascular malformations. Therefore, its proper management warrants precise information on each malformation involved, as well as its severity. Generally, non-invasive studies can confirm the vascular malformation components without difficulty. **b** Whole body blood pool scintigraphy (*WBBPS*) can depict the exact location and severity of coexisting VM lesions throughout the whole body in addition to the left lower extremity itself so that a proper treatment plan can be initiated. **c** Radionuclide lymphoscintigraphy can identify the accurate condition/severity of lymphatic dysfuction caused by a truncular LM lesion so that lymphedema management can be initiated based on this finding. **d, e** MRI study is essential to assess VM and LM together: a honey-comb type image of the soft tissue is the hallmark of chronic lymphedema to confirm clinically observed diffuse swelling of the limb as lymphedema. **f, g** Transarterial lung perfusion scintigraphy (*TLPS*) can rule out any possibility of AVM combined with this condition and reduce the need for unnecessary invasive studies (e.g., arteriography). Only careful evaluation such as this will allow proper management of this complex form of vascular malformation

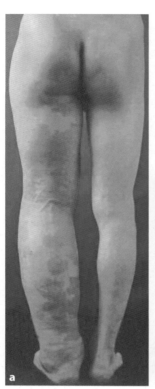

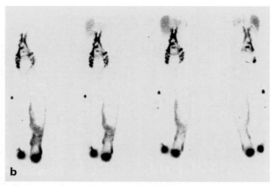

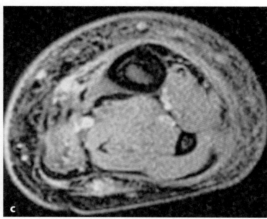

Fig. 29.4. Left lower extremity. **a** Clinical feature of the left lower extremity shows a similarity to common KTS, representing a "hemolymphatic malformation" consisting of LM, VM and CM only, as shown in Figure 29.3. But further clinical evidence based on duplex ultrasonography suggested an additional vascular malformation component: AVM, leading to a diagnosis of Parkes-Weber Syndrome (*PWS*). **b** Initial evaluation with radionuclide lymphoscintigraphy and **c** MRI confirmed a truncular LM lesion as the cause of primary lymphedema while **d** WBBPS confirmed an additional VM component. **e** However, Duplex ultrasonography showed evidence of AVM as the cause of clinically hyperdynamic arterial condition; **f** it was further assessed to 69.3% shunting status by the TLPS. **g** Finally, arteriographic investigation confirmed superficially located multiple micro-shunting AVM lesions scattered through the lower extremity. On the basis of such accurate information, an appropriate treatment strategy can be set up for each involved lesion: LM, VM and AVM (from [40])

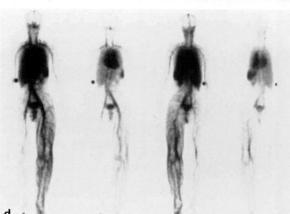

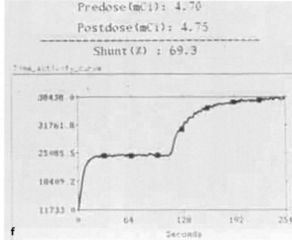

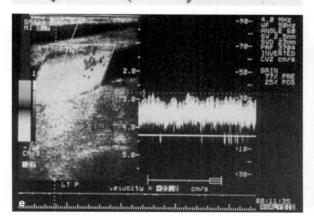

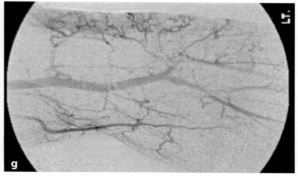

Compared to other CVMs (e.g., VM and AVM), LMs are not life- or limb-threatening. Treatment modalities associated with high morbidity (e.g., absolute ethanol sclerotherapy) should only be considered after lower morbidity treatments have failed [12]. Therapy often begins with safer and less risky treatment methods, such as OK-432. Although these methods carry less risk and morbidity, they are also associated with a higher risk of lesion recurrence. On the other hand, the treatments associated with higher morbidity, such as ethanol, carry a lower risk of lesion recurrence.

LM treatment with sclerotherapy and/or surgical (excisional) therapy should be limited to lesions lo-

cated near vital organs and anatomic structures that threaten vital functions, such as respiration, vision, hearing, or eating (Fig. 29.5). Early treatment should also be considered for lesions with accompanying complications, such as lymph leakage, bleeding (LM lesions with a mixed venous component), or recurrent infections or cellulitis (Fig. 29.6). Symptomatic lesions, with or without cosmetically severe deformities or functional disability, such as of the hand, foot, wrist, and ankle, should also be considered for early therapy (Fig. 29.7) [4, 5, 19, 20].

Definitive treatment in children should be delayed until the child reaches an age at which the risks as-

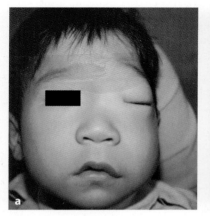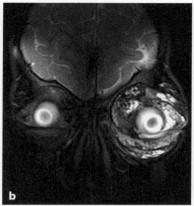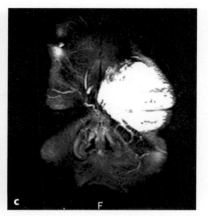

Fig. 29.5. Lymphatic malformation. **a** This young boy was previously known to have moderately puffy eyelids with mild periorbital swelling on the left side due to the infiltrating extratruncular LM, as shown in **b, c** MRI findings. However, sudden massive swelling along the left eye resulted in complete blockage of his vision following mild infection due to this LM lesion. Such an LM lesion is as dangerous, if not more, than an ordinary VM or AVM lesion in terms of acute/urgent necessity and the immediate treatment that was needed to save his vision; this is particularly the case if it occurs in an infant before vision is fully matured

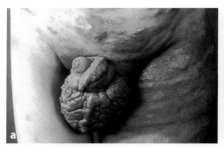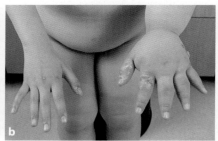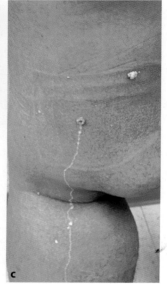

Fig. 29.6. Infection along the lymphatic leakage is the worst combination for the prognosis of LM lesions. **a** The clinical outcome of chronic infection combined with leakage. The LM lesion itself is relatively benign although it extends into the retropelvic structure as a mixed cystic type, but its complication remains a potentially life-threatening condition which may progress to general sepsis. **b** A difficult condition with recurrent ruptures of lymph vesicles on the hand/fingers which is already compromised with lymphedema, which allows the progression of acute skin infection. **c** The leakage of lymphatic fluid from the posterior thigh due to the chylo-reflux from truncular LM lesion; it is further complicated with chylo-ascites by intra-abdominal LM. This patient also has extratruncular LM lesions. These complications as well as morbidities indicate early aggressive care with priority

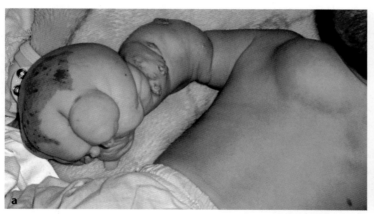
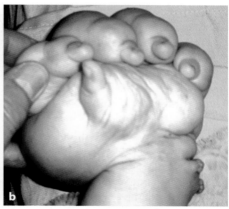

Fig. 29.7. This young baby was born with enormous swelling of the hand and forearm/upper arm caused by an extra-truncular LM lesion; this condition would certainly interfere with normal physical and mental development. Further clinical evaluation revealed another large extratruncular LM lesion affecting the back/shoulder/neck, which also seemed to grow rapidly. In terms of a functional point of view, the hand lesion affecting the fingers presents a daunting task for supporting normal physical and functional development of the hand and fingers. This case, therefore, was of utmost priority for management with no delay

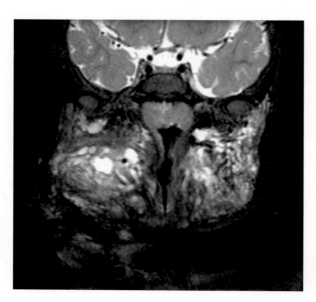

Fig. 29.8. This massive extratruncular LM lesion affecting the entire neck became the source of an acute infection resulting in acute airway obstruction; it required a limited debulking operation to relieve the airway obstruction as an emergency life-saving procedure. The child subsequently underwent a more radical operation to remove an expanding residual lesion along the left side of the neck

sociated with therapy are reduced. Unless the lesion is located at a life- or limb-threatening region, and requires immediate and/or urgent treatment, conservative management, such as compression therapy, should be continued. Conservative management is usually continued in the young pediatric age group until the age of two or older, when the child can better tolerate the treatment.

Emergency life-saving measures may be required, especially in neonatal and young pediatric patients where LM lesions cause acute respiratory or alimentary problems (Fig. 29.8).

When a LM occurs with another CVM, such as an HLM, the decision to treat is usually based on the severity of symptoms associated with the concomitant CVM. AVMs and VMs are clinically more virulent vascular malformations compared with LMs and capillary malformations (CMs) (Fig. 29.9). Treatment of the LM should be addressed after successful management of the VM and/or AVM, when present.

When both extratruncular and truncular LMs occur together, the extratruncular lesion should be treated initially by, for example, excision and/or sclerotherapy. Extreme care should be taken not to risk further damage to the lymph-transporting system that is already jeopardized by the truncular LM lesion causing the chronic lymphedema (Fig. 29.10).

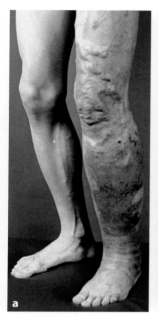

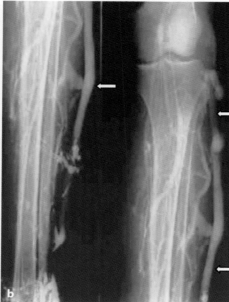

Fig. 29.9. a A left lower extremity was diagnosed as a hemolymphatic malformation consisting of VM, LM and CM. The LM component was further verified for both the extratruncular and also truncular LM lesions. **b** As for the VM component, truncular VM was identified as a "lateral embryonic/marginal vein"; it ran along the lateral aspect of the lower leg and extended to the upper leg as the source of massive venous reflux due to the lack of the venous valves (*arrows*). Chronic venous insufficiency with venous hypertension by the VM lesion is clinically more serious than two LMs combined. Therefore, a marginal vein resection was carried out, bringing an improvement not only to the venous system but also to the lymphatic system

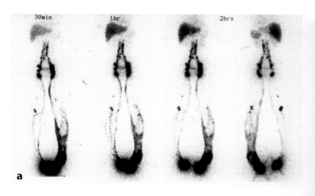

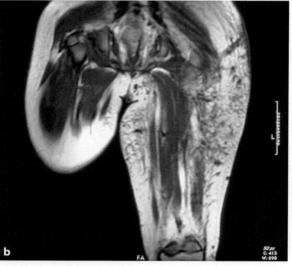

Fig. 29.10. Primary lymphedema. **a** Patient with primary lymphedema affecting the left lower extremity, as confirmed with radionuclide lymphoscintigraphy was found to have another LM lesion of a different type affecting the left buttock. **b** By MRI the lesion along the buttock was confirmed as a diffuse infiltrating extratruncular LM lesion without much evidence of connection to the truncular LM lesion of the lower extremity. Repeated sclerotherapy with ethanol was given to the buttock lesion to control the lymph leakage as the cause of recurrent local cellulitis. Subsequently, the leg swelling/lymphedema rapidly deteriorated, confirmed by lymphoscintigraphy. Hence, the sclerotherapy was stopped and the swelling took more than 6 months to go back to the original level (clinical stage II), while the laboratory/lymphoscintigraphic stage of the lymphedema remained in L-stage II-B

From a treatment priority standpoint, the truncular LM should be treated after the extratruncular LM has been addressed. Truncular LM causes chronic lymphedema that is generally well managed with conservative measures when started early, including manual lymphatic drainage (MLD) based on complex decongestive therapy (CDT) (Fig. 29.11) [21–24].

Surgical treatment for truncular LM, either reconstructive [25, 26] or ablative [27, 28], should be considered as supplemental therapy following aggressive CDT (Figs. 29.12, 29.13). Patients with primary lymphedema have limited indications for reconstructive surgery. Patients who undergo surgery typically experience outcomes that are generally poor compared

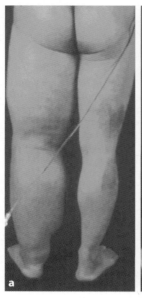
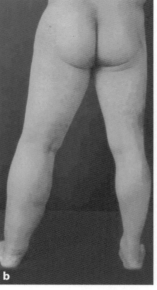

Fig. 29.11. Primary lymphedema. **a** Clinical status of primary lymphedema affecting the left lower extremity before therapy was initiated. This lymphedema is due to a defective lymph-transporting system of the extremity caused by the truncular LM lesion; a hypoplastic condition of lymph nodes and lymph collecting vessels resulted in lymph stasis/obstruction. Therefore, the therapy aims at the relief of lymphatic congestion in the leg utilizing its collateral system. The standard regimen is now based on manual lymphatic drainage-based complex decongestive therapy (MLD-CDT) with/without combined compression therapy. **b** Remarkable relief of the swelling by intense hospital-based treatment; the long-term outcome of the maintenance of such an excellent initial response will totally depend on the patient's compliance with the life-long therapy

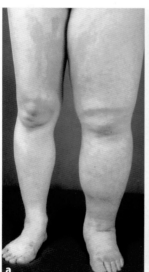
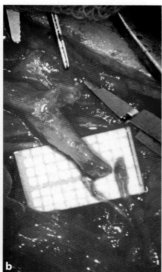
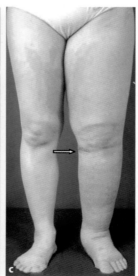

Fig. 29.12. Primary lymphedema. **a** Clinical status of primary lymphedema affecting the left lower extremity before reconstructive surgery was performed. Due to recurrent cellulitis with rapid deterioration of the limb swelling despite aggressive care with CDT for 2 years, reconstructive surgery was chosen as a supplement to improve the efficacy of CDT. **b** Multiple well-functioning lymphatic vessels for the lympho-venous anastomoses. Lymphatic vessels at the popliteal level were selected instead of those at the femoral level for the anastomoses in order to retrieve more functional/non-paralyzed lymphatic vessels for the bypass anastomoses; those lymph vessels with good pulsatile condition were more capable of relieving intense distal swelling to improve lymphatic function. **c** Improvement of the leg swelling by well-functioning anastomoses done at popliteal level (*arrow*); the limb following the reconstructive surgery had a much better response to the physical therapy and this clinical improvement was further confirmed on 6 months follow-up lymphoscintigraphy showing much decreased dermal backflow, etc. (from [4])

to outcomes observed in patients with secondary lymphedema. This difference is likely to be due to the fact that primary lymphedema patients have developmental defects that occur along the lymph-transporting system and present as aplastic, hypoplastic or hyperplastic lesions that are often combined with further defects in lymph nodes producing a complex condition (e.g., lymphangio-lymphadenosodysplasia) [29]. Further

detailed information is found elsewhere [12–15].

Selection of treatment modalites, in addition to the basic conservative treatment regimen with CDT, either surgical or non-surgical (e.g., sclerotherapy), should be made by a multidisciplinary team. Priority for treatment among multiple lesion types should be based on the relative degree, extent and severity of the specific lesion (Fig. 29.14).

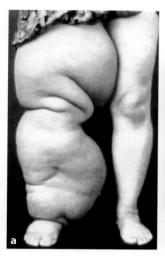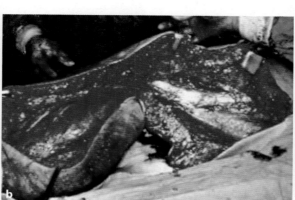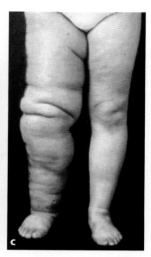

Fig. 29.13. Chronic lymphedema. **a** Very advanced chronic lymphedema of right lower extremity. Such an enormous and grotesquely swollen limb represents the end stage of the lymphedema; the local condition accompanies advanced fibrotic changes through the entire soft tissue and skin: the phenomenon of "lymphodermatofibrosclerosis". It becomes the source of recurrent life-threatening sepsis and there is no longer a salvageable lymphatic system. Proper CDT is virtually impossible due to the disfigured contours, hindering an effective wrapping with compression stocking, which is an essential part of the physical therapy. **b** Therefore, extensive excision of hardened skin and soft tissue was performed along the upper and lower legs in stages with a modified Homans' technique. **c** Immediate outcome of the "excisional" surgery to remove most of the hardened soft tissue; it could reduce the source of infection/sepsis and also provide appropriate CDT/compression therapy postoperatively (from [27])

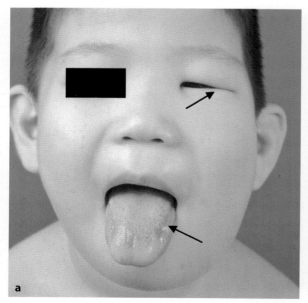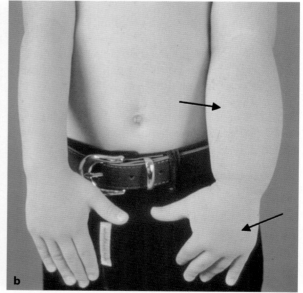

Fig. 29.14. Multiple LM lesions. **a** This young male patient was found to have multiple LM lesions affecting the left periorbital region, mouth and tongue (*arrows*) and **b** left forearm and hand (*arrows*). The lesion affecting the head and oral cavity belongs to an extratruncular LM lesion, while the one affecting the forearm and hand is a truncular lesion. In addition, he was later found to have another two small extratruncular lesions on the back. Among these multiple lesions, the priority for medical attention should be carefully chosen based on clinical significance. Although the oral cavity lesion is more symptomatic, the periorbital lesion is potentially more risky as it may block the vision, especially as there is a recent history of acute cellulitis. Therefore, the evaluation and management of this orbital lesion were initiated and the oral lesion was treated later. The truncular lesion affecting the left upper extremity was handled with a CDT-based life-long regimen as with a primary lymphedema

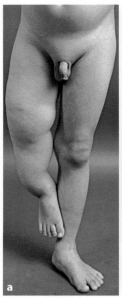
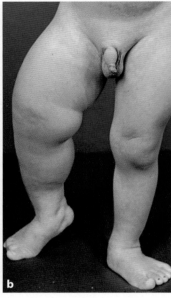
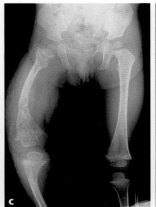
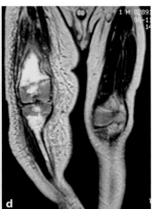

Fig. 29.15. Vascular bone syndrome. **a** This young male patient shows the outcome of unsuccessful management of vascular bone syndrome resulting in an irreparable condition of angio-osteohypotrophy. **b** The child was initially treated as for an ordinary primary lymphedema of his truncular lesion affecting the right lower extremity. However, following subsequent episodes of recurrent pathological fracture, the child was referred for further management. **c, d** The child has an intraosseous LM lesion affecting both the femur and tibia of the right lower extremity in addition to soft tissue truncular LM lesion; this caused severe limb length shortage without normal long bone growth, resulting in uncorrectable leg length discrepancy. It would have been more appropriate to handle this lesion with aggressive sclerotherapy from its earlier stage in order to control the steady expansion of the LM lesion to allow improved new bony tissue growth

Accurate and thorough hemodynamic assessment of the deep venous system of the lower extremity is absolutely required for the safe management of LMs located in the lower extremity. This is especially important when the LM lesion is combined with a VM [30].

LM lesions producing the vascular-bone syndrome (e.g. angio-osteohypotrophy) [31, 32] are best treated early in order to prevent long bone growth discrepancy (Fig. 29.15).

Treatment Modalities

The treatment strategy for extratruncular LM lesions has changed substantially based on observations regarding their embryology. Incomplete excision is followed by inevitable recurrence, such as cystic hygroma, and often becomes a potential source of significant complications and morbidity. Traditional surgical excision has its role in the treatment of LM along with a mutidisciplinary approach combined with endovascular therapy [33].

Surgical excision is no longer considered as a first line therapy or as a sole treatment modality because LMs rarely become life-threatening. Combination of conventional surgical excision with endovascular therapy based on sclerotherapy should be considered initially. Endovascular therapy with either OK-432 and/or ethanol is usually the first treatment option. This is especially true in difficult lesions that are surgically inaccessible [4, 5].

OK-432 Sclerotherapy

OK-432 is the preferred initial treatment for LM lesions. OK-432 is a lymphatic sclerosing agent.

Also known as Picibanil, OK-432 is the lyophilized exotoxin of the low-virulence Su strain of type III group A *Streptococcus pyogenes*. It is produced after removing streptolysin S-producing activity and has a specific affinity for lymphatic endothelium resulting in selective injury via a relatively benign inflammatory process [34].

OK-432 can easily be injected into a macrocystic lesion or cavity. Outcomes are excellent, with minimal morbidity in the majority of cases (Fig. 29.16) [4, 35]. Microcystic cavernous lesions, on the other hand, are virtually impossible to treat/inject. In

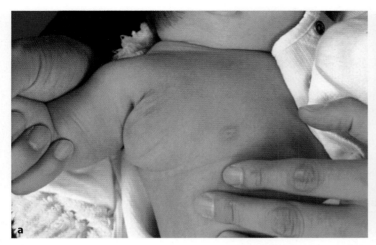
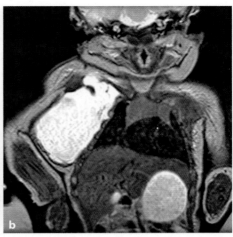

Fig. 29.16. Indications for sclerotherapy with OK-432. **a** This young baby was born with a relatively small soft mass lesion near the right arm pit. However, it grew suddenly in size. **b** MRI study showed a large cystic lesion extending to the root of the right side of the neck with the proximity to the brachial plexus. Therefore, OK-432 was used as a scleroagent to control the lesion very effectively since it was a "macrocystic" lesion with minimal septa

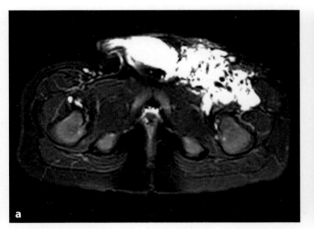
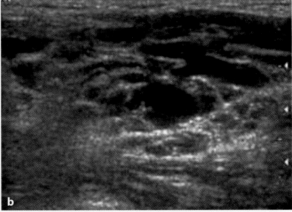

Fig. 29.17. Microcystic LM lesions. **a** Extensive multicystic lesions affecting the left groin extended into the retroperitoneal space, mostly consisting of "microcystic" LM lesions. **b** This was further confirmed with duplex ultrasonography. It became the constant source of local cellulitis. In view of the extensive nature of the lesions with proximity to the iliac-femoral neurovascular structures, OK-432 was selected to minimize the potential risk involved in multiple session therapy. Because of the patient's youth, the procedure was performed under a brief general anesthesia. However, if the recurrent/residual lesion should become a major problem in the future, a combined approach will be considered with surgical excision limited to the critically located lesion and supplemental ethanol sclerotherapy to the other safer part of the lesion after the child is old enough to tolerate such difficult therapy. Ethanol is generally contraindicated for the treatment of microcystic lesions, which also respond poorly to OK-432. However, preoperative OK-432 often hardens the tissue to make local conditions more amenable to later excision

addition, these honey-combed lesions are more likely to communicate with the lymph-transporting system, posing the additional risk of injury to the lymphatic system and peri-lymphatic tissues (e.g., nerves and blood vessels). Compared to other sclerosing agents, OK-432 is relatively safe, even when extravasation occurs.

Multicystic, lobulated lesions are ideal candidates for OK-432 therapy. The risk of extravasation is much lower compared to other scleroagents, especially in a mixed lesion with a microcystic component (Fig. 29.17). These lesions, however, require multiple treatment sessions in order to reduce significant local and systemic reactions.

OK-432 is much less effective than more powerful agents, such as ethanol, but carries a lower risk of complications. It is useful even when sclerotherapy fails. OK-432 thickens the wall of a single-layer endothelial lesion, allowing easier dissection, compared with a primary thin-walled lesion, in situations where subsequent surgical excision is necessary. OK-432 is a sclerosing agent with minimal potential for collateral damage, and acceptable recurrence rates. It is the ideal sclerosing agent for treatment of relatively benign LM lesions compared to the more virulent VM and AVMs. It is relatively free of significant complications and morbidity that is associated with the more powerful sclerotherapeutic agents [4].

When a LM lesion occurs with a VM lesion (which is easily confirmed by the presence of blood mixed with lymph on the aspiration) OK-432 is totally useless. In these situations, the more powerful sclerotherapy agents such as ethanol are required to control the lesion.

We generally recommend OK-432 for initial treatment of all de novo LM lesions. Repeat treatment of recurrent LM lesions that have failed OK-432 therapy is also recommended, especially in situations where treatment with ethanol carries unacceptable risk.

Ethanol Sclerotherapy

Ethanol is an excellent sclerotherapeutic agent for treatment of a "macro-cystic" LM lesions. In experienced hands, ethanol therapy is associated with minimum morbidity and almost zero recurrence. This agent is an excellent substitute for OK-432 therapy and has better long-term results. In the treatment of a "microcystic" LM lesion, ethanol sclerotherapy is associated with high complication rates and significant morbidity. Significant collateral tissue necrosis often occurs during treatment of this relatively benign malformation (e.g., nerve damage) (Fig. 29.18).

The general principles of ethanol sclerotherapy should be applied to the treatment of LM lesions: the minimal effective dose of ethanol should be used during each treatment session to minimize the risk of complications [36].

We recommend that ethanol sclerotherapy be limited to the treatment of macrocystic LM lesions occurring in anatomically safe/deep locations. We strongly urge limited use of ethanol for the treatment of microcystic or mixed LM lesions. Recurrent symptomatic lesions, failed OK-432 sclerotherapy, a mixed LM lesion occurring with a VM lesion, and a surgically inaccessible lesion are indications for ethanol sclerotherapy (Fig. 29.19) [4, 5].

Post Sclerotherapy Care of the Lesion/Patient

Post procedure fever is common after OK-432 sclerotherapy and is well managed with antipyretic therapy (acetaminophen or ibuprofen). Pediatric patients often require a short hospitalization post procedure.

Ethanol sclerotherapy patients require close perioperative monitoring for pulmonary hypertension;

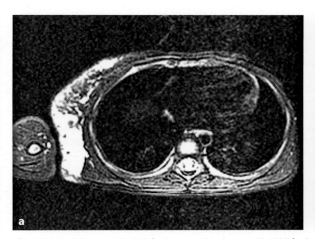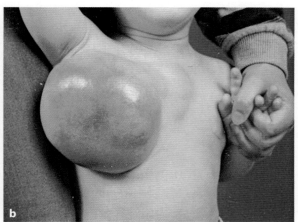

Fig. 29.18. Microcystic LM lesions. **a** A microcystic LM lesion shown by MRI is not a good candidate for ethanol sclerotherapy. However, following repeated failure with OK-432 sclerotherapy, ethanol was carefully combined with OK-432; its injection was carried out under ultrasonographic guidance and limited to the lesion which had the best cystic condition to allow safe injection with the least risk of extravasation. **b** However, the outcome was alarmingly: tremendous swelling, but without skin necrosis. Following such difficult conditions which cannot be controlled by the conventional sclerotherapy, the lesion was subsequently surgically excised

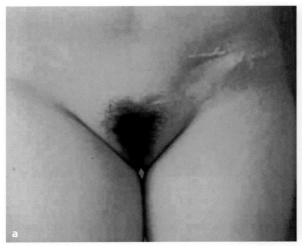 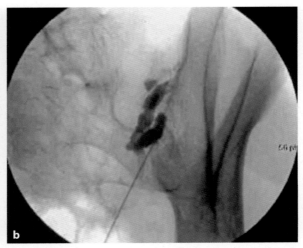

Fig. 29.19. Recurring lesions. **a** There are multiple operation scars along the left lower abdomen following surgical excisions. However, due to their embryologic nature, the extratruncular lesions recurred despite multiple operations to remove them completely. **b** Subsequently, MRI and duplex ultrasonography easily identified a few residual lesions located deeply along the pelvic wall. Under the fluoroscopic guidance, ethanol sclerotherapy was given to these "recurrent" but mostly "macrocystic" and deep-seated lesions; this ethanol therapy potentially cured the lesion (5 year follow-up with no evidence of recurrence on sonography)

this is continued post operatively. These patients also require post procedure pain control and close observation of the treated areas for local tissue reaction and edema. However, post procedure compression therapy is controversial at best, with a higher chance of harmful versus beneficial effect following ethanol therapy.

Treatment outcomes are best assessed by duplex ultrasonography performed within a week of treatment and just before additional therapy.

Surgical/Excisional Therapy

Surgical therapy in the treatment of LM lesions is limited due to the significant risk and morbidity associated with the radical procedure [4, 5]. The majority of LM lesions occur as mixed lesions containing both macrocystic and microcystic components. The presence of the microcystic component limits the effectiveness of OK-432. Ethanol therapy of these mixed lesions is associated with significant morbidity. In addition, many microcystic LM lesions often occur with VM lesions. In this situation, complications associated with ethanol therapy preclude its use, while OK-432 has no effect on VM lesions. Therefore, this lesion type is best treated with surgical excision with or without preoperative OK-432 sclerotherapy (Fig. 29.20).

Certain lesions that cannot be treated effectively with sclerotherapy (such as neck lesions that extend into the deep mediastinal structures) may require surgical excision because of mass effect and extensive involvement of surrounding anatomical structures (Fig. 29.21). The risk of injury to adjacent vessels and nerves during dissection may be prohibitively high and associated with significant life-long morbidity. This is especially true in the pediatric population [2, 3, 19, 20]. The approach to treatment in these situations has changed over the years. Incomplete excision, sparing vital anatomic structures, is an acceptable alternative to radical resection, which results in significant morbidity. LM lesions are rarely life-threatening compared to VM or AVM lesions, and can often be managed with a less aggressive surgical approach.

The role of surgical therapy in the treatment of LM has been well defined and is now fully integrated with endovascular therapy (sclerotherapy) [4, 5]. Surgical excision is especially useful in the treatment of macro- and microcystic mixed LM lesions. These lesions can be effectively controlled with preoperative sclerotherapy followed by surgical excision (Fig. 29.21).

There is no well defined optimal time for surgical excision. Surgical resection should be delayed for as long as possible. Partial excision of an easily accessible lesion is acceptable as the first stage of a multi-stage approach. It allows a better chance for later excision of the residual lesion. Emergency procedures should be limited to decompressive surgery designed to relieve acute symptoms until a later, more definitive treatment can be planned.

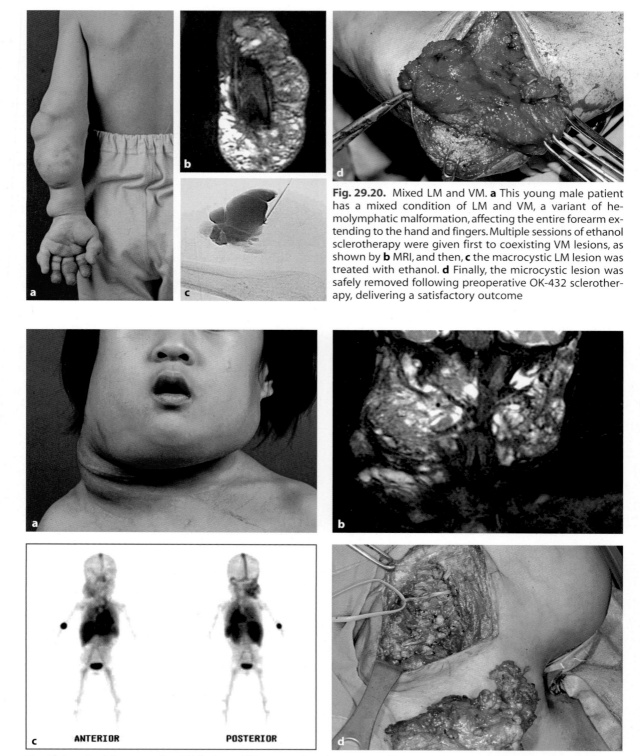

Fig. 29.20. Mixed LM and VM. **a** This young male patient has a mixed condition of LM and VM, a variant of hemolymphatic malformation, affecting the entire forearm extending to the hand and fingers. Multiple sessions of ethanol sclerotherapy were given first to coexisting VM lesions, as shown by **b** MRI, and then, **c** the macrocystic LM lesion was treated with ethanol. **d** Finally, the microcystic lesion was safely removed following preoperative OK-432 sclerotherapy, delivering a satisfactory outcome

Fig. 29.21. Rapidly expanding LM lesion. **a** This young female patient underwent limited resection of a LM lesion along the right lateral neck, and was referred with a rapidly expanding lesion. **b** MRI showed a potentially life-threatening condition with high risk of upper airway obstruction. **c** WBBPS showed a significant abnormal blood pool coexisting with the VM lesion along this histologically-proven extratruncular LM lesion. **d** OK-432 sclerotherapy was therefore ruled out due to this coexisting VM lesion and surgical excision was carried out to relieve the rapidly expanding LM lesion from the right lateral neck. However, limited ethanol sclerotherapy was added to moderately cystic VM and LM lesions preoperatively to reduce subsequent surgical morbidity

Clinical Experiences – Predominant (Truncular and Extratruncular) LM Lesions

Among the various sclerotherapy agents (such as polidocanol, bleomycin, tetracycline, cyclophosphamide), two agents, ethanol and OK-432, have been shown to be useful in the management of LM lesions and have become our sclerotherapy agents of choice for the treatment of LMs.

As previously published [4, 5], ethanol gives excellent results when used as a sole treatment modality for recurrent or deeply seated lesions, preferably the macrocystic types. Superficial lesions treated independently with OK-432 also respond well in most cases.

Microcystic/cavernous lesions, when treated independently, generally do not respond well. When possible, microcystic lesions are treated with pre- and peri-operative sclerotherapy combined with surgical excision. However, results of this approach are mixed and success is limited.

Among a total of 1,203 CVM patients, 393 patients were confirmed to be predominantly LM: 271 had a truncular LM and 122 had an extratruncular LM. LM was combined with VM as HLM in 108 of 1,203 CVM patients. Of 122 patients with predominantly extratruncular LM, 89 had the macrocystic type with a predilection for the head, neck and thorax (63/122). Of the 271 patients with truncular LM, 247 had an aplastic and/or obstructing type with a predilection for the extremities (253), mostly of lower extremity (224).

Extratruncular Lesion: Lymphangioma

Ninety-seven patients received endovascular treatments: sclerotherapy with OK-432 (89/97) or ethanol (8/97) as independent therapy (82/97) or adjunct therapy (15/97). Thirty-five patients underwent surgical excision, either independently (20/35) or with preoperative OK-432 and/or ethanol sclerotherapy (15/35).

Independent OK-432 sclerotherapy was given over 169 sessions and delivered excellent results in the majority of macrocystic type lesions (51/61) and limited success in the microcystic type (5/10); with a minimum follow-up of 32 months.

Of eight patients with recurrent lesions, independent absolute ethanol sclerotherapy delivered excellent results (6/8) over 12 sessions, but also significant complications (4/8). Preoperative OK-432 sclerotherapy and subsequent surgical excision (n = 15) have shown excellent to good results in a majority of patients (12/15), with a minimum fol-

low-up of 49 months. Independent surgical therapy (n = 20) showed satisfactory results in 13 patients, with four recurrences.

Truncular Lesion: Primary Lymphedema

CDT and/or compression therapy were given as main treatment to a total of 275 patients. These patients were divided according to their clinical stages: with 54 in clinical stage I, 142 in stage II, 58 in stage III and 21 in stage IV.

Clinical response was excellent to good in the majority of clinical stage I and II patients (171/196), with decreased improvement in stage III and IV (42/79), with a minimum of 2 years to a maximum of 4 years for follow up.

Long-term results of the treatment based on self-initiated home-maintenance care were totally dependent on patient compliance.

Surgical therapy was added to the CDT-based management as a supplement to failing CDT: reconstructive surgery with lympho-venous anastomoses [37] in 19 patients in clinical stage I and II, free lymph node transplant surgery [38] in 13 patients in clinical stage II and III, and ablative (excisional) surgery in 33 patients in clinical stage III and IV.

Long-term maintenance of initially successful surgical results was totally dependent on the patients' compliance: three of 19 lymphatic reconstructions and 18 of 33 ablative surgeries maintained good results during the follow-up period (minimum 2 years to maximum 4 years).

Management of LM Belonging to HLM

LM is a component of the HLM. Its management is different from the management of LM alone due to the interrelationship with the other vascular malformations: truncular and/or extratruncular VM and/or AVM.

Definitive diagnosis and assessment of a concomitant VM can be further strengthened with whole body blood pool scintigraphy (WBBPS) [39], while the diagnosis of an AVM can be confirmed with transarterial lung perfusion scintigraphy (TLPS) [40]. General assessment of the degree of severity and extent of all "low-flow" lesions should be made with magnetic resonance imaging (MRI) [41]. Accurate staging of the lymphedema should also be made with lymphoscintigraphy [42].

Treatment of this complex HLM should be based on the treatment of the VM component (either truncular or extratruncular forms) with a priority to the LM component.

Treatment of the concomitant VM often results in a transient worsening of the lymphatic dysfunction due to the interrelated venous and lymphatic systems. This often occurs following surgical resection of a marginal or lateral embryonic vein (e.g., increased lymphatic leakage and/or sepsis of lymphatic origin) (Fig. 29.22) [43]. When the deep venous system is involved in VM, such as in deep vein hypoplasia, further care/support of an already compromised lymphatic system is essential to prevent associated complications, such as recurrent cellulitis (Fig. 29.23).

Infrequently, HLM lesions have both truncular and extratruncular LM components, which make clinical management more complicated. When extratruncular and truncular LM lesions occur together where surgical excision is required, a staged approach should be taken. This approach should minimize its impact on an already poorly functioning lymphatic system. Aggressive MLD should prevent further deterioration of lymphatic function.

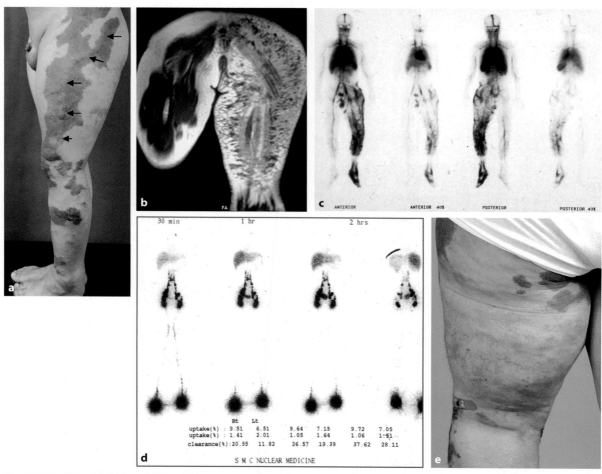

Fig. 29.22. VM with LM and CM. **a** This young male patient was confirmed as having a hemolymphatic malformation consisting of a VM and LM in addition to CM. **b, c** Truncular VM was confirmed as a marginal vein and an extratruncular LM lesion was confirmed in infiltrating conditions along the buttock as shown by MRI. **d** There was no evidence of extratruncular VM on WBBPS or truncular LM by lymphoscintigraphy. Therefore the patient underwent successful one stage excision of the marginal vein, leaving a scar running along the lateral aspect of the thigh; chronic venous insufficiency by severe venous reflux was finally controlled. **e** However, immediately following the VM excision, the extratruncular LM lesion affecting the posterior upper thigh showed rapid deterioration with increased leakage and more severe/frequent local cellulitis often extending to systemic sepsis. It took many months until moderate compensation was achieved to adjust to the new venodynamic as well as lymphodynamic condition

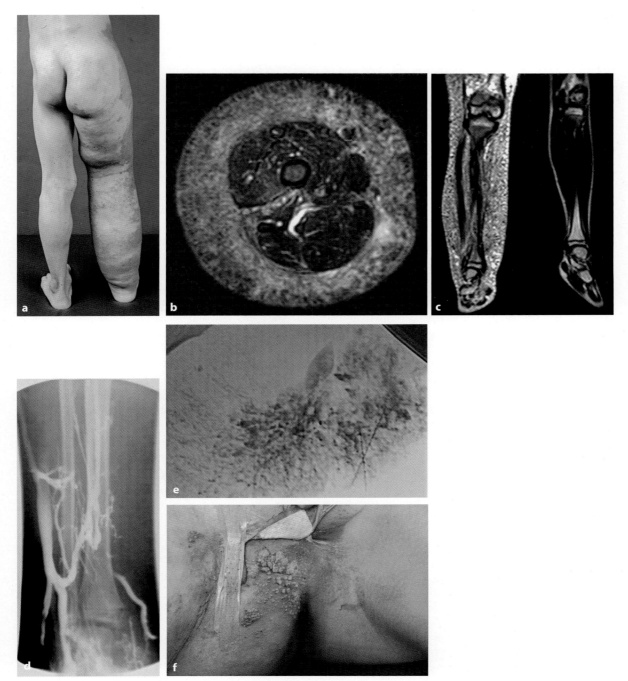

Fig. 29.23. Multiple lesions. **a** This male child was initially diagnosed only with primary lymphedema by truncular LM as shown by **b, c** MRI. **d** However, further investigation identified a marginal vein running along the lateral aspect of the lower extremity as a truncular VM lesion, shown in ascending phlebography. **e** Percutaneous direct puncture lymphangiography confirmed an infiltrating extratruncular LM lesion along the buttock as a LM component of the HLM, in addition to truncular LM. Due to marginal capacity of the deep vein system because of its hypoplastic condition, the marginal vein was confirmed as a major venous drainage route. Therefore, it was decided to leave this marginal vein untreated and conservative care with compression therapy was given. However, the swelling rapidly increased with recurrent sepsis along the perineum, so that the sclerotherapy to these perineal LM lesions was initiated with ethanol/OK-432 due to the mixed condition with VM. **f** Local sepsis was controlled but the lymphatic leakage worsened, forcing further LM treatment to halt. There has not yet been any practical solution in this case

Clinical Experiences – HLM lesion

Among 108 patients with HLM, 61 were confirmed to have at least one "clinically significant" VM and/or LM lesion that required appropriate treatment. Sixty-one patients had a total of 79 LM lesions altogether: 37 extratruncular LM lesions and 42 truncular LM lesions. Among 37 extratruncular LM lesions, 29 were confirmed as major lesions with clinical significance while eight had a minor component (Fig. 29.24).

Among 29 patients with major extratruncular LM lesions, ten were able to receive appropriate treatment to control lymphatic leakage and/or local/systemic sepsis with ethanol/OK-432 sclerotherapy (6/10) or a surgical excision (4/10) but 19 patients were neither indicated (11/19) nor suitable (8/19) for currently available therapy for various reasons, such as location-proximity to nerve, age, and/or severity.

Four of six patients who underwent ethanol/OK-432 sclerotherapy showed excellent response with satisfactory outcome, with a follow-up of 3.3 years.

Another four who underwent surgical excision had excellent results with no evidence of recurrence, with a follow-up of 3.1 years.

Forty-two patients with truncular lesions received conservative management of primary lymphedema, with CDT and/or compression therapy to prevent further progression/ deterioration. Thirty of the patients showed good compliance, with a maintenance of satisfactory conditions, while 12 noncompliant patients deteriorated during the follow-up period (3.1 years).

Prospects

The future of the clinical management of LM is now brighter than ever, with new concepts and approaches based on the correction of defective lymphangiogenesis [44, 45]. There has been substantial progress made in the quest to localize and characterize the responsible genes and mutations.

Exogenous growth factor administration will open a new chapter to effective gene and gene product therapy; recently anti-VEGFR-3 neutralizing antibody has been confirmed as having the capacity to completely and specifically inhibit lymphatic vascular regeneration.

The cloning of the gene responsible for lymphangiogenesis and identification of the defective genes involved in abnormal lymphangiogenesis will eventually lead to prenatal diagnosis and ultimately mutational screening of at risk populations.

The correction of defective lymphangiogenesis will become a major tool for the future management of 'primary' lymphedema, as well as lymphangioma. Theoretically, timely detection of defective genes during embryonic development and appropriate correction could prevent lymphatic defects at birth, and gene modification could also compensate for abnormal functions in adult patient group. However, the feasibility of these therapeutic implementations is still far from reality and only a few steps have been made toward these goals.

Conclusion

Extratruncular LM lesions can be treated with different sclerotherapy agents as the primary mode of therapy. The macrocystic type is well treated by sclerotherapy with excellent results and minimum risk of recurrence. Surgical excision with and without perioperative sclerotherapy may be considered a better option in the treatment of the localized microcystic lesion and carries a reduced risk of recurrence.

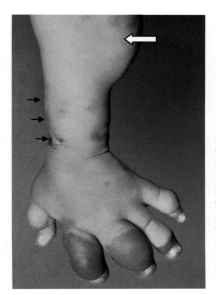

Fig. 29.24. Before a large microcystic extratruncular LM lesion was excised along the radial side of the distal forearm (*arrows*), the potential risk of worsening the lymphatic function along the distal part by the excision was assessed since the lesion was located close to the main lymphatic channel, starting from radial aspect of the wrist. Lymphedema/swelling of the hand and fingers immediately got worse following the excision due to the disrupted lymphatic transport system with transient blockage of compensatory lymphatic drainage through the surgical area. It took over 6 months to relieve this worsened swelling and get the hand and fingers back to the preoperative state. Therefore, further plans to proceed with excision of the mass lesion located on the ulnar side of the upper forearm, proximal to the previous excision site (*white arrow*), were delayed until full compensation of the previously inflicted surgical lymphedema was achieved

References

1. Belov St (1990) Classification of congenital vascular defects. Int Angiol 9:141–146
2. Alqahtani A, Nguyen LT, Flageole H et al (1999) 25 years' experience with lymphangiomas in children. J Pediatr Surg 34:1164–1168
3. Orvidas LJ, Kasperbauer JL (2000) Pediatric lymphangiomas of the head and neck. Ann Otol Rhinol Laryngol 109:411–421
4. Lee BB, Kim YW, Seo JM et al (2005) Current concepts in lymphatic malformation (LM). J Vasc Endovasc Surg 39(1):67–81
5. Lee BB (2005) Lymphedema-Angiodysplasia syndrome: a prodigal form of lymphatic malformation (LM). Phlebolymphology 47:324–332
6. Lee BB, Kim DI, Huh S et al (2001) New experiences with absolute ethanol sclerotherapy in the management of a complex form of congenital venous malformation. J Vasc Surg 33:764–772
7. Lee BB (2003) Current concept of venous malformation (VM). Phlebolymphology 43:197–203
8. Mattassi R (1990) Surgical treatment of congenital arteriovenous defects. Int Angiol 9:196–202
9. Lee BB, Do YS, Yakes W et al (2004) Management of arterial-venous shunting malformations (AVM) by surgery and embolosclerotherapy. A multidisciplinary approach. J Vasc Surg 39:590–600
10. Jacob AG, Driscoll DJ, Shaughnessy WJ et al (1998) Klippel-Trenaunay syndrome: spectrum and management. Mayo Clin Proc 73:28–36
11. Lee BB (2005) Statues of new approaches to the treatment of congenital vascular malformations (CVMS) – single center experiences – (editorial review). Eur J Vasc Endovasc Surg 30:184–197
12. Lee BB (2005) Current issue in management of chronic lymphedema: personal reflection on an experience with 1065 Patients. Lymphology 38:28–31
13. Lee BB, Kim DI, Whang JH, Lee KW (2002) Contemporary management of chronic lymphedema – personal experiences. Lymphology 35 [Suppl]:450–455
14. Lee BB (2004) Chronic lymphedema, no more stepchild to modern medicine! Eur J Lymphol 14:6–12
15. Lee BB (2005) Current issue in management of chronic lymphedema: Personal Reflection on an Experience with 1065 Patients. Commentary. Lymphology 38:28–31
16. Bastide G, Lefebvre D (1989) Anatomy and organogenesis and vascular malformations. In: Belov St, Loose DA, Weber J (eds) Vascular malformations. Einhorn-Presse Verlag GmbH, Reinbek, pp 20–22
17. Woolard HH (1922) The development of the principal arterial stems in the forelimb of the pig. Contrib Embryol 14:139–154
18. Lee BB (2004) Critical issues on the management of congenital vascular malformation. Annals Vasc Surg 18:380–392
19. Al-Salem AH (2004) Lymphangiomas in infancy and childhood. Saudi Med J 25:466–469
20. Stromberg BV, Weeks PM, Wray RC Jr (1976) Treatment of cystic hygroma. South Med J 69:1333–1335
21. Lee BB, Kim HH, Mattassi R et al (2003) A new approach to the congenital vascular malformation with new concept-Seoul Consensus. Int J Angiol 12:248–251
22. Lee BB, Mattassi R, Loose D et al (2004) Consensus on controversial issues in contemporary diagnosis and of congenital vascular malformation–Seoul Communication. Int J Angiol 13:182–192
23. Casley-Smith, Judith R, Mason MR et al (1995) Complex physical therapy for the lymphedematous leg. Int J Angio 4:134–142
24. Hwang JH, Kwon JY, Lee KW et al (1999) Changes in lymphatic function after complex physical therapy for lymphedema. Lymphology 32:15–21
25. Baumeister RGH, Siuda S (1990) Treatment of lymphedemas by microsurgical lymphatic grafting: what is proved? Plastic and Reconstructive Surgery 85:64–74
26. Campisi C, Boccardo F, Zilli A et al (2001) Long-term results after lymphatic-venous anastomoses for the treatment of obstructive lymphedema. Microsurgery 21:135–139
27. Kim DI, Huh S, Lee SJ et al (1998) Excision of subcutaneous tissue and deep muscle fascia for advanced lymphedema. Lymphology 31:190–194
28. Auchincloss H (1930) New operation for elephantiasis. Puerto Rico J Publ Health & Trop Med 6:149
29. Papendieck CM (2002) Lymphangiomatosis and dermoepidermal disturbances of lymphangioadenodysplasias. Lymphology 35[Suppl]:478
30. Lee BB, Mattassi R, Choe YH et al (2005) Critical role of duplex ultrasonography for the advanced management of a venous malformation (VM). Phlebology 20:28–37
31. Mattassi R (1993) Differential diagnosis in congenital vascular-bone syndromes. Sem Vasc Surg 6:233–244
32. Kim YW, Do YS, Lee SH, Lee BB (2006) Risk factors for leg length discrepancy in patients with congenital vascular malformation. J Vasc Surg 44:545–553
33. Lee BB, Bergan JJ (2002) Advanced management of congenital vascular malformations: a multidisciplinary approach. Cardiovascular Surgery 10:523–533
34. Ogita S, Tsuto T, Deguchi E et al (1991) OK-432 therapy for unresectable lymphangiomas in children. J Ped Surg 26:263–270
35. Kim KH, Kim HH, Lee SK, Lee BB (2001) OK-432 intralesional injection therapy for lymphangioma in children. J Korean Asso Ped Surg 7:142–146
36. Lee BB, Do YS, Byun HS et al (2003) Advanced management of venous malformation with ethanol sclerotherapy: mid-term results. J Vasc Surg 37:533–538
37. Krylov V, Milanov N, Abalmasov K (1982) Microlymphatic surgery of secondary lymphoedema of the upper limb. Ann Chir Gynaecol 71:77–79

38. Becker C, Hidden G, Pecking A (1990) Transplantation of lymph nodes: an alternative method for treatment of lymphedema. Progr Lymphol 6:487–493
39. Lee BB, Mattassi R, Kim BT et al (2004) Contemporary diagnosis and management of venous and AV shunting malformation by whole body blood pool scintigraphy (WBBPS). Int Angiol 23:355–367
40. Lee BB, Mattassi R, Kim BT, Park JM (2005) Advanced management of arteriovenous shunting malformation with Transarterial Lung Perfusion Scintigraphy (TLPS) for follow up assessment. Int Angiol 24:173–184
41. Lee BB, Choe YH, Ahn JM et al (2004) The new role of MRI (Magnetic Resonance Imaging) in the contemporary diagnosis of venous malformation: can it replace angiography? J Am Coll Surg 198:549–558
42. Lee BB, Bergan, JJ (2005) New clinical and laboratory staging systems to improve management of chronic lymphedema. Lymphology 38:122–129
43. Kim YW, Lee BB, Cho JH et al (2007) Haemodynamic and clinical assessment of lateral marginal vein excision in patients with a predominantly venous malformation of the lower extremity. Eur J Vasc Endovasc Surg 33:122–127
44. Szuba A, Skobe M, Karkkainen MJ et al (2002).Therapeutic lymphangiogenesis with human recombinant VEGF-C. FASEB J 16:1985–1987
45. Bridenbaugh E (2005) Literature Watch. Lymph Res Biol 3:87–92

Treatment of Vascular Malformations in Newborns and Infants

30

Géza Tasnádi

Abstract

There is little information on the physiological features of the circulation in the newborn and infant. The first haemodynamic change which may induce the development of latent vascular malformations appears when the umbilical cord is cut. Stopping the maternal-neonatal contact also produces important hormonal and metabolic changes. All these effects appear complex in case of already avoidable vascular malformations. At the same time, the vascular malformations have a great influence on the systemic circulation and on the development of the extremity, particularly in this age group. We can prevent the serious sequelae of vascular defects by beginning treatment at the appropriate time – even in neonates and infants – and providing well-planned treatment. Indications for therapy and treatments according to the type of vascular malformation are described in this chapter.

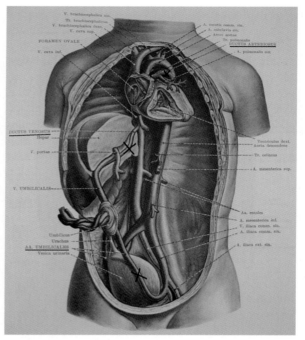

Fig. 30.1. Foetal circulation. Occluded shunts after birth. Reproduced from [1], with permission

Introduction

When treating vascular malformations in newborns and infants, one must take into consideration the physiological features of the circulation.

The first haemodynamic change which may induce the development of latent vascular malformations appears when the umbilical cord is cut (Fig. 30.1). During this time the shunted circulation changes, and from this point it takes part completely in the systemic circulation.

Compared to later ages, in newborns and infants there is increased perfusion of the extremity; high venous pressure; small oxygen consumption for the metabolism, high pO_2 and high lactate dehydrogenase (LDH) activity.

In rare cases, the foramen ovale, ductus venosus or ductus arteriosus fail to close after birth, causing heart and vascular disorders.

Stopping maternal-neonatal contact produces important hormonal and metabolic changes. The high and variable estradiol value in neonates, physical, hydrostatic changes after standing up, and later hormonal changes in adolescence may also influence the circulation [2–4] These effects appear complex in cases of already avoidable vascular malformations.

R. Mattassi, D.A. Loose, M. Vaghi (eds.), *Hemangiomas and Vascular Malformations*.
© Springer-Verlag Italia 2009

At the same time the vascular malformations have a great influence on the systemic circulation and on the development of the extremities, particularly in this age group. In predominantly arteriovenous (AV) defects of the lower extremities, total blood flow increases; LDH activity increases; oxygen consumption decreases, pO_2 and venous pressure increase, there is hypoxic hypoxia in the tissues, and a real hypertrophy of the extremity because of parasitic circulation. All of these factors further increase the cardiac circulatory load.

In predominantly venous malformations, stagnant hypoxia in the tissues is significant. In cases of venous malformations (aplasia, hypoplasia, stenosis, dilatation of deep veins), reduced circulation, decreased or delayed blood flow and diffuse ischaemia – stagnant hypoxia – cause the hypotrophy of tubular bones. In some forms of venous malformations (aplasia, hypoplasia of deep veins), bone hypertrophy is noticeable at the age of 6–10 years. In these cases of venous malformation in childhood, bone hypertrophy is noticeable only in association with AV fistulae. The pathogenic connection between the decompensated venous reduction and the opening of short circuits mostly occurs at 6–10 years of age [3–11].

We can prevent the serious sequelae of vascular defects by beginning treatment at the appropriate time – even in neonates and infants – and providing well-planned treatment.

Indication for Therapy and Treatments

The indication for therapy and treatments differs according to the type of vascular malformation.

Arterial Malformations

Truncular Forms

Truncular forms of arterial malformations include aplasia or obstruction (hypoplasia, stenosis) and dilatation.

Coarctation of the Aorta Descendens

Coarctation of the aorta descendens is a congenital narrowing or complete obstruction of its lumen in a limited area. The narrowing is usually found at the junction of the aortic arch and the descending thoracic aorta.

Indications for Therapy

Since the blood stream meets resistance, the left ventricle experiences systolic overstrain and hypertrophies. Arterial pressure may reach 250–300 mmHg in the upper extremities but be low or absent in the lower extremities.

Coarctation of the aorta descendens in newborns must be operated on if symptoms of serious decompensation are present, otherwise operation during infancy is sufficient.

Techniques

Techniques for treating coarctation of the aorta descendens include ductus ligature and reconstruction, resection and end-to-end anastomosis, patch plasty, bypass, downturning of subclavia, resection and end-to-end Teflon replacement (Fig. 30.2).

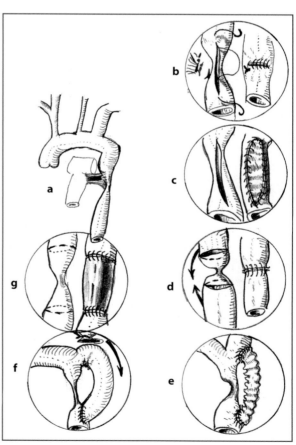

Fig. 30.2. Aorta descendens malformations (coarctation, stenosis). **a** Coarctatio aortae et ductus Botalli persistens. **b** Ductus ligature and reconstruction. **c** Patch plasty. **d** Resection and end to end anastomosis. **e** Bypass. **f** Downturning of subclavia. **g** Resection and end to end Teflon replacement. Reproduced from [12], with permission

Arterial Aneurysms

Arterial aneurysms may be congenital or acquired (Table 30.1). Two basic causes of congenital arterial aneurysm can be identified: developmental arrest of the vessel and anomalous maturation of the mesenchymal cell components. The failure of development is confined to all three layers or only to

Table 30.1. Classification of arterial aneurysms [13]

I. Congenital

II. Aquired

    1. Media's degeneration
       – Ehlers-Danlos syndrome
       – Marfan syndrome
       – Sclerosis tuberosa

    2. Arteritis
       – Kawasaki's disease
       – Takayasu's disease
       – Giant cell arteritis
       – Polyarteritis nodosa

    3. Fibromuscular dysplasia (adrenalis)

    4. Septic aneurysm

    5. Pseudoaneurysm

the medial layer of the vascular walls. This may be part of a general infection – septic, mycotic aneurysm – but injury or trauma can also cause them (pseudoaneurysms).

Indications for Therapy

The indication for operative management of arterial aneurysms remain poorly defined but relates to the size of the aneurysm. Aneurysms of more than 2 cm diameter can rupture.

Techniques

Aneurysms in which all three layers are involved (congenital aneurysms) can be solved by surgery: in most cases by reconstruction with autogenous tissue. Aneurysms that develop as a consequence of the degeneration of the medial layer can rarely be cured by surgery. In the future endovascular intervention should achieve impressive results.

    Surgical or interventional treatment of dilatations as a consequence of arteritis are indicated only after unsuccessful medical therapy (Figs. 30.3–30.5).

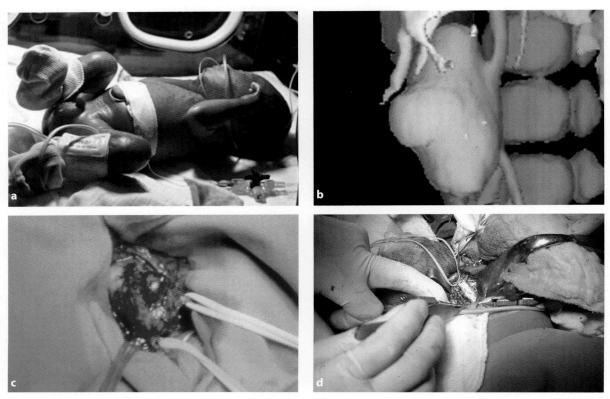

Fig. 30.3. Saccular aorta abdominal aneurysm. **a** A 6 month old infant. Congenital ichthyosis. **b** Computed axial tomography. **c, d** Patch plasty

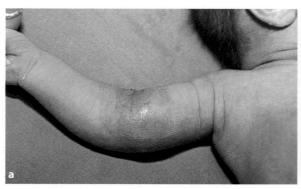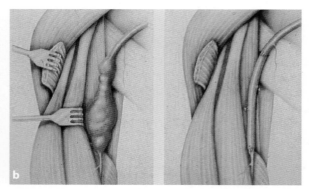

Fig. 30.4. Fusiform brachial aneurysm. **a** Pulsating aneurysm in an 8 month old infant. **b** Resection and venous replacement. Figure 30.4b is reproduced from [12], with permission

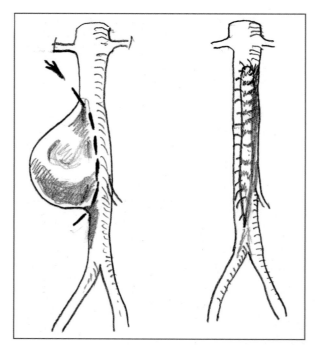

Fig. 30.5. Operation method for aneurysms in infants and children. Lateral resection and patch plasty. Reproduced from [12], with permission

Extratruncular Forms

Extratruncular forms of arterial malformations include infiltrating and limited types.

Port-Wine Stains (PWS), Salmon Patch – Nevus Flammeus

Port-wine stain and various teleangiectasias – Rendu-Osler-Weber syndrome (hereditary haemorrhagic teleangiectasia), ataxia-teleangiectasia, generalised essential teleangiectasia – are best included under the broad heading of vascular malformations. They are present at birth and present with no involution.

Port-wine stains may be present in conjunction with other vascular anomalies: on the trunk or the extremities (Klippel-Trenaunay syndrome) with venous and lymphatic malformations; on the posterior thorax (Cobb syndrome) – with AV malformation of the spinal cord; on the facial with unilateral AV malformation of the retina and intracranial optic pathway (Bonnet-Dechaume-Blanc syndrome); on the face (V2 and/or V3 trigeminal area), choroids and ipsilateral leptomeninges (Sturge-Weber syndrome).

The pink colour, characteristic of infancy, gradually darkens to a red shade during middle age. The surface of the port-wine stain becomes raised and studded with nodular lesions.

Nevus Flammeus Neonatorum (Nevus Teleangiectaticus Medialis)

Nevus flammeus neonatorum stains are pink, macular and irregularly outlined. They blanch completely with pressure and become suffused when the infant cries. Of affected newborns, 40.3% had neonatal staining in the following distribution: 81% of had stains on the on the nape (nuchae), 45% on the eyelids, and 33% on the glabella. There is a remarkable tendency for these lesions to vanish within the first year of life, leaving no residual evidence.

Indication for Therapy

Indications for therapy include prevention of the progression of the nevi, conjugate malformations and psychogenic problems.

Techniques

Initially, argon laser showed promise in the treatment of vascular disorders, but the incidence of scarring is now considered too common.

The pulse-dye laser has proven reliability in treating PWS.

In our experience, intense pulsed light has also proven highly effective and safe for treating PWS. It is imperative to institute early laser therapy to counteract detrimental psychological and physical forces, and to continue therapy based on the response to the treatment and the tolerance and desire of the patient and family towards further cycles of therapy (Figs. 30.6, 30.7).

Venous Malformations

Truncular forms

Truncular forms of venous malformations include aplasia or obstruction (hypoplasia, stenosis) and dilatation.

Aplasia or Obstruction, Dilatation of Deep Veins

Venous malformations cause obstruction to the blood flow and stagnation in the main deep veins. The anomaly of the deep veins is mainly encountered among boys (62%) and for the most part on the lower extremities (54%). The disease is unilateral.

The syndrome is characterised by three signs: vascular stains, varicosity (phlebectasy) and hypo- or hypertrophy (Klippel-Trenaunay syndrome). The vascular stains are inconstant, being encountered in approximately 40% of cases, and are found from birth. In some cases there are dark coloured skin growths 0.1–0.3 cm in diameter over the vascular stains – these growths are easily injured and bleed. Varicosity of the superficial veins may not be pronounced at birth but may become evident in the first years of life. The prevalent location of the varicosities is the lateral surface of the extremity (lateral-embryonal or marginal veins). Hypertrophy or hypotrophy of the diseased extremity is the most common sign of this anomaly and becomes evident only at 6–10 years of age.

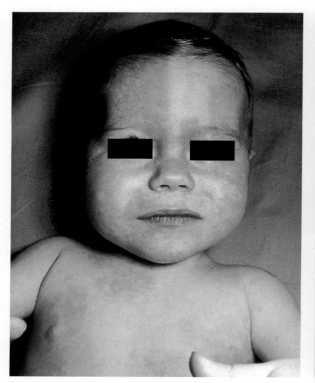

Fig. 30.6. Salmon patches and buphthalmus (glaucoma). Capillary malformation. Therapy is dye-laser or Vasculight (intense pulsed light [IPL])

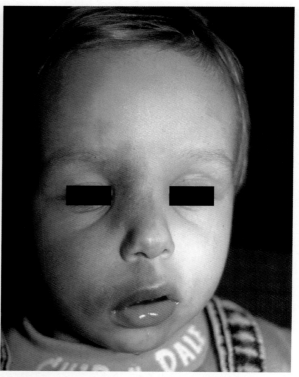

Fig. 30.7. Port wine stain (PWS). Sturge-Weber syndrome. Capillary malformation. Therapy is dye-laser or Vasculight (IPL)

Indications for Therapy

Indications for therapy include prevention of the varicosity (the venous hypertension), the hypo- or hypertrophy (opening of AV shunts), and trophic disorders.

Techniques

In aplasia of a main vein the only method for normalizing the flow of blood is replacement of the affected vascular segment with a venous autograft. Very rarely is conservative compressive treatment effective.

In hypoplasia of deep veins, early compressive treatment for 5–6 years with bandages is important, followed by step-by-step marginal vein resection ("derivation").

In dilatation of deep and marginal veins the operative method is valve replacement, and resection of marginal veins.

The difference in the length of the healthy and diseased limbs gradually reduces with the child's growth and in some cases may disappear entirely.

The above indicates that the anomaly must be detected and treated as early as possible. The most suitable age for the operation is 3–5 years (Figs. 30.8–30.11).

Treatment of Discrepancy in the Length of Lower Limbs

Transitory epiphyseodesis with staples with Blount's technique on the distal extremity of the femur, associated with a similar procedure on the proximal extremity of the tibia is nowadays the procedure of choice to correct discrepancies of less than 4 cm in lower limbs. It is indicated in children above 8 years of age, with open epiphyseal cartilage and no axial deviation of the limbs.

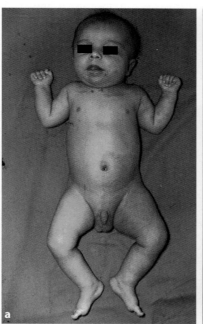
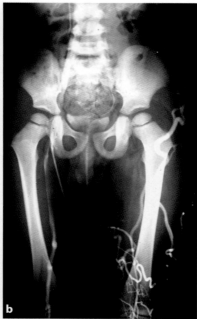
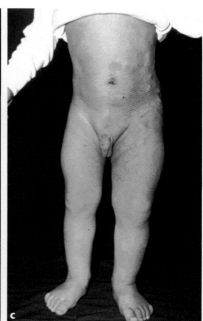
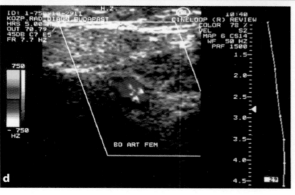

Fig. 30.8. Aplasia of the vena femoralis superficialis. **a** A 4 month old infant (nevus, phlebectasia). **b** Phlebography. **c** A 4 year old with nevus, varicosity and hypertrophy (Klippel-Trenaunay syndrome). Therapy is conservative compressive treatment. **d** Color Doppler Duplex

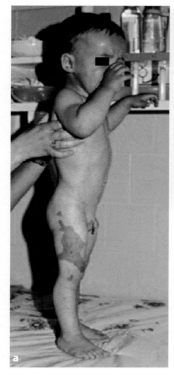

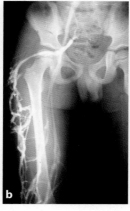

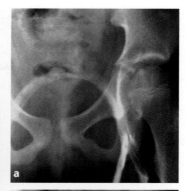

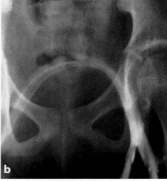

Fig. 30.9. Hypoplasia of the vena femoralis superficialis. **a** A 12 month old infant (nevus, phlebectasia). **b** Phlebography. Therapy is conservative compressive treatment (bandage) and at 5–6 years old, a marginal vein resection ("derivation")

Fig. 30.10. Aplasia of femoral-iliac veins. **a** Phlebography I. Intrauterine reparation: "Spontaneous Palma". **b** Phlebography II. Therapy is "Palma arc" resection and vena saphena valve replacement at 5–7 years old

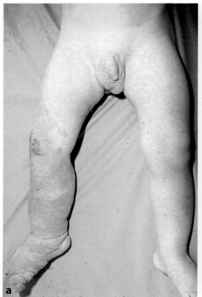

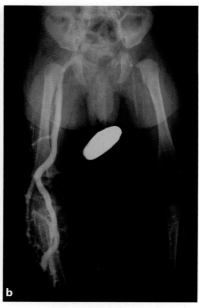

Fig. 30.11. Dilatation of deep and superficial veins with absence of valvulae. **a** A 6 month old infant. Nevus, phlebectasia and hypotrophy (Klippel-Trenaunay syndrome). **b** Phlebography. Therapy is a valve replacement and resection of marginal vein

Elongation of Limbs with the Ilizarov Technique

The external tutor consists of a series of metal rings connected to each other by means of screwed bars and fixed to the limb by tensile wires. The instrument can be used for osseus distraction in discrep-

ancies of limb length that can only be solved by elongation of the shorter limb, whether or not there are axial deviations. It is indicated above 10–12 years of age.

The monolateral strut of the Orthofix or Wagner types is more comfortable to wear but not as versatile.

Obstruction of Inferior Vena Cava – "Cava Membrane Disease" (Budd-Chiari Syndrome)

Budd-Chiari syndrome (BCS) consists of hepatic venous outflow obstruction, regardless of the cause, with the obstruction being either within the liver or the inferior vena cava (IVC) between the liver and the right atrium. Functional hepatic venous flow obstruction caused by congestive heart failure is not considered BCS. Membranous obstruction of IVC is the most common cause of BCS (43%).

The first symptoms may appear already in infancy and develop completely by the age of 2–3 years.

Indications for Therapy

Medical management is rarely effective and surgical treatment is considered as soon as the child's general condition allows it (normally less than 3–5 years of age).

Techniques

If the IVC is obstructed by membrane (web), membranectomy (angioplasty) is a good method. If the IVC is obstructed or very narrow, surgery consists of porto-pulmonal or mesoatrial shunt. In certain children, it is also possible to envisage percutaneous transluminal angioplasty with a balloon dilatation catheter for segmental obstruction of the IVC or limited stenosis of a hepatic vein. Liver transplantation may be successful if there is no other surgical possibility. Surgery provides good results in many instances (Fig. 30.12).

Venous Aneurysms and Aneurysms of Vena Jugularis Interna

Dilatation of the venous lumen in a limited area is a rather rare occurrence. Aneurysms of the jugular veins are of most interest. Unilateral lesions of the internal jugular vein are encountered most frequently.

The disease usually manifests at 3–5 years of age. The parents notice a swelling that appears on the side of the child's neck when he shouts, cries or strains himself and disappears as soon as straining ceases.

Indications for Therapy

In addition to the cosmetic defect, serious complications may be caused by congenital aneurysms of the jugular veins. Cases with thrombosis of veins and spontaneous rupture of the aneurysm have been described.

Techniques

Congenital aneurysms of the jugular veins are treated by surgery. Excision of the aneurysm is the method of choice when there is involvement of the superficial neck muscles. Management of aneurysm of the internal jugular vein consists of reinforcing the vascular wall with an allograft or fascial sheet (Fig. 30.13).

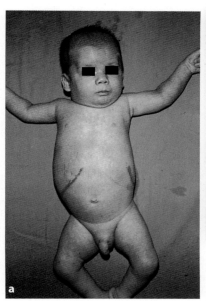
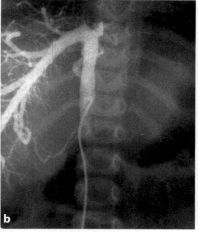
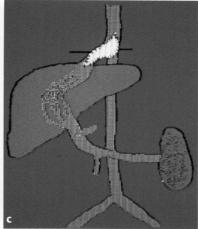

Fig. 30.12. Obstruction of vena cava inferior. "Cava membrane disease". **a** A 7 month old infant. Budd Chiari syndrome. **b** Cavography. **c** Membranectomy plus patch plasty – at 2–3 years old

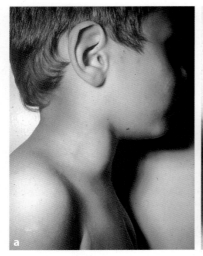
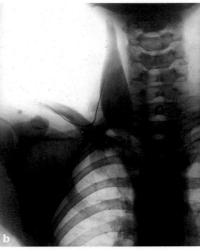
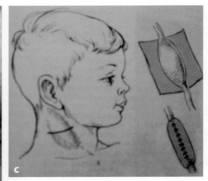

Fig. 30.13. Aneurysm of vena jugularis interna. **a** A 4 year old boy. **b** Phlebography. **c** Therapy is Muff plasty

Extratruncular Forms: Infiltrating and Limited Venous Malformations

Cutaneous, Subcutaneous and Muscular Infiltrating Venous Malformations ("Glomovenous Malformations")

The malformation is evident at birth or in the first months of life. The parents notice a tumour-like structure (on the extremities for the most part) which becomes larger with the gradual growth of the child. Subjective complaints are absent at first. With the child's growth and increase in physical strain a sensation of heaviness is felt in the involved extremity and fatigability occurs. Continuous excruciating pain appears gradually, making the child reluctant to move. The overlying skin is thin, atrophic, blue and cyanotic. In combination with affected superficial veins and that of the vessels of the underlying tissues, the "sponge" sign is demonstrated. Phlebectasia in children with developmental anomalies of the superficial veins differs from adults. The lesions in children are characterised by their diffuse character, varied locations and distributions, which are not usually linked with any of the main systems of the superficial veins, as is the case in adults.

Scout radiography of the diseased extremity demonstrates atrophy of the muscles, thin distorted and sometimes shortened bones (osteoporosis), and abnormal contours of the articular sufaces. Spherical shadows of various size and density are often seen in the subcutaneous fat and muscles along the dis-

tribution of the vessels (phleboliths, Bockenheimer's syndrome, Maffucci's syndrome).

Indication for Therapy

Diffuse lesions with involvement of the underlying tissues are marked by atrophy of the muscles, which is particularly noticeable when the extremity is raised. The skeleton also suffers in such cases. Limited movements at the joints, deformity and delayed growth of bones may be found.

Techniques

Surgery is indicated in developmental anomalies of the superficial, cutaneous veins. The best age at which to perform the operation is at 2 or 3 years old. The operation consists of a step-by-step removal of the dilatations with excision of the most affected skin areas. The role of sclerotherapy has been slowly expanded for this venous lesion. A sclerosing agent may also be used, depending on the extent of the superficial infiltrating venous malformation. In smaller cutaneous "glomangiomatosis", PhotoDerm DL Flashlamp treatment may be successful.

At later ages, in childhood the subcutaneous venous malformation can be skeletonised, preserved and resected or extirpated afterwards with application of ultrasonic energy (Sonotom).

In cases of deep, muscular venous malformations, magnetic resonance imaging (MRI) and contrast-guided sclerotisation with ethanol are used (Figs. 30.14–30.16).

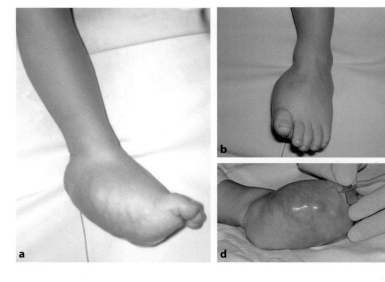

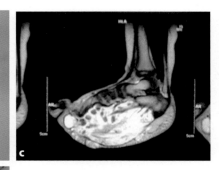

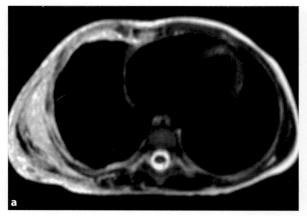

Fig. 30.14. Subcutaneous and muscular venous malformation in the leg. "Glomovenous malformation". **a, b** A 5 month old infant. **c** Magnetic resonance imaging (MRI). **d** MRI and contrast guided sclerotisation with ethanol

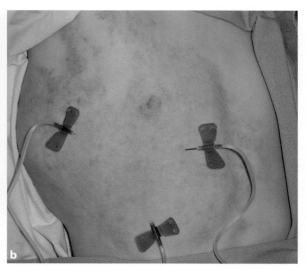

Fig. 30.15. Subcutaneous and muscular venous malformation of the thoracic wall. **a** MRI. **b** MRI and contrast guided sclerotisation with ethanol

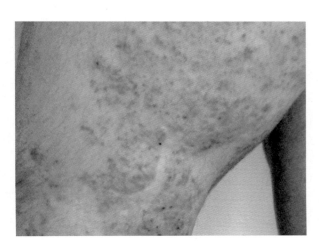

Fig. 30.16. Cutaneous and subcutaneous venous malformation. Dark blue hue of the skin. Therapy is ultrasound (US) aspirator or Nd:Yag laser

Limited Venous Malformation

The tumour-like venous malformation is a limited "venous cavity" with an endothelial-wall. These may be superficial (cutaneous, subcutaneous) and deep (muscular, visceral).

The overlying skin is thin, translucent and blue in colour. In deep forms there may be pain, thrombophlebitis or – in cases of intestinal localisation – invagination

Indication for Therapy

Indications for therapy include prevention of rupture, phlebitis and treatment of complications (invagination etc.).

Techniques

The techniques used are excision: resection with Sonotom (US dissector) and extirpation after sclerotisation (Fig. 30.17).

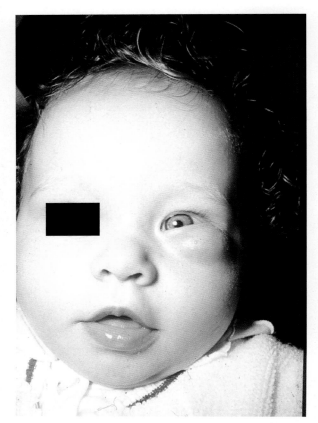

Fig. 30.17. Limited venous malformation ("glomangioma"). A 10 month old infant. Therapy is excision

Lymphatic Malformations

The majority of lymphatic malformations have their origin in infancy, although some may not become clinically symptomatic until adolescence. Secondary lymphatic anomalies (acquired) are uncommon in children.

Truncular Forms

Truncular forms include aplasia or obstruction (hypoplasia, stenosis) and dilatation.

Lymphoedema – Aplasia or Obstruction (Hypoplasia, Stenosis) of Lymphatic Vessels

These truncular malformations are manifested mainly by stable, continuously progressive oedema. In this hard form the oedema and thickening of the skin do not disappear. Pressure fails to produce pitting. The lymphoedema is discovered at birth or in the following years. It may be sporadic or hereditary. The non-familial early lymphoedema, frequent in girls, is painless and involves the foot or leg. Congenital familial lymphoedema (None-Milroy's disease) is usually present from birth, is cyclic, more often in the lower limbs, and is related to the X-chromosome.

Indications for Therapy

Indications for therapy include aplasia, hypoplasia or complete absence of patency of lymph vessels in a progressive disease. The developing trophic changes in the skin lead to chapping of the skin from time to time, and a recurrent inflammatory process.

Techniques

Techniques for treatment include conservative therapy as early as in infancy. The four main steps of the treatment are: manual lymph-drainage; compression bandage; special circulation corrective exercises and mechanical compression treatment with a modern compression machine.

With infants, manual lymph-drainage is predominantly used. The earliest we can start making children accustomed to the compression bandage treatment is at about the age of 6–7 months, in accordance with the infant's movement development and limits of endurance. In the beginning it is worth putting the bandage on only for the night, so that the child can get used to it more easily without it interfering with their movement. In early childhood the child can be taught the basics of the circulation corrective exercise. In most cases we use a combination of these two treatments.

Regarding lymphoedema in childhood, the machine is used exclusively in cases accompanied by dilatation after a thorough preparation over 5–6 months (manual lymph-drainage). Mechanical compression only supplements manual and bandage treatments, but does not replace them.

If we carry out conservative treatment continuously, progression can be significantly reduced and we can achieve recovery by the age of 5–7 years: the role of the missing (aplastic) or hypoplastic lymphatics is taken over by the venous system. In this case we cannot remove the dilated, superficial venous system, and we must not carry out varicectomy (Fig. 30.18).

Soft Lymphoedema – Dilatation of the Lymphatics

In soft lymphoedema the skin can be gathered in a fold and small depressions (pitting) form on the skin from pressure. The radiological image shows many dilated and winding lymphatic vessels, which are insufficient because of unsatisfactory valves.

There are two different forms: unilateral and bilateral hyperplasia.

In the unilateral form chylous reflux occurs frequently.

In the case of the bilateral form of hyperplasia, the lumbar lymphoglandulae, the thoracic duct and the cisterna chyli show narrowing and cause progressive accumulation of the lymph. As a consequence of this narrowing and reflux, lymph gathers in the limbs and in the cavities of the abdomen and thorax (chylascites, chylothorax).

Indications for Therapy

The indication for therapy is to prevent difficult consequences. Papillomatous growths, vesicles filled with yellowish fluid, and fissures appear relatively early (in 1–2 year olds), with findings on the skin. Lymphorrhoea constantly recurs from fistulae. In cases of chylascites, chylothorax serum-like fluid passes from the bloodstream through the dilated lymph vessels to the abdomen/thorax. This fluid bathes the cells and provides them with oxygen and nutrients. The loss of chyle leads to cachexia and circulatory disturbances in infants and children.

Techniques

Techniques for treating soft lymphoedema are regular manual lymph-drainage, followed by instrumental lymph-drainage and a night time bandage.

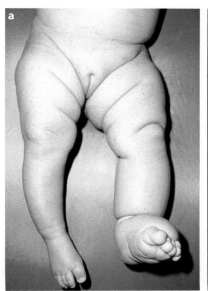
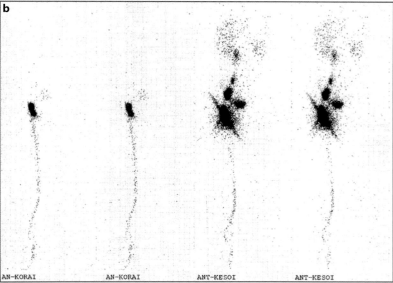

Fig. 30.18. Lymphoedema – as an aplasia of lymphatic vessels. **a** A 4 month old infant (Nonne-Milroy disease) **b** Lymphoscintigraphy. Therapy is compressive treatment (bandage) and at over 5 years old, a subcutaneous excision

In cases of chylous reflux we perform ligation of refluxing vessels and/or installation of a lymphovenous shunt, bypassing the distal lymph vessels into the proximal intact lymph vessels or into veins. In the small infant the best results are obtained by shunting with the Niebolowitz-Olszewski technique.

Computed tomography (CT) and radionuclide lymphangiography have been used to identify large, dilated lymphatics and the chyle reflux (Fig. 30.19).

Chylous Ascites

Chylous ascites may occur early in life. It is usually a result of absent connections (obstruction) of the mesenteric lymphatics to the thoracic duct. Chylous ascites is reflux of chyle into the abdomen from intestinal or mesenteric lymphatics.

Rupture of dilated intestinal lymphatics into the intestinal lumen can occur with subsequent enter-

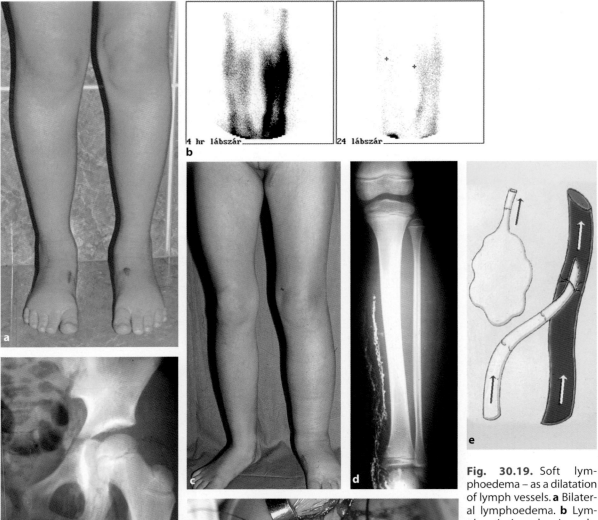

Fig. 30.19. Soft lymphoedema – as a dilatation of lymph vessels. **a** Bilateral lymphoedema. **b** Lymphoscintigraphy. Lymphangiectasia. **c** Unilateral lymphoedema. **d** Lymphography. Lymphangiectasia. **e** Therapy is a lympho-venous shunt. End to side anastomosis. **f** Reflux – lymphorrhea ex vulvae. **g** Therapy is reflux ligature. Figure 30.19e reproduced from [12], with permission

al loss of protein and fat (protein-losing entero-pathy).

Indications for Therapy

The loss of chyle leads to cachexia and circulatory disturbances in infants or children. Chylus ascites is unrelenting and can be fatal. Death results from mal-nutrition, hypoproteinemia, dehydration and sepsis.

Techniques

Non-operative treatment consists of total parenteral nutrition (TPN) or of a medium-chain triglyceride (MCT) diet.

Laparatomy is indicated if a correctable lesion is suspected. In these instances, radionuclide lym-phangiography may be a useful method of demon-strating the approximate location of the leak within the abdomen or obstruction of lymphatics. Some chyle leaks may be identified during surgery and then ligated. An operative direct lympho-venous shunt may be curative in lymphatic obstruction.

In a few cases a localised lymphatic obstruction in a small segment of bowel may cause diarrhoea, vomiting and loss of protein. A short intestinal re-section may be curative in these cases.

Draining the stagnating lymph and gathered lymph with different shunt instruments away from the dilated vessels – just as from lymph accumulations – may have good results. A Denver shunt has a pump-like reservoir and a one-way valve. As a consequence there is bypassing of the lymph into a vein. Howev-er, the Denver shunt-implantation should be used in cases where the operative direct lympho-venous shunt connection or chyle leaks ligation cannot be carried out, in order to save time (Fig. 30.20 a, b).

Congenital Chylothorax

Congenital chylothorax presents as effusion of chyle in one or both pleural cavities. The cause of this problem can be rupture of dilated lymph ves-sels (chyle leak), communication failure, minimal re-absorption of lymph, abnormalities of the pulmonary

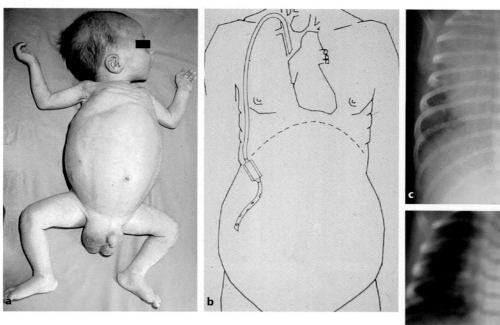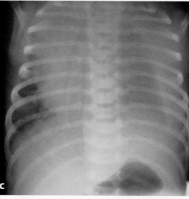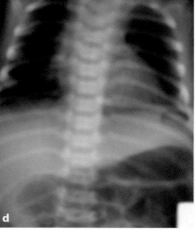

Fig. 30.20. Chylascites and chylothorax. **a** A 4 month old infant. Chylascites. **b** Therapy is a lympho-venous (Denver) shunt implantation. **c** A 2 month old infant. Chylothorax. **d** After treatment with bleomycin, intrapleural sclerotisation. Figure 30.20e reproduced from [12], with permission

lymphatics or injury in the newborn during a difficult delivery.

A pleural effusion may develop prenatally or at birth. The fluid may appear serous, but a fluid cell count with more than 60% lymphocytes is diagnostic of chylothorax. The protein content averages 40 g/l, and electrolyte and glucose levels are similar to plasma levels.

Indications for Therapy

The pleural effusion causes compression of the underlying lung, leading to breathing difficulty and cardiac load.

Techniques

Treatment consists of repeated thoracocentesis and thoracic drainage to expand the lungs. The oral feeding consist an elemental diet with MCT. If fluid reaccumulates, TPN may be required. If drainage persists for 3–4 weeks, local hyperosmolar dextrose solutions or intrapleural Bleomycin (1 mg/kg) injection repeated weekly may be successful. Rarely, the surgical ligation or thoracoscopic sclerotisation of chyle leaks may be necessary (Fig. 30.20 c, d).

Extratruncular Forms: Infiltrating and Limited Lymphatic Malformations

Lymphangiomas

Lymphangiomas are malformations of the lymphatic system characterised by multiple communicating lymphatic channels and cystic spaces of varying size. Lymphangioma simplex – composed of small capillary-sized lymphatic channels – involves all layers of the skin and subcutaneous tissue, lymphangioma cavernosum comprises dilated lymphatic channels, often with a fibrous covering.

It may be inconspicuous at birth but is usually obvious by the age of about 2 years.

The multicystic lesion usually grows slowly, enlarging proportionately with the growth of the child. Spontaneous regression is very rare.

Lymphangiomas are commonly seen in the tongue, cheek, chest, buttocks, extremities and peritoneal cavity. They may also involve the skeletal system (disappearing bone syndrome).

Indications for Therapy

Indications for therapy include disfigurement, extreme size, chronic leakage of lymph fluid and frequent bouts of infection.

Techniques

Surgical treatment is rarely successful in order to completely remove a lymphangioma. Partial resection is necessary in at least one third of the cases. Ultrasound-guided bleomycin injection is effective.

Cystic lesions have been treated by injection of OK-432, a monoclonal antibody produced by incubation and interaction of *Streptococcus pyogenes* and penicillin. Small cutaneous lymphangiomas, as well as portions of weeping, larger cutaneous lesions, may be effectively treated with serial CO_2 laser therapy.

Injection of ethanol as a sclerosing agent has been of benefit for the treatment of bone-lymphangiomatosis (in disappearing bone syndrome) (Fig. 30.21).

Cystic Hygroma

Cystic hygroma presents as a multicystic mass with a thin, almost transparent wall. Hygromas usually are bound to large veins and lymphatic ducts, such as are found in the neck, axilla, abdomen and groin.

Most hygromas are first noted shortly after birth and enlarge gradually.

Indications for Therapy

When lesions extend into deep tissues or vital structures, the major, prominent portion of the hygroma should be removed.

Techniques

Total removal by surgical treatment is rarely possible, partial resection may be enough for life-threatening airway obstruction.

Staged resection and bleomycin injection is the best treatment method.

For smaller, inoperable cysts there have been good results with ultrasound-guided bleomycin (Figs. 30.22, 30.23).

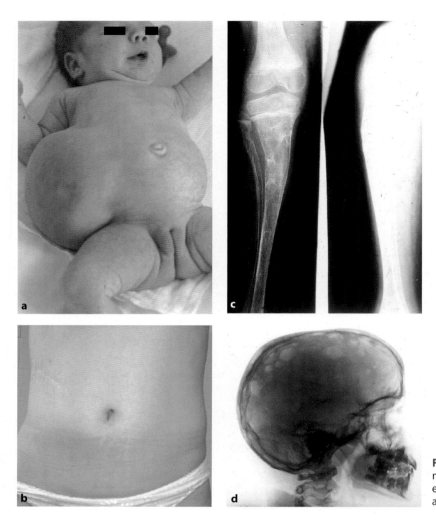

Fig. 30.21. Lymphangioma. **a** A 3 month old infant. **b** Therapy is radical excision. **c** Disappearing bone I. **d** Disappearing bone II

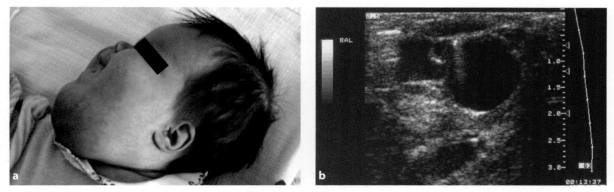

Fig. 30.22. Cystic hygroma. Lymphangioma colli, infiltrating form. **a** A 3 month old infant. **b** US guided sclerotisation with OK-432 (directly into the cyst)

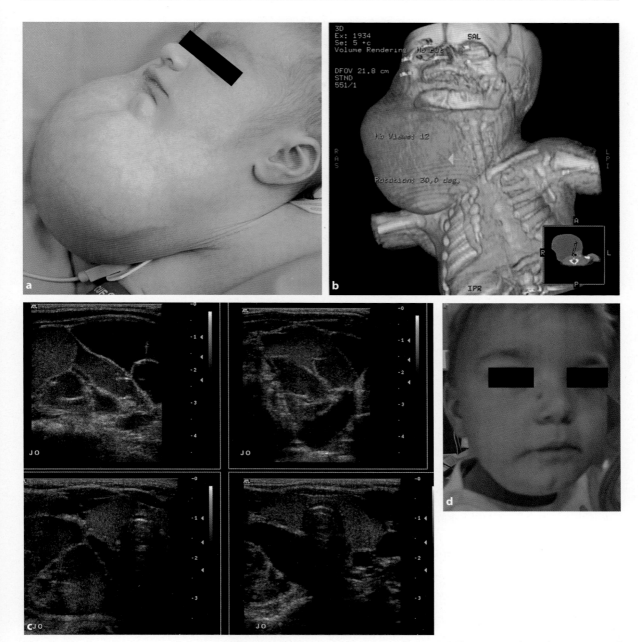

Fig. 30.23. Cystic hygroma. **a** A 2 week old newborn. Giant lymphangioma. **b** CT. **c** US. Therapy is subtotal resection and US guided bleomycin sclerotisation pre-and postoperatively. **d** After treatment

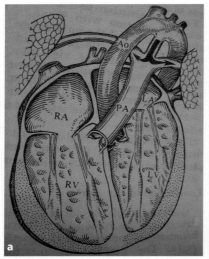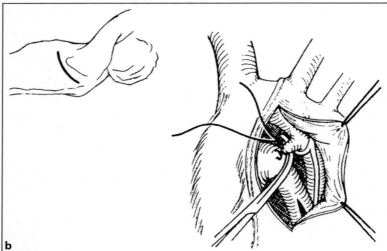

Fig. 30.24. Deep, direct AV shunt. **a** Patent Ductus Arteriosus (Botalli). **b** Ductus Botalli operation

Arteriovenous Malformations

Arteriovenous malformations are manifest from birth or in the first months of life.

The character and degree of the signs are determined for the most part by the number, size, localisation, and distribution of the abnormal communications between arteries and veins.

Truncular Forms: Deep and Superficial AV Fistulae

Ductus Arteriosus Botalli (Deep, Direct (Central) AV Shunt)

Anatomically, a ductus arteriosus Botalli is a short vessel connecting the aorta and the pulmonary artery.

Ductus arteriosus induces a number of haemodynamic disorders. The degree of changes in the body is determined by several factors: the patient's age, the diameter of the duct, the volume of blood shunted from the aorta into the pulmonary artery, the resistance of the vessels of the pulmonary circulation, and the reserves of the heart muscle. The additional volume of blood leads to hypertrophy of the left ventricles, dilatation of its cavity and development of sclerotic changes in the vessels of the lungs.

Indications for Therapy

Operation must be undertaken before irreparable changes develop in the pulmonary circulation.

Techniques

The operation consists of ligating the ductus arteriosus by suturing and dividing it (Fig. 30.24).

Superficial, Indirect (Peripheral) AV Shunts (Parkes-Weber Syndrome)

Local and general symptoms of Parkes-Weber syndrome include: the skin on the involved limb is abnormal in colour due to the presence of either a pigmented spot or flat teleangiectasia; varicosity of the veins may be hardly noticeable in the initial stages of the disease but becomes fully manifest with the child's growth; and hypertrophy of the involved organ. The degree of hypertrophy is always directly dependent on the size and number of the communications.

Changes are also found in cardiac activity: compensatory tachycardia, increase in arterial pressure and hypertrophy first of the right and then of the left heart (hyperkinetic circulation).

Indication for Therapy

The indication for therapy is to prevent cardiac load, varicosity, hypertrophy and trophic disturbances – from early in infancy.

Techniques

Complete surgical cure is possible only in cases with abnormal communication between the main vessels: lig-

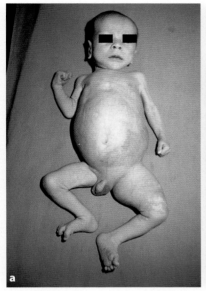
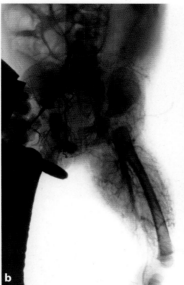
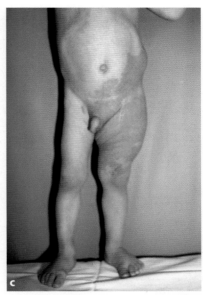

Fig. 30.25. Superficial, indirect AV shunt. **a** A 3 month old infant, nevus, phlebectasy, hypertrophy plus thrill (Parkes Weber syndrome). **b** Angiography. Therapy is shunt embolisation with polyvinyl alcohol and ligature. **c** At 3 years old – after operation

ation of the fistulae and separation of the artery from the vein make it possible to correct this severe anomaly.

Later in childhood in some patients who are poor surgical candidates or who refuse surgery, periodic embolisation without surgical excision has provided a significant measure of palliation (Fig. 30.25).

Extratruncular Forms: Infiltrating and Limited AV Fistulae

Infiltrating Multiplex AV, Microcommunications (Parkes-Weber Syndrome)

There are many diffuse AV microcommunications possible on the leg. The signs are present after birth: telangiectatic naevi, increased skin temperature and minimal hypertrophy on the leg. In the first 6 months the symptoms speed up: varicosity, hypertrophy. After 2–3 years the severe circulatory disorders encountered in AV fistulae induce grave trophic disturbances as a rule. Hyperkeratosis and hyperhidrosis may develop.

Indication for Therapy

The indication for therapy is to prevent serious consequences.

Techniques

In the first 6 months cortisone therapy may be effective. Compression bandage treatment can begin at about 6–7 months of age. In childhood, periodic embolisation can be the elective method (Fig. 30.26).

Limited Tumour Form AV Malformation

In some newborn/infants the arteriovenous "aneurysma" or abnormal vascular networks formed in limited areas are seen as soft elastic tumours which pulsate and hardly collapse upon compression.

Indications for Therapy

Indications for therapy are rapid growth, cardiac load, ulceration and bleeding.

Techniques

Techniques used include complete excision, and preoperative embolisation is often desirable 24–48 hours before surgery (Fig. 30.27).

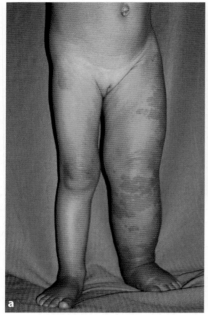

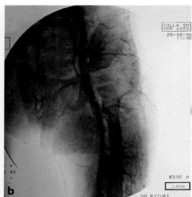

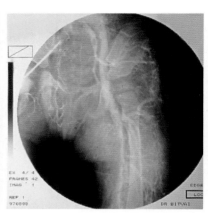

Fig. 30.26. Infiltrating multiplex AV malformation. **a** A 2 year old girl. Nevus, phlebectasy, hypertrophy (Parkes Weber syndrome). **b** Angiography. Therapy is embolisation with polyvinyl alcohol and conservative compressive treatment

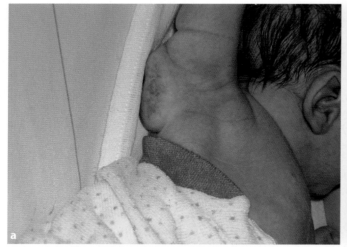

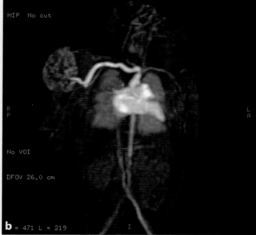

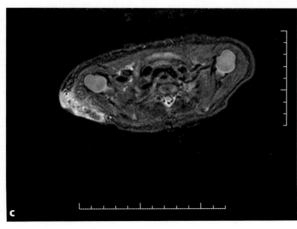

Fig. 30.27. Limited, tumour-form AV malformation. **a** A 3 month old infant with an AV humeroscapularis malformation (Plexus paresis) **b, c** MRI. Therapy is embolisation with polyvinyl alcohol and ligature plus excision

Combined Vascular Malformations

Congenital vascular malformation involves two or more elements of the vascular system: arteries, veins, lymphatics and haemolymphatics. The haemolymphatics are congenital cutaneous or deep vascular malformations, containing combined lymphatic and blood vascular elements.

Combined vascular malformations have very few symptoms in newborns. These are recognisable only at the later age of 1–2 years. The symptoms are characteristic of dominant elements of the vascular system.

Indication for Therapy

The indication for therapy is to prevent serious consequences.

Techniques

Techniques used are conservative and/or surgical and radiological interventions, according to the dominant elements of the vascular system (Figs. 30.28–30.30).

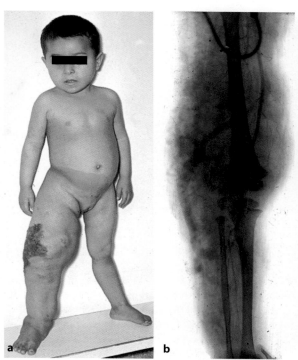

Fig. 30.28. Combined arterial and venous malformation. **a** A 5 year old girl with a nevus varicosity and hypertrophy (Klippel-Trenaunay-Parkes-Weber syndrome). **b** Angiography (aplasia of deep veins, persisting marginal vein, microcommunication AV). Therapy is conservative compressive treatment

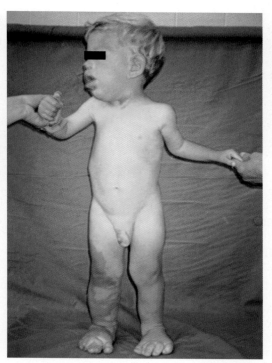

Fig. 30.29. Combined haemolymphatic malformation. A 16 month old girl. Nevus, phlebectasy, lymphangio capillary dysplasia, macropodia or macrodactilia, segmental corporal hemihypertrophia primary deep venous anomaly (Klippel-Trenaunay-Servelle syndrome). Therapy is surface therapy

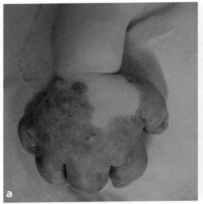
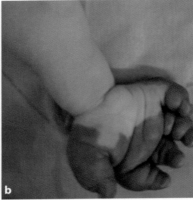
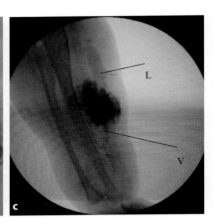
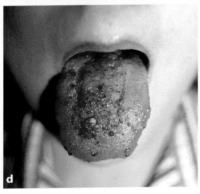

Fig. 30.30. Combined infiltrating haemolymphatic malformation. **a, b** A 12 month old infant, lympho-capillary-venous malformation of the hand. **c** Lympho-phlebography: extreme dilatated lymph (*L*) and venous (*V*) vessels. Therapy is contrast-guided sclerotisation with bleomycin. **d** A 3 year old girl. Lympocapillary malformation of the tongue (linguae)

References

1. Kiss F, Szentágotai J (1984) Anatomischer Atlas des Menchlichen körpers. Ed Medicina, Budapest
2. Tasnádi G (1977) Clinical examinations of venous dysplasias of infant and childhood. Dissertation, University of Budapest
3. Wang Z (1998) Congenital defects of the inferior vena cava causing Budd-Chiari syndrome. In: Selected sc. papers of Zhong Gao Wang. Int Academic Publishers, Beijing, pp 360–367
4. Wong WH, Pyk J (1976) Blood flow and venous distensibilities in the upper and lower extremity of newborns and infants. Acta Paed Uppsala 65:571–576
5. Belov S (1990) Hemodynamic pathogenesis of vascular bone syndromes in congenital vascular defects. Int Angiol 9:155–162
6. Mattassi R, Belov S, Loose DA, Vaghi M (2003) Malformazioni vascolari ed emangiomi. Springer-Verlag Italia, Milano
7. Soltész L (1965) Contribution of clinical and experimental studies of the hypertrophy of the extremities in congenital a-v fistulas. Proceedings of the 7th Congress of the International Cardiovascular Society, Philadelphia. J Cardiovasc Surg (Suppl 6):260–262
8. Tasnádi G (1989) Parkes-Weber Syndrome on the lower extremity and retroperitoneal angiolipomatosis. In: Belov S, Loose DA, Weber J (eds) Vascular malformations. Periodica Angiologica 16. Einhorn-Presse Verlag, Reinbek, pp 226–229
9. Tasnádi G (1989) Phlebangiomas and their treatment. In: Belov S, Loose DA, Weber J (eds) Vascular malformations. Periodica Angiologica 16, Einhorn-Presse Verlag, Reinbek, pp 183–187
10. Tasnádi G (1992) Clinical investigations in epidemiology of congenital vascular defects. In: Balas P (ed) Progress in angiology. Edizioni Minerva Medica, Torino, pp 391–394
11. Tasnádi G, Mattassi R (1998) Chyledema of a limb and chylothorax treated successfully with a Denver shunt. Lymphology 31:381–385
12. Acsady GY, Nemes A (2005) Az érbetegségek Klinikai és mütéttani atlasza. Ed. Medicina Budapest
13. Sarkar R (1991) Arterial aneurysms in children. Clinicopathologic classification. J Vasc Surg 13:147

Part IV
TREATMENT PROBLEMS ACCORDING TO SPECIFIC LOCALIZATIONS

Introductory Remarks

31

Raul Mattassi

The principles of treatment that are discussed in the previous chapters are useful for all peripheral vascular malformations. However, in some areas of the body, anatomical peculiarities and specific functions may create approach difficulties. In case of surgical indication, a multidisciplinary approach may be necessary, while embolisation or sclerosis may require great skill and experience.

In the face, aesthetic and functional problems need to be considered. It is in this area that the largest group of specialists may become involved: plastic surgeons, dermatologists, ophtalmologists, otorhinolaryngologists, maxillofacial surgeons and radiologists. Surgeons must avoid visible scars and damage to branches of facial nerves; ophtalmologists must avoid eye damage; and radiologists, the creation of ulcers and fistulas.

The thorax wall is an anatomical structure with a large surface covered by different layers of flat muscles, where surgery may be difficult, particularly in cases of infiltrating forms. Sclerosis and embolisation may be good alternative therapies although not necessarily always possible.

The limbs are cylindrical structures with bones, long muscles, nerves and vessels in specific positions. Infiltrating malformations may involve one or more tissues contemporaneously, creating approach difficulties.

The hand is a very peculiar organ; fine and high functions are located in small spaces. Therapeutic approaches demand a high degree of skill and knowledge of anatomy and function.

The foot has also different small spaces filled with muscles, bones, nerves and vessels. The function is not as fine as in the hand, but the anatomy should be well known if a surgical approach is planned.

The joints are structures with a specific anatomy and function. Involvement of joints by vascular malformations may create severe damage and demand treatment. Specific orthopaedic techniques are used in this area.

Bones have extended vascularisation. Their involvement by vascular malformations requires specific treatment techniques.

Chapters 32–38 should provide some concepts of the specific techniques needed to approach these particular areas.

R. Mattassi, D.A. Loose, M. Vaghi (eds.), *Hemangiomas and Vascular Malformations*.
© Springer-Verlag Italia 2009

Management of Head and Neck Vascular Malformations: an Overview

32

Jonathan A. Perkins

Abstract

Head and neck vascular malformations (HNVM) arise from different types of vessels. All can adversely affect function, depending on their size and location. A primary concern is preserving or restoring normal breathing, vision, speech and eating. After the impact of the HNVM on function has been determined, an accurate diagnosis of the lesion must be obtained with history, exam and imaging studies; occasionally, a biopsy is necessary to solidify the diagnosis. Once the diagnosis is established, a variety of intradisciplinary treatment modalities are necessary for HNVM management, as often HNVM can be recalcitrant to cure. Paramount in any treatment is the need to preserve function and not induce further morbidity (i.e., motor nerve injury, etc.). In general, localized HNVM can be treated successfully, whereas more extensive lesions need long-term management.

Long-term HNVM management needs to be focused on chronic problems that can be associated with these lesions. These malformations can have intermittent swelling that is painful or induces functional compromise. Medical therapy directed at reduction of swelling and pain is essential. When functional compromise is present, therapeutic intervention may be required. Occasionally, these lesions become infected or reduce normal infection barriers predisposing patients to infection (i.e., meningitis from skull base erosion): judicious use of antibiotics is necessary in these circumstances. Chronic problems induced by HNVM morbidity and possibly by treatment complications can have significant adverse psychosocial impact on patients: this must be addressed when caring for affected individuals.

Introduction

What is a Vascular Malformation?

When examining a head and neck vascular lesion, it is helpful to remember that there are three types of vascular vessels in humans: arterial, venous and lymphatic [1]. Each of these vessels transports a unique fluid, a function that is reflected in their structure. These factors affect the clinical appearance of a vascular lesion composed of one or more of these vessel types. Arteries carry blood at high pressure and velocity but do not leak. As a result, vascular lesions composed predominantly of arteries are often pulsatile and warm, requiring diagnostic tests that detect rapid blood flow and rapid venous filling. Occasionally, increased blood flow through an arterial vascular lesion can cause high output cardiac failure. Veins carry blood passively at low velocity and are leaky. Venous malformations are non-pulsatile, but they swell with increased blood volume or venous blockage. Diagnostic studies used for venous malformations detect slow blood flow and characteristics unique to abnormal veins (i.e., phleboliths). Venous malformations are frequently associated with pain thought to be secondary to lesion expansion. Lymphatic vessels transport lymph at slow rates, enlarge with inflammation, and are very leaky. Purely lymphatic malformations transilluminate and swell with inflammation, but diagnostic studies show no fluid movement (Fig. 32.1). Determining the predominant vessel type in vascular lesions through imaging is important for accurate diagnosis, treatment planning and prediction of treatment outcomes [2].

R. Mattassi, D.A. Loose, M. Vaghi (eds.), *Hemangiomas and Vascular Malformations*.
© Springer-Verlag Italia 2009

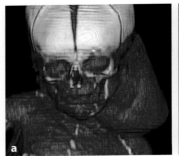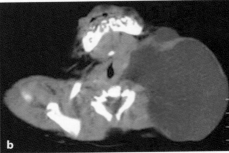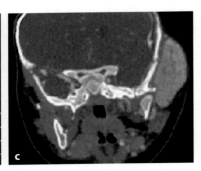

Fig. 32.1. Imaging characteristics of vascular anomalies. **a** Three-dimensional computerized tomography image of non-enhancing lymphatic malformation. **b** Axial section of same malformation. **c** Coronal section of pericranial hemangioma

Vascular Malformation and Vascular Tumors

Vascular malformations have been separated from other vascular anomalies (Table 32.1) [3]. Vascular tumors are lesions composed of vessels that demonstrate neoplastic growth. In the head and neck, this is most often a hemangioma of infancy [4]. While this discussion is limited to vascular malformations of the head and neck, many of the diagnostic and therapeutic dilemmas present in head and neck vascular tumors are also present in vascular malformations. Vascular malformations are masses of abnormal vessels that can be present at birth or occur at any time during life. These abnormal vessels can have abnormal connections with other types of vessels, as seen in "arteriovenous" malformations (AVMs). In this situation, arteries are connected to veins prior to reaching capillaries. In lymphovenous malformations, there are abnormal connections between venous and lymphatic channels, thought to be a result of arrested separation of veins and lymph vessels. Venous and/or lymphatic malformations are often present at birth and can be detected in utero. Following detection, these lesions enlarge with the patient throughout their life. AVMs are usually detected later in life and also slowly enlarge. Local trauma to the lesion or hormonal changes during puberty can be associated with rapid malformation growth. As in any region of the body, head and neck vascular malformations can be difficult to treat due to size and location.

Considerations in Head and Neck Vascular Malformation Treatment

During evaluation and treatment of HNVMs, the impact of the lesion on fundamental head and neck function must be considered. Of greatest importance is airway preservation [5]. Airway compromise from vascular lesions is most commonly seen in

Table 32.1. Vascular Anomaly Classification*

Vascular Malformation	Vascular Tumor
Single Vessel Type	Hemangioma
Capillary	Hemangioma of Infancy
Venous	Congenital Hemangioma
Lymphatic	Rapidly Involuting Congenital Hemangioma (RICH)
Arteriovenous	Non-Involuting Congenital Hemangioma (NICH)
Combined/Complex Malformations	Vascular Neoplasm
Lymphaticovenous	Kaposiform Hemangioendothelioma
Capillary-venous	Angiosarcoma
Capillary-lymphaticovenous	Hemangiopericytoma
Capillary-arteriovenous	Miscellaneous
	Tufted Angioma
	Pyogenic Granuloma

* Binary classification system adopted by the International Society for the Study of Vascular Anomalies (ISSVA) in 1996

hemangiomas of infancy (Fig. 32.2). However, vascular malformations can distort or compress any aspect of the upper airway, inducing acute airway compromise or chronic sleep disturbed breathing. Evaluation of HNVM should always include a thorough assessment of the upper airway and trachea, as any malformation swelling can induce airway compromise.

Intracranial vascular malformations are often associated with HNVM [6]. Occasionally, these lesions have direct intra-extracranial communication (Fig. 32.3). These communications can compromise cerebral function and HNVM treatment can induce cerebral injury via these communications. This is especially apparent in orbital malformations, which can impair visual function, with and without treatment. Skull base defects from the malformation or its treatment can cause leakage of cerebrospinal flu-

id, increasing the possibility of meningitis. Evaluation of HNVM with high resolution imaging techniques can detect malformations that are high risk for neurologic compromise.

The pharynx and larynx provide us with swallowing and speech capabilities which can be affected by HNVM. Again, this can be due to the HNVM itself or to its treatment. Assessment of these functions is essential in the management of HNVM, as changes in lesion size can adversely affect swallowing and speech, necessitating treatment. One of the most problematic areas is the tongue, which can be affected by any malformation.

Our ability to interact with others in society is dependent on many factors; one of these is our physical appearance. In addition to causing functional changes, HNVM and their treatment often severely

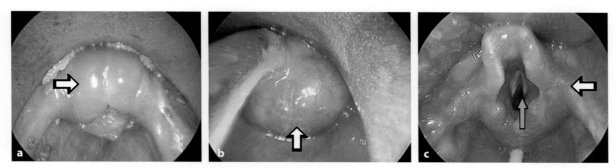

Fig. 32.2. Laryngeal involvement by vascular anomalies. **a** Epiglottis (*arrow*) swollen by lymphatic malformation in patient with bilateral upper neck lymphatic malformation. **b** Posterior laryngeal involvement by venous malformation (*arrow*). **c** Mucosal laryngeal involvement by hemangioma (*white arrow*), and subglottic narrowing by deep hemangioma (*green arrow*)

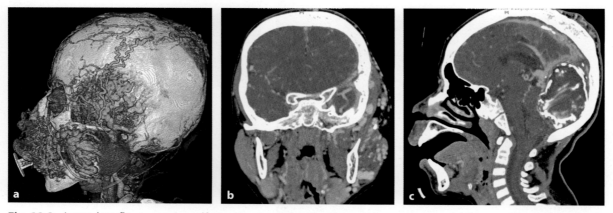

Fig. 32.3. Large low flow venous malformation involving the face and posterior cranial fossa. **a** Three-dimensional computerized tomography. **b** Coronal computerized tomography section demonstrating masticator muscle and skull base involvement. **c** Sagittal computerized tomography section demonstrating large posterior cranial fossa venous malformation

distort appearance (Fig. 32.4). This can have a major impact on an affected individual and their family. In evaluation and management of HNVM, it is essential to monitor and treat the psychological aspects of an individual's condition.

In addition to history and physical examination, HNVM need to be assessed with state of the art imaging techniques, such as computerized angiography and/or magnetic resonance imaging (MRI), to determine the full extent and physiology of the malformation (Fig. 32.5).

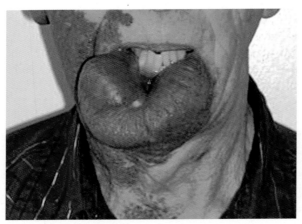

Fig. 32.4. Capillary malformation with progressive hypertrophy of soft tissue

Specific HNVM

Lymphatic Malformations

The most common large HNVMs are lymphatic [5]. These malformations are clinically apparent at birth approximately 70% of the time and frequently occur in the posterior neck. The other 30% occur at any time in life in association with infection or trauma. Lymphatic malformations are low flow lesions usually not associated with any syndrome, with the rare exception of Gorham Stout, where there is skull erosion. Depending on the lymphatic malformation location, they are variably associated with soft and bony tissue hypertrophy that can adversely impact breathing, swallowing and speech (Fig. 32.6). Oropharyngeal and/or laryngeal involvement of the malformation can cause airway narrowing that is persistent or intermittent, as the malformation can swell intermittently with infection. When the malformation is in the orbit or near the skull base, any swelling can cause discomfort and potentially compromise function. Macroglossia is frequently associated with mandibular hypertrophy, both of which impair normal speech and swallowing function (Fig. 32.7).

In addition to clinical exam findings, lymphatic malformations are diagnosed with imaging studies

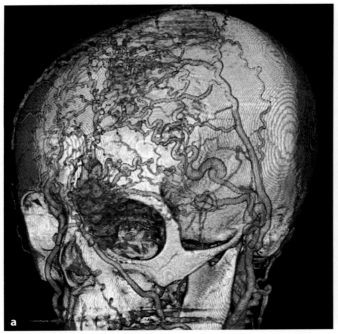

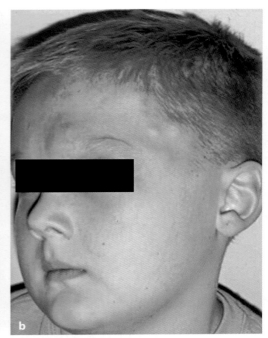

Fig. 32.5. High flow AVM of forehead, eyelid and orbit. **a** Three-dimensional computerized angiography of AVM. **b** Oblique clinical photo of affected patient

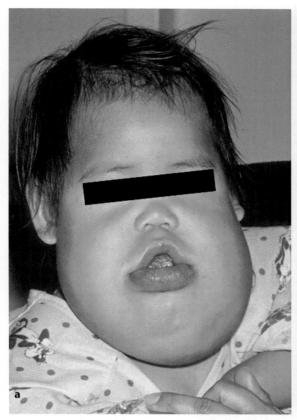 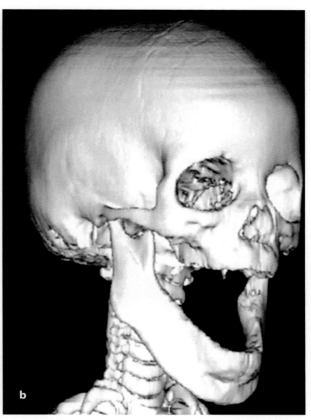

Fig. 32.6. Mandibular hyperplasia in setting of large bilateral upper neck lymphatic malformation. **a** Bilateral upper neck/oral lymphatic malformation. **b** Three-dimensional CT of mandibular hyperplasia

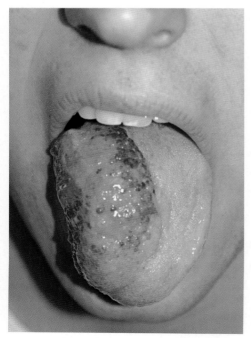

Fig. 32.7. Macroglossia from microcystic lymphatic malformation

that describe the extent and radiographic characteristics of the lesion. More extensive lesions involving the upper neck and oral cavity are more difficult to treat. Lesions can predominantly consist of large cystic spaces (i.e., macrocystic), small cysts (i.e., microcystic), or a mixture of both (Figs. 32.1, 32.8) [7]. Extensive lesions often have a significant venous component. Determination of lesion extent and radiographic characteristics is essential in treatment planning and patient counseling.

Treatment of lymphatic malformations is guided by the presence of functional compromise, lesion extent and characteristics. When vision or breathing is affected by the malformation, orbital/ocular and/or oropharyngeal/laryngeal surgery may be necessary. For the common posterior neck lymphatic malformations, the major concerns are appearance and, occasionally, shoulder function. Malformations in this area can be cured with either sclerotherapy or surgery [8, 9]. However, if the malformation is in the oral cavity and upper neck, frequently treatment is partially effective and

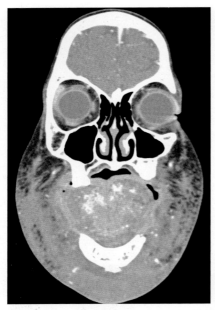

Fig. 32.8. Computerized tomography of microcystic lymphatic malformation. Coronal image of microcystic lymphatic malformation involving the tongue and perimandibular tissues

lesion management, as opposed to cure, is necessary [10]. Management consists of partial surgical resection, medical therapy (i.e., antibiotics, steroids) to treat intermittent malformation inflammation, good oral hygiene and monitoring of immune function [11].

Venous Malformations

Venous malformations are present in the head and neck at birth and involve any location in this region. Most commonly, they are in muscle tissue, where they temporarily enlarge and become painful with muscle use or trauma [12, 13]. These lesions consist of low-flow, blood-filled vessels. Just like lymphatic malformations, venous malformations can cause functional compromise based on their location. In the head and neck, venous malformations most commonly involve the mucosal surfaces, orbicularis oris and muscles of mastication (Fig. 32.3); less frequently, they involve skin and neck. On occasion, they involve the facial bones and skull. Venous lesions next to skull bone can have direct communication with dural sinuses. When bone is involved, the venous malformation treatment can be complicated by bleeding. Tissue surrounding a venous malformation is

frequently enlarged so that dental occlusion and facial symmetry are affected. In lesions that are incurable, long-term management must consider venous malformation persistence and the psychosocial aspects of this problem.

Treatment of venous malformations is performed to alleviate functional compromise and improve appearance. Airway narrowing from a swollen venous malformation often requires staged procedures to avoid tracheotomy. Any mucosal surface in the upper aerodigestive tract can be involved, swell and cause airway compromise. Most of these areas can be treated endoscopically through a combination of sclerotherapy, excision and interstitial laser treatment. When the venous malformation is near the upper airway and a general anesthesia is required, careful induction of anesthesia and airway control are necessary, since the malformation will frequently swell with recumbency and the vasodilatory effect of some anesthetic agents. This can be accomplished with awake and upright intubation. When there is pain associated with the venous malformation, treatment is necessary. Pain frequently occurs in adolescence when vessels within the malformation are occluded with thrombi. If this is a persistent problem, antiplatelet therapy or anticoagulation can be used for treatment. Surgical excision and chemical or laser sclerotherapy of the involved area can also be performed when the symptomatic area is well localized. When surgery is considered, preoperative occlusion of the malformation with glue is very helpful in reducing hemorrhage. Skin that is involved with venous malformations can be treated with excision and transcutaneous and interstitial laser therapy. Often, this does not completely solve the problem. In this situation, long-term management strategies must be employed.

Arteriovenous Malformations

AVMs can involve any region of the head and neck [14]. Most frequently, they involve the auricle (Fig. 32.9). These lesions are thought to arise from a nidus of blood vessels that have abnormal connections between arteries and veins. Due to excessive blood flow through these channels, surrounding blood vessels become dilated. Consequently, AVMs are pulsatile, may have a bruit, and slowly enlarge. During periods of hormonal change (i.e., puberty, pregnancy) or trauma, these lesions can enlarge rapidly. Due to the expansion of AVMs, soft and bony tissue in the head and neck can become compromised. Intracranial AVMs can cause

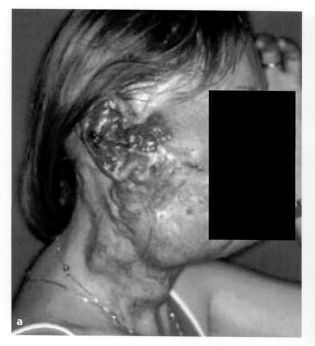

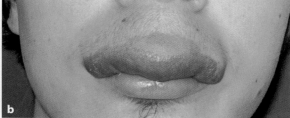

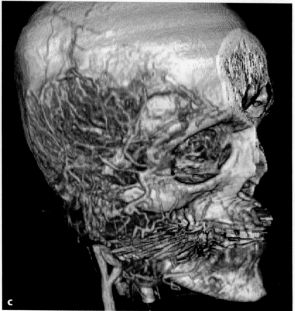

Fig. 32.9. Extensive AVMs. **a** AVM of ear and **b** face. **c** Computerized tomography angiography of AVM involving ear and face

life-threatening bleeding. Most extracranial AVMs do not communicate with intracranial vasculature, but this is always possible. Large untreated AVMs can induce high output cardiac failure due to increasing vascular area.

AVM treatment is determined by lesion extent, location and functional compromise. Conceptually, treatment centers on complete excision of the lesion nidus. In reality, it is difficult to determine when the nidus has been completely removed, and as a consequence, surgical excision and reconstruction may be extensive. Small localized lesions can be treated with surgical excision alone. Larger AVMs are removed with a combination of preoperative embolization and surgery. Embolization is done to reduce intraoperative blood loss. Long-term follow-up is necessary to detect lesion recurrence. For large, unresectable lesions, periodic embolization may be necessary to control bleeding. Intraosseus AVMs can be controlled with endovascular placement of biologically tolerated glue.

Capillary Malformations

Capillary malformations, also known as port wine stains, frequently involve the dermatomes of cranial nerve five [15]. When these lesions involve the V1 and V2 it is necessary to make sure the vascular malformation does not involve the meninges. When meningeal involvement is present with a capillary malformation, Sturge Weber syndrome is diagnosed. Capillary malformations progressively thicken for unclear reasons (Fig. 32.4) [16]. Soft and bony tissue around these malformations also hypertrophies (Fig. 32.10). It is thought that the skin nodules that develop in these lesions are neural hamartomas, reflecting a deficiency in neural control of capillary diameter. Occasionally, capillary malformations can be on the surface of AVMs, so careful assessment of all malformations is necessary (Fig. 32.11).

Treatment of capillary malformations is directed reduction of skin discoloration with serial pulsed dye laser treatments (Fig. 32.12). For extensively thickened lesions and nodules, surgical excision can be performed.

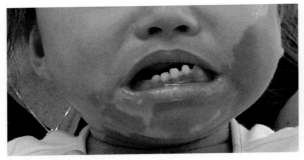

Fig. 32.10. Capillary malformation with mandibular overgrowth

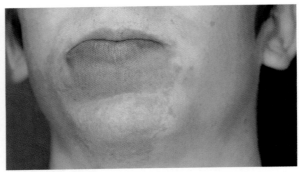

Fig. 32.11. Lip AVM with capillary malformation

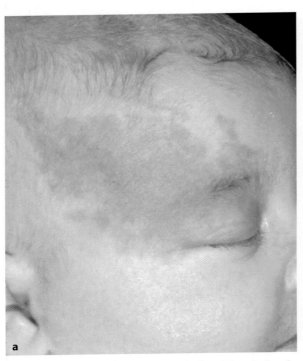
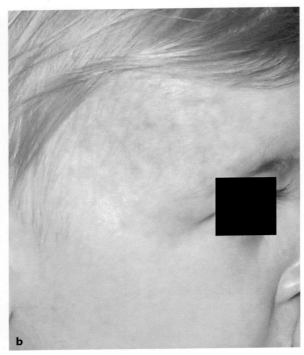

Fig. 32.12. Capillary malformation before (**a**) and after four pulse dye laser treatments (**b**)

References

1. North PE, Waner M, Buckmiller L et al (2006) Vascular tumors of infancy and childhood: beyond capillary hemangioma. Cardiovasc Pathol 15:303–317
2. Konez O, Burrows PE (2004) An appropriate diagnostic workup for suspected vascular birthmarks. Cleve Clin J Med 71:505–510
3. Enjolras O (1999) Vascular tumors and vascular malformations: are we at the dawn of a better knowledge? Pediatr Dermatol 16:238–241
4. Frieden IJ, Haggstrom AN, Drolet BA et al (2005) Infantile hemangiomas: current knowledge, future directions. Proceedings of a research workshop on infantile hemangiomas, April 7–9, 2005, Bethesda, Maryland, USA. Pediatr Dermatol 22:383–406
5. Bloom DC, Perkins JA, Manning SC (2004) Management of lymphatic malformations. Curr Opin Otolaryngol Head Neck Surg 12:500–504
6. Burrows PE, Robertson RL, Mulliken JB et al (1998) Cerebral vasculopathy and neurologic sequelae in infants with cervicofacial hemangioma: report of eight patients. Radiology 207:601–607
7. Burrows PE, Mason KP (2004) Percutaneous treatment of low flow vascular malformations. J Vasc Interv Radiol 15:431–445

8. Claesson G, Kuylenstierna R (2002) OK-432 therapy for lymphatic malformation in 32 patients (28 children). Int J Pediatr Otorhinolaryngol 65:1–6

9. Riechelmann H, Muehlfay G, Keck T et al (1999) Total, subtotal, and partial surgical removal of cervicofacial lymphangiomas. Arch Otolaryngol Head Neck Surg 125:643–648

10. Raveh E, de Jong AL, Taylor GP, Forte V (1997) Prognostic factors in the treatment of lymphatic malformations. Arch Otolaryngol Head Neck Surg 123:1061–1065

11. Tempero RM, Hannibal M, Finn LS et al (2006) Lymphocytopenia in children with lymphatic malformation. Arch Otolaryngol Head Neck Surg 132:93–97

12. Hein KD, Mulliken JB, Kozakewich HP et al (2002) Venous malformations of skeletal muscle. Plast Reconstr Surg 110:1625–1635

13. Lee A, Driscoll D, Gloviczki P, Clay R et al (2005) Evaluation and management of pain in patients with Klippel-Trenaunay syndrome: a review. Pediatrics 115:744–749

14. Kohout MP, Hansen M, Pribaz JJ, Mulliken JB (1998) Arteriovenous malformations of the head and neck: natural history and management. Plast Reconstr Surg 102:643–654

15. Orten SS, Waner M, Flock S et al (1996) Port-wine stains. An assessment of 5 years of treatment. Arch Otolaryngol Head Neck Surg 122:1174–1179

16. Sanchez-Carpintero I, Mihm MC et al (2004) Epithelial and mesenchymal hamartomatous changes in a mature port-wine stain: Morphologic evidence for a multiple germ layer field defect. J Am Acad Dermatol 50:608–612

Surgical Treatment of Vascular Malformations in the Hand

33

Piero Di Giuseppe

Abstract

As the hand is an organ of many different structures, located in a small space, with a high functional value, congenital vascular malformations (CVM) may easily involve many tissues, presenting complex clinical pictures that are difficult to treat. Surgical treatment is possible but general principles of hand surgery should be followed. Skin incisions should be carefully planned to save hand function. Bleeding is reduced by the use of a tourniquet. Magnification with a microscope during surgery is crucial for a precise dissection and recognition of neurovascular pedicles. In case of nerve involvement, external neurolysis is the first choice, as interfascicular treatment is a risky procedure. Total or partial resection of infiltrated muscles should be carefully performed, according to their function. Intraosseous arteriovenous (AV) malformations are best treated by direct occlusion through alcohol or glue injection, avoiding surgery.

Introduction

The hand has a very complex function strictly related to its particular anatomy: its sensorial and motor functions are interdependent [1]. Congenital vascular malformations (CVM) in the hand may involve any structure, and are often atypically distributed [2]. As many different tissues of high functional value are located in a small space, clinical pictures can be extended and complex and can involve skin, bones, nerves, muscles and tendons, posing special therapeutic problems. To surgically treat CVMs in the hand, the fourth principle of Belov should be followed: a functional radical operation should be performed, meaning as radical as possible, to avoid recurrences, and as sparing as feasible in order to preserve or restore hand function [3, 4].

Surgical strategies can consist of single or multiple stage surgery, alone or associated with other procedures, such as sclerotherapy, embolization or laser treatment [5–7].

Surgical techniques should respect general principles of hand surgery, including skin incisions and skin undermining and the selection criteria of structures to be resected according to their function. Techniques and timing of hemostasis and postoperative bandage should also be performed correctly.

General Principles of CVM Surgery in the Hand

Skin Incisions

The skin in the hand works like a distinct organ with its own passive motor function. The dorsal skin of the hand is more elastic, while the palmar skin is more adherent and sensitive. The elasticity of the skin in the web spaces allows independent movements of the fingers; scar contracture precludes mobility even if all the other structures are normal. When skin incisions are planned scar lines should be mainly at the level of skin creases in order to avoid scar contracture.

There are some typical incisions in hand surgery. Each of these incisions can be performed alone or combined with others. CVMs may be sometimes difficult to approach through conventional incisions; atypical incisions may sometimes be necessary.

Incisions for hand surgery should respect some basic principles:

1. Limited skin undermining and preparing of flaps that offer large exposure of the deep structures should be planned.

R. Mattassi, D.A. Loose, M. Vaghi (eds.), *Hemangiomas and Vascular Malformations*.
© Springer-Verlag Italia 2009

2. Web spaces and joint creases should be respected by broken incisions to avoid scar contracture (Fig 33.1a).
3. Scars from previous surgery influence the choice of new incisions. A flap should not be performed with a previous scar at its base. Incisions should be planned in order to permit extensions, when necessary. Drawing the contour of the CVM mass on the skin before marking the incision lines is helpful in order to better approach the malformation (Fig. 33.2a).

Skin Sparing Technique

Skin sparing is possible by subdermal undermining, which should be carefully done with a scalpel to preserve subdermal vascular networks. This allows minimal blood loss and saves skin flaps for coverage (Fig. 33.1b). It is best performed under a microscope or with loupe magnification.

Use of a Tourniquet

A tourniquet reduces bleeding and is useful for microsurgical techniques, especially in venous malformations. In arteriovenous (AV) malformations, a tourniquet is best applied after preparation of the fistulous area, as fistulae may be difficult to recognize during ischemia [8].

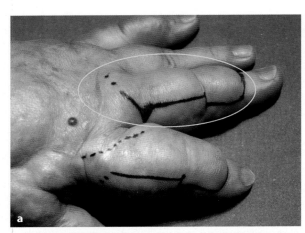
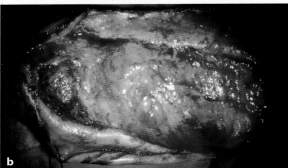
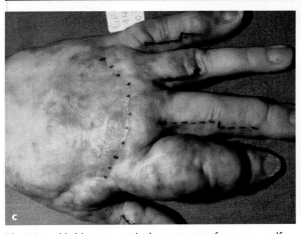

Fig. 33.1. Multistage surgical treatment of venous malformation of the hand. **a** Marking of incisions on the dorsolateral aspect of the middle finger. **b** Subdermal surgical undermining under microscope shows the avascular plane and exposition of the involved tissue (skin sparing technique). **c** Late result showing scars from previous operations at the time of index finger surgery. Figures 33b, 33c reproduced from [8]

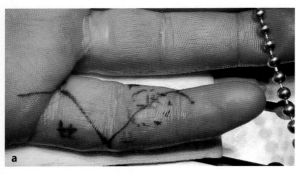
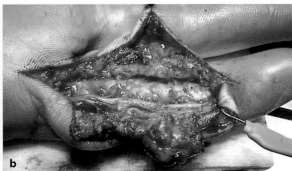

Fig. 33.2. Arteriovenous malformation in the volar aspect of the little finger. **a** Two fistulae areas guided the choice of a Brunner incision. **b** Neurovascular bundles used as a guide for the dissection of the malformed tissue. Tourniquet and microscope control reduced bleeding and resulted in a safe radical excision

Microscope

CVMs often enclose nerves and a direct approach may be difficult and risky for the patient. In these cases microsurgical techniques permit neurovascular pedicles to be isolated with extreme precision, following their course inside the vascular lesion. The resulting dissection is then much more precise and permits not only the integrity of the nerves to be respected, but can also be used as a guide during the dissection of CVM (Figs. 33.1b, 33.3b, c).

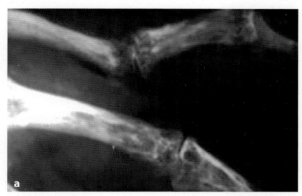
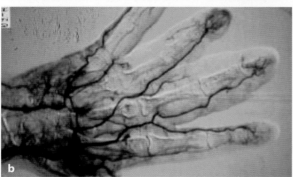
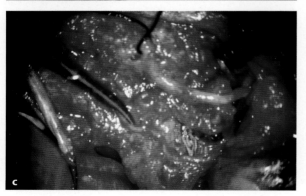

Fig. 33.3. Venous malformation. **a** Important bone involvement with proximal interphalangeal (PIP) joint instability mainly in the ring finger. **b** Angiography shows multiple digital artery damage during previous operations. **c** Dissection of nerves and arteries is more accurate and safe under microscope magnification

This technique lengthens surgery time but allows a precise dissection which is essential in difficult cases [8].

Tissue Involvement: Clinical Pictures and Surgical Treatment

One of the main challenges in this surgery is the involvement of surrounding structures, such as bone, nerves, muscle, tendons, ligaments and skin. CVM inside tissues may cause infiltration or compression [9].

Skin Involvement

In venous CVM, the skin is thinned by compression. A subdermal dissection is possible, preserving skin flaps and reducing bleeding ("skin sparing technique") (Fig. 33.1) [10].

In AV CVM, the subcutaneous tissue is involved and the skin is damaged by ischemia or direct infiltration.

In lymphatic CVM, the subcutaneous tissue is firmly infiltrated and fatty tissue is hypertrophic. The best procedure is an en bloc resection of the CVM after a precise skin drawing of involved areas with a correct orientation of final scars (Fig. 33.4).

However, the involvement of other tissues is the main challenge in surgical treatment of VM of the hand: the most difficult to treat areas are bones and nerves. Tendons are seldom affected, while synovia and muscles are commonly involved.

Bone Involvement

Bones can be affected in venous, AV and also in lymphatic CVMs.

Standard radiograms are the best diagnostic method and should be always performed before surgery of CVMs (Figs. 33.3a, 33.5b). Percutaneous direct bone puncture and intraosseous pathological vessel occlusion by ethanol or glue injection seems to be the best treatment. In many cases these procedures should be performed before surgery (Fig. 33.5a–c) [11].

Nerves

Nerves may be surrounded or infiltrated by a CVM. The main dilemma is to choose between resection

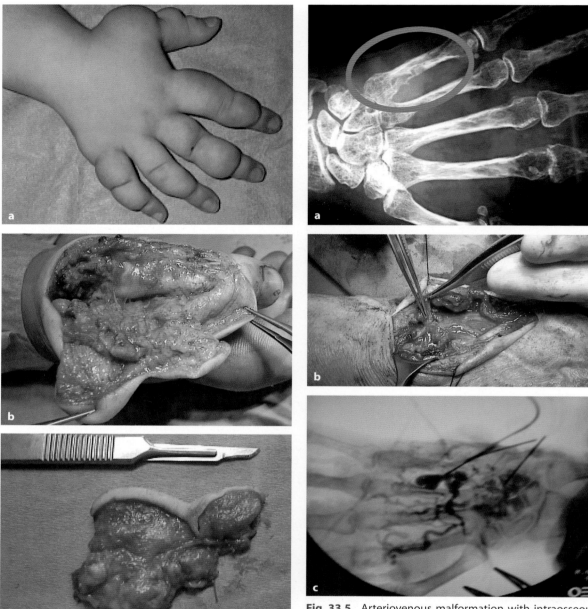

Fig. 33.4. En bloc excision of lymphatic malformation in the thumb of a young girl. **a** Clinical picture. **b** Radical resection of a planned segment of skin and underlying hypertrophic subcutaneous tissue. **c** Specimen of the removed tissue

Fig. 33.5. Arteriovenous malformation with intraosseous fistulae. **a** Radiogram shows the extent and site of bone involvement (*red circle*). **b** Subcutaneous AV fistulae have been removed and communicating vessels to the bone are clearly seen. **c** Direct alcoholization of bone fistulae reduced the malformed tissue in a few minutes

of surrounding malformed vessels only, or to extend surgery inside the nerve. In our experience, external decompression should be the first procedure used to reduce symptoms (Figs. 33.2, 33.6).

Internal interfascicular neurolysis is a risky procedure and may lead to irreversible nerve damage, immediately or later as a result of scarring. Selective resection and nerve grafting should be the final

option, performed only in case of severe pain and after failure of external resection of CVMs.

In case of nerve damage during surgery, immediate repair by suture or graft should be performed. To prevent damage, the best procedure is to follow the nerves as a guide through the malformation starting from a non involved area (Fig. 33.2). A direct approach can be risky.

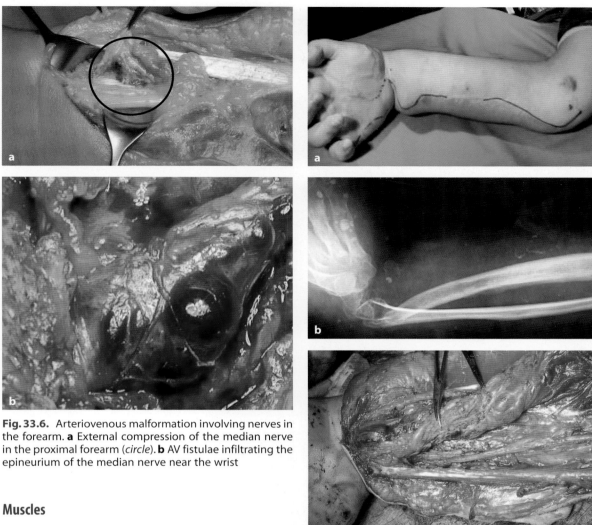

Fig. 33.6. Arteriovenous malformation involving nerves in the forearm. **a** External compression of the median nerve in the proximal forearm (*circle*). **b** AV fistulae infiltrating the epineurium of the median nerve near the wrist

Muscles

Total resection of expendable muscles is a common procedure (Fig. 33.7), especially when they are extensively infiltrated. Partial resection of an important muscle or a group of muscles is also possible according to the severity of infiltration and the possibility of maintaining or restoring function. Non resectable infiltrated muscles can be treated by foam sclerotherapy, direct alcohol injection or echoguided lasertherapy [9].

Tendons

Tendons are generally not involved directly by CVMs. However, tendon sheets are frequently involved; synovectomy is a safe and effective operation (Fig. 33.8).

Attention must be paid to important structures such as pulleys of flexor tendons and complex extensor digital systems.

Fig. 33.7. Extended venous malformation with secondary deformities of bones mainly at the wrist, wrist stiffness and flexor muscle contracture following several operations and sclerotherapy. **a** Incision along the ulnar side of the forearm. **b** X-ray shows wrist bones deformity and phlebolites. **c** Dissection of the ulnar nerve from the elbow to the wrist. Flexor carpi ulnaris muscle entirely removed and flexor digitorum superficialis elongated

Conclusion

Surgical treatment of CVM of the hand is feasible. If properly planned, it can be effective and safe. A multi-stage and multidisciplinary approach is recommended. Some technical devices such as the microscope and tourniquet can be used. Both devices allow a bloodless and accurate dissection of malformed tissues to be performed, particularly in the

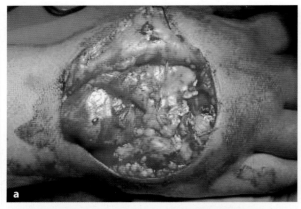
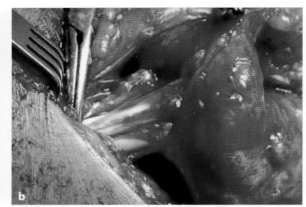
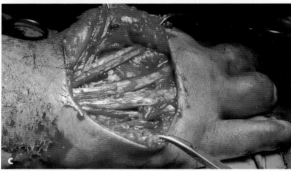

Fig. 33.8. Venous malformation of extensor tendons sheet. **a** Malformed tissue well delimited within the tendon sheet permits an easy skin undermining. **b, c** Limited invasion of the tendons allows a synovectomy with minimal bleeding to be performed

treatment of venous anomalies, which are the most common CVM. Nerves can be used as a guide for dissection of CVMs and skin can be saved by a careful subdermal undermining.

Tissue involvement of VM is a major problem in the hand. The more difficult challenge is infiltration of nerves and bones. For nerves, external neurolysis is our first choice, for bones direct sclerotherapy is useful. Muscles are frequently involved and can be totally resected if judged expendable. Tendons are seldom affected, but if the synovial sheet is involved it can easily be removed.

References

1. Levame J-H, Durafourg MP (1987) Reeducation des traumatises de la main. Maloine, Paris
2. Mattassi R (1993) Differential diagnosis in congenital vascular-bone syndromes. In: Semin Vasc Surg 6:233
3. Belov S (1989) Classification, terminology and nosology of congenital vascular defects. In: Belov S, Loose DA, Weber J (eds) Vascular malformations. Einhorn-Presse Verlag, Reinbek, pp 25–30
4. Belov S, Loose DA (1990) Surgical treatment of congenital vascular defects. Int Angiol 9:175–182
5. Mattassi R (1993) Diagnosis and treatment of venous malformations of the lower limbs. In: Mattassi R (ed) Proceedings of the international conference on vascular surgery. Beijing, China, October 21–24, International Academic Publishers, p 397
6. Lee BB, Do YS, Yakes W et al (2004) Management of arteriovenous malformations: a multidisciplinary approach. J Vasc Surg 39:590–600
7. Lee BB (2002) Advanced management of congenital vascular malformations (CVM). Int Angiol 21:209–213
8. Di Giuseppe P (2003) Principi di trattamento delle malformazioni vascolari della mano. In: Mattassi R, Belov S, Loose DA, Vaghi M (eds) Malformazioni vascolari ed emangiomi. Springer-Verlag, Milano, pp 160–165
9. Hein KD, Mulliken JB, Kozakewich HPW et al (2002) Venous malformations of skeletal muscle. Plast Reconstr Surg 110:1625–1635
10. Breugem CC, Maas M, Breugem SJM et al (2003) Vascular malformations of the lower limb with osseous involvement. J Bone Loint Surg 85:399–405
11. Di Giuseppe P (2006) Le angiodisplasie venose della mano ed il coinvolgimento dei tessuti. Riv Chir Mano 43:102–105

Management of Vascular Malformations in the Thorax Wall

34

Francesco Stillo, Giuseppe Bianchini

Abstract

Vascular malformations of the thoracic wall are relatively rare but highly disabling as they cause severe functional and aesthetic disorders. Treatment of thorax vascular malformations is extremely difficult and dangerous for the patient. Therapeutic strategy must be planned for each patient on the basis of clinical and instrumental findings, considering the site, morphology, extent and the hemodynamics of the malformation. Treatment options differ depending on the various types of thoracic vascular malformation: venous, lymphatic or arteriovenous. The most common surgical and endovascular procedures carried out in the treatment of thorax vascular malformations are discussed and described in this chapter, with particular reference to the therapeutic problems and risks in this specific anatomical region.

Introduction

Vascular malformations of the thoracic wall are relatively rare but highly disabling as they cause severe functional and aesthetic disorders [1].

The treatment of thoracic vascular malformations is extremely difficult and dangerous for the patient because the malformations are often very large with diffuse tissue infiltration and involvement of the central vessels.

The aims of treatment are partial or complete regression of the malformation, reduction or disappearance of clinical symptoms and functional rehabilitation.

The therapeutic strategy must be planned for each patient on the basis of the clinical and instrumental findings, with particular reference to the site, morphology, extent and hemodynamics of the malformation.

Treatment options differ depending on the type of thorax vascular malformation: venous, lymphatic or arteriovenous [2].

Venous Malformations

Thoracic venous malformations are located on the anterior, lateral or posterior thorax wall. These malformations are congenital but may show a progressive volume increase in children and young patients. Venous malformations are usually very large and deep with diffuse involvement of the thoracic wall muscles, including the intercostals, latissimus dorsi and trapezium. It is sometimes possible to observe costal bone or pleuric involvement (Fig. 34.1) [3].

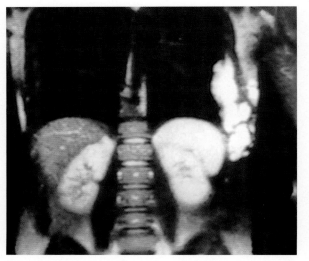

Fig. 34.1. Venous malformation of the thorax wall with pleuric involvement

R. Mattassi, D.A. Loose, M. Vaghi (eds.), *Hemangiomas and Vascular Malformations*.
© Springer-Verlag Italia 2009

Surgery is the elective choice for small and superficial venous malformations located on skin and subcutaneous tissue. Excision should be carried out by micro-invasive techniques, using a spiral purse string suture where possible. When the malformation is very large a double stage approach is preferable, performing the implant of a skin expander in the first step and the removal of the malformation followed by a limb reconstruction in the second step [4]. The best positioning of skin expanders depends on the site of the malformation. In many cases it is useful to implant the skin expander on the anterior abdominal or lumbar area and to perform a rotational flap after the exeresis of the thorax wall malformation.

Sclerotherapy is useful in very extensive venous malformations with muscle or bone involvement, when total surgical removal is not possible. It is recommended that schlerotherapy be performed under radioscopic guidance because these malformations often show direct drainage in the azygos, hemiazygos, brachiocephalic or superior cava veins. An intraoperative direct puncture phlebography allows the injection site and the diffusion of the sclerosing mixture to be controlled (Fig. 34.2). A number of different sclerosing agents are used. The choice depends on the morphological characteristics, and the anatomical site and extent of the malformation. For small-caliber venous malformations it is possible to use 2–3% polydocanol or 0.2–3% sodium-tetradecyl-sulphate solution [5]. For large-caliber venous malformations it is preferable to use 95% ethanol because a more powerful sclerosant is necessary in these cases. The dosage of the sclerosing agent will be established in proportion to the size of the malformation, up to a maximum dose of 2 ml/kg body weight

[6]. In any case, it is preferable to inject the sclerosant by multiple direct punctures of the malformation in different sites on the chest wall (Fig. 34.3). After sclerotherapy of thorax venous malformations a low-molecular heparin and steroid treatment is recommended, in order to prevent thrombophlebitis, skin necrosis or nerve damage.

A combined treatment is the preferred option in the majority of cases. Combined percutaneous and surgical treatment offer the best clinical, morphological and functional results. In cases of extensive thorax venous malformations it is necessary to perform multiple sequential surgical or endovascular procedures in order to obtain a complete regression [7].

Lymphatic Malformations

Thoracic lymphatic malformations are usually cystic hygromas arising from the subclavian or axillary regions with involvement of the thorax wall. These malformations induce severe clinical symptoms because they are often large and expansive and tend to gradually grow over the years, especially in concomitance with hormonal, traumatic or infective events [8]. Early treatment is recommended to avoid the risk of a pleuric or mediastinal events with compression of vital structures such as the trachea or central veins.

Surgical removal is considered the best cure for thorax lymphatic malformations [9]. When the cystic sac is very large and deep with infiltration of muscle and peripheral nerves it is very difficult to achieve complete surgical extirpation. In these cases it is possible to perform a surgical excision in stages, thus

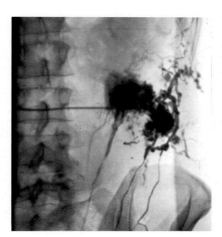

Fig. 34.2. Intraoperative direct puncture phlebography before scleroembolization of a thorax wall venous malformation

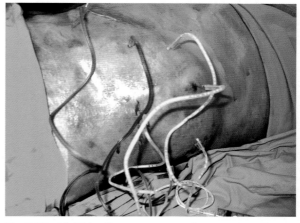

Fig. 34.3. Multiple direct punctures of a venous malformation in different sites on the chest wall

reducing the risk of hemorrhage or nerve injury [10].

Pecutaneous sclerotherapy is accepted as a safe and satisfactory treatment for small lymphatic malformations of the thorax, particularly in pediatric patients. Intralesional injection of sclerosants is a low-invasive procedure which gives good clinical results with marked or complete shrinkage of the cystic mass and minimum recurrence (Fig. 34.4) [11]. The size of the malformation dictates the choice of sclerosing agent. Sodium-tetradecyl-sulphate is preferred for circumscribed forms. Ethanol is more effective in larger lymphatic malformations of the thorax, but induces a considerable risk of pleuric reactions or brachial plexus injuries. OK-32 is a good alternative scleroagent in these malformations because it allows mass shrinkage with a moderate inflammatory reaction to be achieved [12]. Recently cystic lymphatic malformations have been treated by transthoracic bleomycin injection. In this case several sessions of sclerotherapy are required to obtain a complete reduction of the mass and to reduce complications or recurrence. For very large and deep forms it is useful to perform percutaneous ultrasound-guided sclerotherapy. If possible, the sclerosing injection should be followed by selective locoregional compression.

A combined treatment is also very useful in thorax lymphatic malformations. Intralesional sclerotherapy may be a preliminary treatment before performing the surgical excision of the lymphatic mass.

Arteriovenous Malformations

Thoracic arteriovenous malformations originate from the intercostal arteries or from the subclavian artery branches. Involvement of the thoracic wall muscles, including the pectorals, intercostals, serratus and latissimus dorsi, is frequent. In many cases costal bone infiltration is observed. These malformations are extremely dangerous because their natural history shows rapid growth and a high incidence of cardiac failure [13].

For these reasons the treatment of thorax arteriovenous malformations is extremely difficult and controversial. The current literature does not provide scientific evidence in this field. Furthermore, inappropriate therapy can be responsible for rapid growth of the malformation. The therapeutic strategy should be a multidisciplinary decision, taking into consideration the type, extent and localization of the malformation [14].

Surgery is indicated in tight-nidus and low-flow arteriovenous malformations of the thoracic wall, especially in superficial forms [15]. Extensive ligation of all fistulas in the chest wall and skeletization of the feeding artery from its proximal to its distal extent may obtain good early results but carry a high risk of late recurrence. Total excision of arteriovenous fistulas and niduses with surrounding soft tissues is recommendable when technically feasible (Fig. 34.5). A double stage approach is also useful in these malformations, with an implant of a skin expander performed first in order to allow easier reconstruction [16]. Surgery of thoracic arteriovenous malformations carries a very high risk of hemorrhage because it is not possible to carry out adequate intraoperative compression. For this

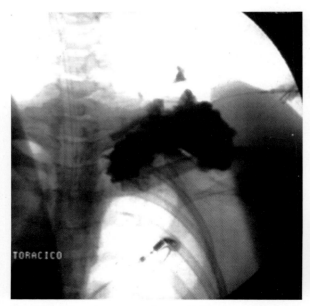

Fig. 34.4. Percutaneous scleroembolization of a cystic lymphatic malformation of the thorax wall

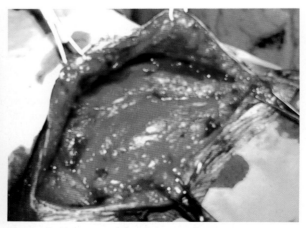

Fig. 34.5. Treatment of a thorax wall arteriovenous malformation by total excision of arteriovenous fistulas and niduses with surrounding soft tissues

reason it is recommended that a preliminary tissue infiltration by saline solution be performed, and bleeding control be achieved with the use of an autotransfusion system.

Endovascular treatments are preferred in large-nidus and high flow arteriovenous malformations, particularly in deep infiltrating forms, using transcatheter or direct puncture techniques. The choice of different procedures or embolic materials for thoracic embolization depends on the anatomic configuration and hemodynamic patterns of the arteriovenous malformations [17].

Embolization of the afferent arteries by highly selective catheterization is a good choice for fistulous type arteriovenous malformations, showing a small number of large-caliber feeding arteries (Fig. 34.6).

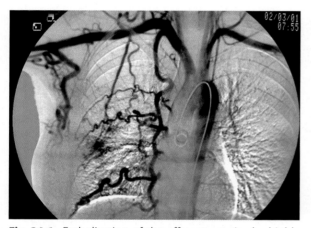

Fig. 34.6. Embolization of the afferent arteries by highly selective catheterization in a thorax fistulous type arteriovenous malformation

In these cases it is possible to release nidus fluid or solid agents, such as polyvinyl alcohol, N-butyl-2-cyanoacrylate glue and tungsten coils into the malformation. Embolization in the thorax presents special problems related to the risk of inadvertent occlusion of important branches of the thoracic aorta, such as the spinal arteries. In some cases, when superselective catheterization is difficult or dangerous, it may be useful to perform surgical access to the afferent arteries on the thoracic wall.

Retrograde venous sclerotherapy is an alternative approach to treat the micro-fistulous type arteriovenous malformations, which are very frequent in the thorax region [18]. These malformations arise from multiple low-caliber feeding arteries and consequently an anterograde approach cannot be performed. The obliteration of dominant out-flow veins is successfully obtained by direct puncture or transcatheter injection of ethanol or sodium-tetradecyl-sulphate. Vein occlusion using a balloon catheter may be helpful during the procedure [19].

Early results of endovascular treatment are satisfactory with significant regression of the malformation and improvement of clinical features. The long-term follow-up shows a high recurrence rate. Furthermore, skin ulcerations are relatively frequent complications in the scleroembolization of thorax arteriovenous malformations.

Combined treatment is recommended to improve results and to reduce injuries. In many cases arterial embolization may be a preliminary procedure to reduce the fistulous flow before subsequent treatment by venous retrograde sclerotherapy or surgery. In any case, the most appropriate therapeutic strategy should be based on the clinical and instrumental picture of each individual case.

References

1. Waldo RT (1991) Chest wall vascular malformations. Chest 100:887–888
2. Arneja JS, Gosain AK (2006) An approach to the management of common vascular malformations of the trunk. J Craniofac Surg 17:761–766
3. Demos TC, Posniak HV, Pierce KL,et al (2004) Venous anomalies of the thorax. AJR Am J Roentgenol 82:1139–1150
4. Bianchini G, Nicodemi EM, Stillo F (2003) Thoraco-abdominal venous malformations: diagnostic and therapeutic strategies. International Angiology 22(2 supp 1):69
5. O'Donovan JC, Donaldson JS, Morello FP et al (1997) Symptomatic hemangiomas and venous malformations in infants, children, and young adults: treatment with percutaneous injection of sodium tetradecyl sulfate. AJR Am J Roentgenol 169:723–729
6. Shireman PK, McCarthy WJ, Yao JS, Vogelzang RL (1997) Treatment of venous malformations by direct injection with ethanol. J Vasc Surg 26:838–844
7. Agus GB, Allegra C, Antignani PL et al (2005) Guidelines for the diagnosis and therapy of the vein and lymphatic disorders. Int Angiol 24:107–168
8. Daya SK, Gowda RM, Gowda MR, Khan IA (2004) Thoracic cystic lymphangioma (cystic hygroma): a chest pain syndrome. Angiology 55:561–564
9. Shahriari A, Odell JA (2001) Cervical and thoracic components of multiorgan lymphangiomatosis managed surgically. Ann Thorac Surg 71:694–966

10. Papagiannopoulos K, Van Raemdonck DE, De Boeck K, Lerut T (2004) Pediatric thoracic lymphangiomatosis: is chest wall resection too radical? Ann Thorac Surg 77:695–697

11. Duman L, Karnak I, Akinci D, Tanyel FC (2006) Extensive cervical-mediastinal cystic lymphatic malformation treated with sclerotherapy in a child with Klippel-Trenaunay syndrome. J Pediatr Surg 41:e21–e24

12. Greinwald JH JR, Burke DK, Sato Y et al (1999) Treatment of lymphangiomas in children: an update of Picibanil (OK-432) sclerotherapy. Otolaryngol Head Neck Surg 121:381–387

13. Itano H, Lee S, Kulick DM et al (2005) Nontraumatic chest wall systemic-to-pulmonary artery fistula. Ann Thorac Surg 79:e29–e31

14. Salo JA, Ketonen PS (1988) Congenital arteriovenous fistulas in the chest wall. Scand J Thorac Cardiovasc Surg 22:7–10

15. Uchida Y, Kawano H, Koide Y et al (2003) Arteriovenous fistula of internal thoracic vessels. Intern Med 42:987–990

16. Laurian C, Diner P, Enjolras O et al (1996) Surgical treatment of superficial vascular malformations. Indications for tissue expansion. J Mal Vasc 21:31–35

17. Hartnell GG (1993) Embolization in the treatment of acquired and congenital abnormalities of the heart and thorax. Radiographics 13:1349–1362

18. Yakes WF, Rossi P, Odink H (1996) How I do it. Arteriovenous malformation management. Cardiovasc Intervent Radiol 19:65–71

19. Jackson JE, Mansfield AO, Allison DJ (1996) Treatment of high-flow vascular malformations by venous embolization aided by flow occlusion techniques. Cardiovasc Intervent Radiol 19:323–328

Joint Involvement in Patients with Vascular Malformations. Destructive Angiodysplastic Arthritis

35

Jürgen Hauert, Dirk A. Loose, Florian M. Westphal

Abstract

Intra-articular vascular malformations are mainly seen in the knee. The evolution of a joint with this disease is a progressive destructive angiodysplastic arthritis, with destruction of synovia, cartilage, menisci and Hoffa's fat pad. To avoid this progression, early treatment is based on arthroscopic coagulation and/or debridement, open arthrolysis or joint replacement in severe cases.

Introduction

Orthopaedic features are commonly seen in patients with congenital vascular malformations. In our patient selection (n = 1,304) reviewed between 1970 and 2007, there were 322 patients (25%) with orthopaedic pathologies (leg length discrepancy, contractures, osteolytic lesions, osseous involvement), 52 of whom showed joint involvement of lower limb (4%). The distribution according to the Hamburg Classification [1] was: n = 49 predominantly venous, extratruncular, infiltrative; n = 2 predominantly arteriovenous (AV), extratruncular, infiltrative; and n = 1 Jaffe-Lichtenstein.

The vast majority (n = 48) had affected knee joints, followed by ankles (n = 2) and hip joints (n = 2). We published our early experiences on this clinical picture of destructive angiodysplastic arthritis in 2000 [2]. The comparatively few publications found in the literature on this subject concentrate on the knee joint [3–6].

The destructive intra-articular changes evolve from the infiltrative growth of the malformations (Fig. 35.1) with destruction of synovial membrane, cartilage, menisci and Hoffa's fat pad. As this dis-

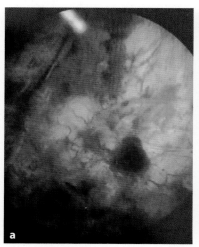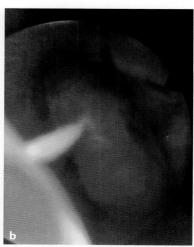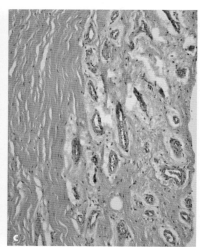

Fig. 35.1. Transarthroscopic view on the medial capsule of the knee joint. **a** Small capsular defect with the malformation pushed extra-articularly by water pressure. **b** Same region with water pressure turned off – the malformation infiltrates the knee joint. **c** Histological aspect of malformations (*right* part of the panel) adjacent to meniscal tissue (*left* part of the panel) – (HE stain, ×25)

R. Mattassi, D.A. Loose, M. Vaghi (eds.), *Hemangiomas and Vascular Malformations*.
© Springer-Verlag Italia 2009

ease pattern is of a progressive nature, the therapeutic approach should be performed in early stages to prevent further damage to the joint. The clinical symptoms consist of joint swelling, pain and restriction of joint movement. These features can easily be misinterpreted and referred to the malformation itself. Therefore, careful clinical and radiological examination by X-ray and magnetic resonance imaging (MRI) [7] should be performed to diagnose and treat intra-articular pathologies at early stages.

Classification and Therapeutic Approach of Joint Pathologies

As the joint pathologies in patients with vascular malformations are of a (partially) rapid progressive nature, we recommend a graded classification, which allows a defined therapeutic approach.

Destructive Angiodysplastic Arthritis – Stage 1

In this early stage the clinical symptoms are mild and are shown by X-ray. The pathbreaking findings are seen by MRI (Fig. 35.2a). The therapeutic approach should be transarthroscopic with coagulation of infiltrative malformations and/or debridement of impaired tissues (Fig. 35.2b, c). In nearly all cases it was also necessary to extirpate extra-articular vascular malformations by vascular surgery. In our patient selection (n = 8) we found good clinical results with partly non-progressive radiological findings at follow-up.

Destructive Angiodysplastic Arthritis – Stage 2

In this stage the clinical symptoms are more severe, particularly with more pronounced limitations in range of movement. The X-ray examination shows early destructive changes (cysts, joint space narrowing) and the therapeutic approach is mainly transarthroscopic in combination with vascular surgery. In cases of an extension deficit we recommend a redressing brace post-operatively. The use of external fixation for redressing contractures is not recommended due to the comparatively higher risk of this invasive procedure, bearing in mind that relapse of contractures is not uncommon.

Open arthrolysis should be reserved for recrudescence and cases with an extension deficit greater than 60 degrees, where arthroscopic access is highly limited.

Our patients (n = 18) benefited from minimal invasive surgery with so far no further joint intervention necessary; a case of a 29 year old female with progressive gonalgia and an extension deficit of 10 degrees is shown (Figs. 35.3, 35.4). After arthroscopic debridement and medial microfracturing an excellent result with pain only at extensive sporting level was seen at 5 years follow-up.

Destructive Angiodysplastic Arthritis – Stage 3

This final stage with radiologically severely damaged joints is characterised by severe arthralgia. Due to the partly rapid progressive course of the disease, com-

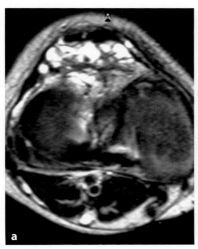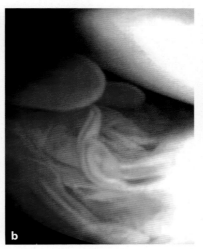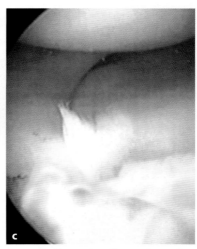

Fig. 35.2. a MRI showing infiltrative subpatellar malformations. **b** Intra-operative view of infiltrated malformation. **c** Early destructive changes of tibial plateau

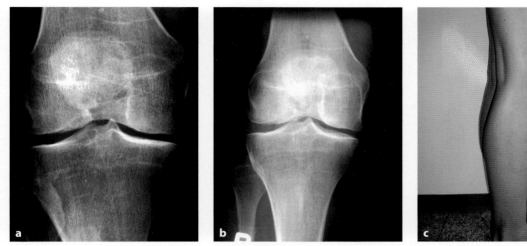

Fig. 35.3. a Pre-operative X-ray showing bone cysts and joint space narrowing. **b** X-ray at five years follow-up – no progressive changes visible. **c** Lateral view at five years follow-up – residual extension deficit of 5 degrees

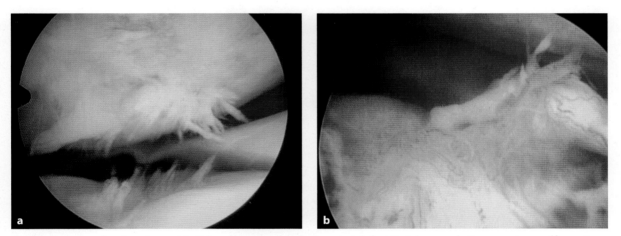

Fig. 35.4. Intra-operative view. **a** Medial compartment with chondral defect 3–4 degrees. **b** Overgrowing malformations with chondral defect at the trochlear region

pletely destroyed joints appear independent of age (Fig. 35.5). Despite the vast destructive changes, arthroscopic debridement leads to surprisingly good results (n = 12) compared to degenerative joint diseases [8].

If arthroscopic surgery does not lead to satisfying results, joint replacement can be indicated (n = 3 in our patient selection).

Careful planning in cooperation with the vascular surgeon is required with an individual approach. Depending on the extent of vascular involvement, specialized techniques of vascular treatment may be required (Fig. 35.6).

If the dorsal capsule is infiltrated and excessive bleeding is encountered, the implantation has to be modified by leaving a small bony ridge of the dorsal tibial plateau in order to protect malformed vessels against damage in the popliteal region (Fig. 35.7).

Conclusion

Joint pathologies are common and often underdiagnosed in patients with vascular malformations. To prevent progressive intra-articular destruction, early intervention – in cooperation with the vascular surgeon – should be performed.

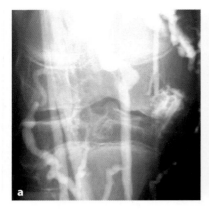
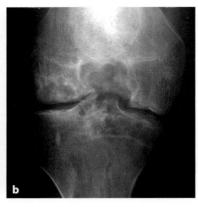

Fig. 35.5. Nineteen year old male presenting with severe gonalgia. **a** Radiograph at 15 years without major destructive changes and with malformed veins. **b** Radiograph at 19 years old with completely destroyed joint

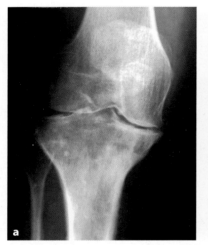
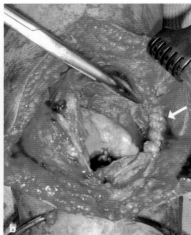
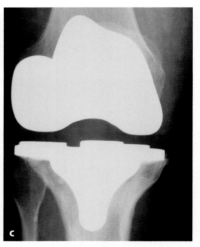

Fig. 35.6. **a** Pre-operative X-ray showing progressive, destructive changes. **b** Intra-operative view – soft tissue with malformed veins handling according to the technique of Belov IV (*arrow*) **c** Post-operative X-ray

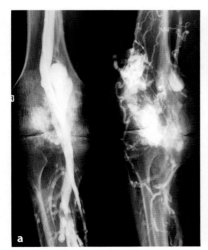
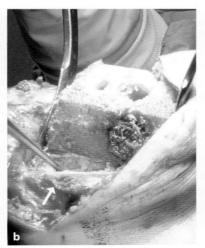
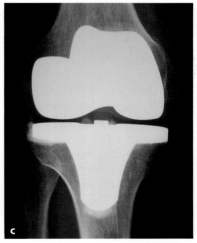

Fig. 35.7. **a** Phlebography showing the predominantly venous malformations. **b** Intra-operative view – bony ridge left to protect the popliteal region. **c** Post-operative X-ray

Our diagnostic and therapeutic algorithm for Hauert's disease is illustrated in Table 35.1. In contrast to the current literature, we prefer minimal invasive surgery by arthroscopy rather than open arthrolysis.

In cases of open procedures, interdisciplinary cooperation, especially with the vascular surgeon, is mandatory and should be handled in specialised centres only.

Table 35.1. Diagnostic and therapeutic algorithm for Hauert's disease

	Stage 1	Stage 2	Stage 3
Clinical feature	No/mild pain, joint swelling Mild decrease of ROM*	Mild to severe pain Pronounced decrease in ROM	Mild to severe pain Severe restriction in ROM
Radiographic findings	X-ray: no changes MRI: infiltrative malformation	X-ray: early destructive changes MRI: also involvement of constitutional changes	X-ray: advanced destructive changes MRI: not necessary
Orthopaedic surgical	Transarthroscopic	Transarthroscopic (open resection) w or w/o redressing brace	Transarthroscopic, (open resection) w or w/o redressing brace joint replacement

ROM, range of motion

References

1. Belov S (1989) Classification, terminology and nosology of congenital vascular defects. In: Belov S, Loose DA, Weber J (eds) Vascular malformations. Einhorn-Presse Verlag, Reinbek, pp 25–30
2. Hauert J, Betthäuser A, Loose DA (2000) Vascular malformation arthritis – Transarthroscopic treatment – Communication at the 13th Workshop of the International Society for the Study of Vascular Anomalies 10–13 May, Montreal, Canada
3. Laurian C (2002) Malformazioni venose intraarticolari del ginocchio. In: Mattassi R, Belov S, Loose DA (eds) Malformazioni vascolari ed emangiomi. Testo atlante di diagnostica e terapia, pp 176–179
4. Enjolras O, Ciabrini D, Mazoyer E (1997) Extensive pure venous malformations in the upper or lower limb: a review of 27 cases. J Am Acad Dermatol 36:219–225
5. Breugem CC, Maas M, Breugem SJ et al (2003) Vascular malformations of the lower limb with osseous involvement. J Bone Joint Surg Br 85:399–405
6. Bonaga S, Bardi C, Gigante C, Turra S (2003) Synovial involvement in hemangiomatosis. Arch Orthop Trauma Surg 123:102–106
7. Breugem CC, Maas M, Reekers JA, van der Horst CM (2001) Use of magnetic resonance imaging for the evaluation of vascular malformations of the lower extremity. Plast Reconstr Surg 108:870–877
8. Moseley JB, O'Malley K, Petersen NJ et al (2002) A controlled trial of arthroscopic surgery for osteoarthritis of the knee. J Fam Pract 51:813

Surgical Approach to Congenital Vascular Malformations (CVM) in the Foot

36

Giacomo Pisani, Dirk A. Loose

Abstract

The foot is a special localisation for all different forms of vascular malformations. The step-by-step diagnostics contain the assessment of the clinical picture and the functional disturbances of the foot. It is mandatory to get precise diagnostic information about the involvement of the four compartments of the foot. This is the basis for the access surgery to the different regions. Eight main accesses have been developed. Incisions should be traced out to suit the loading zones of the foot. The treatment may have to be performed in a stepwise fashion.

Arteries

The vascular contribution to the foot (Fig. 36.1) is assured by the anterior tibial (*a4*), posterior tibial (*a3*) and peroneal arteries (*a14*). These are tributaries of the popliteal (*a*), which bifurcates into the anterior and posterior tibials just below the arch of the soleus.

The anterior tibial runs between the anterior tibial muscle and the extensor digitorum longus. At the tibiotarsal interline, it continues as the dorsalis pedis (*b*). Its collaterals are the anterior lateral (*c*) and anterior medial (*d*) malleolar arteries; the lateral anastomoses with the perforating branch of the peroneal artery forms part of the malleolar lateral network (*e*), the medial forms part of the malleolar medial network (*f*).

The dorsalis pedis runs dorsally to the tarsus between the hallucis longus and brevis extensors as far as the base of the first intermetatarsal space where it branches off into the deep plantar branch (*g*) and then continues into the dorsal metatarsal artery I (*h*).

It gives rise to two or three medial tarsal arteries (*i*) which join the tarsal medial network (*l*) and anastomose with the medial plantar artery (*m*), and also with the lateral tarsal artery (*n*), which runs under the extensor digitorum brevis towards the base of the fifth metatarsal and anastomoses with the lateral end of the arcuate artery (*o*) to form the tarsal dorsal network (*p*). The arcuate artery (*o*) is the main distal branch. It runs laterally from its origin near the first intermetatarsal space to the base of the metatarsals and then anastomoses with the lateral tarsal artery. It gives rise to dorsal metatarsal arteries II, III and IV (*q*), each of which then bifurcates into dorsal digital arteries (*r*) for the opposite sides of the corresponding toes. These in turn give rise to posterior perforating branches (*s*) between the bases of the metatarsals, and smaller, inconstant anterior branches between their heads. These branches then anastomose with the corresponding branches of the plantar metatarsal arteries (*u*). The deep plantar branch runs to the plantar region, descends proximally into the first intermetatarsal space and anastomoses with the deep plantar arch (*v*).

The dorsal metatarsal artery I runs forward dorsally to the interosseus dorsalis muscle I and provides the dorsomedial digital branch of the second toe and the dorsolateral digital branch of the first toe. One of its perforating branches becomes the medial plantar artery of the second toe and the lateral plantar of the great toe (*a1*). It also anastomoses with the medial plantar digital of the great toe (*a2*).

The posterior tibial artery (*a4*), is localized medial to the Achilles tendon, then runs behind and below the tibial malleolus to pass between the two leaflets of the ligamentum laciniatum, where it bifurcates into its terminal branches; namely the medial (*m*) and lateral (*a5*) plantar arteries. Its collateral branches include the medial anterior malleolar artery (*a6*), which

R. Mattassi, D.A. Loose, M. Vaghi (eds.), *Hemangiomas and Vascular Malformations*.

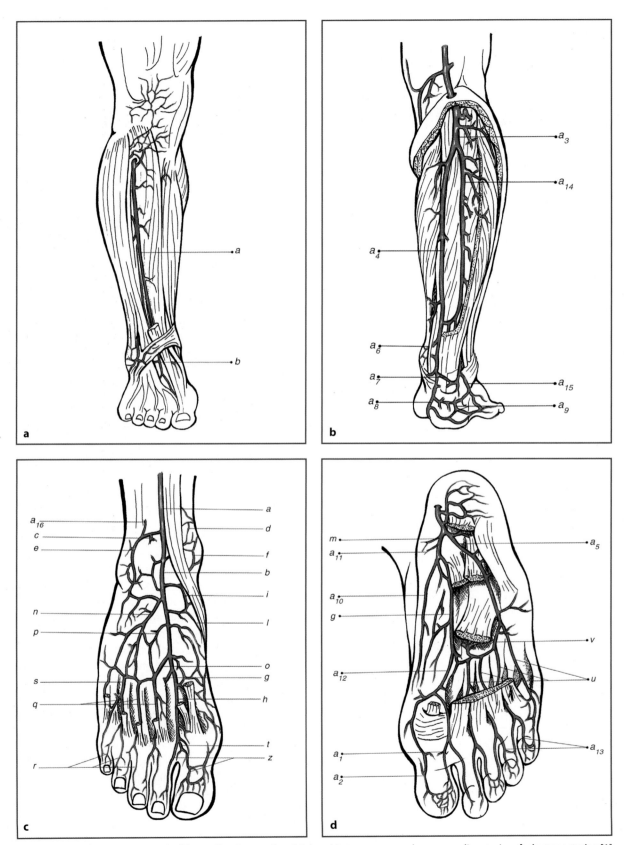

Fig. 36.1. Arteries. **a** Anterior tibial; **b** popliteal, posterior tibial and interosseous; **c** dorsum pedis arteries, **d** plantar arteries [1]

runs to the malleolar medial network; a communicating branch (*a7*) anastomoses with the corresponding branch of the peroneal and the medial calcaneal branches (*a8*) that run to the calcaneal tuberosity network (*a9*).

The medial plantar artery initially runs between the two leaflets of the ligamentum laciniatum within the superior compartment, and then passes between the abductor hallucis and the quadratus plantae, where it bifurcates into deep (*g*) and superficial (*a10*) branches. It then runs along the medial edge of the flexor hallucis longus alongside the medial septum between the adductor hallucis and the tendon of the flexor digitorum longus. It puts out deltoid branches (*a11*) before dividing.

After putting out branches for the abductor hallucis, the superficial branch proceeds along the medial border of the foot to the base of the great toe. The deep branch runs in the sulcus between the abductor hallucis and the flexor digitorum brevis and then between the two bellies of the flexor hallucis brevis to anastomose with the plantar metatarsal artery I (*a12*) or the medial plantar digital artery of the great toe.

The lateral plantar artery runs between the flexor digitorum brevis and the quadratus plantae and is directed distally and laterally towards the base of the fifth metatarsal. It then proceeds medially to form the arcus plantaris (*V*), which passes below the oblique head of the adductor hallucis along the plane of the interossei and the bases of the second, third and fourth metatarsals.

The plantaris arch anatomoses with the deep branch of the dorsalis pedis. It is the origin of the plantar metatarsal arteries which receive the perforating branches of the corresponding dorsales and end in two plantar digital arteries (*a13*) for the opposite inferior side of two contiguous toes. The artery for the medial border of the great toe is usually provided by the plantar metatarsal artery I; the lateral marginal artery of the fifth toe provides a termination for the lateral planar artery.

The peroneal or fibular artery (*a14*) is a proximal collateral branch of the posterior tibial. It runs alongside the interosseous membrane and the capsuloligamentous structures of the ankle. Its calcaneal branches (*a15*) form part of the calcaneal network. It gives rise to a perforating branch (*a16*; Fig. 36.1c) that passes through the membrane just proximal to the syndesmosis, anastomoses with both the anterior and the lateral posterior malleolar artery and contributes to the malleolar lateral and calcaneal network. It also sends a communicating branch to the posterior tibial artery.

Veins

A distinction is drawn between the deep and the superficial venous circulation (Fig. 36.2).

The deep veins are mostly duplicates of the arteries whose course they follow (Fig. 36.1). They are provided with numerous valves whereby blood is drained from the deep to the superficial veins as opposed to the superficial to deep drainage seen in the leg.

In the sole of the foot, (Fig. 36.2a) plantar digital veins (*a*) pass back to form the plantar metatarsal veins (*b*), the many perforating branches of which partly convey blood from the deep to the superficial veins of the dorsum pedis, and partly debouch into the plantar venous arch (*c*). They are also the origin of the lateral plantar veins that combine with the lateral plantar veins to form the posterior tibial veins, which also receive the peroneal veins. The small (*d*) and the great (*e*) saphenous veins receive anastomotic branches from the lateral and the medial plantars, respectively.

The few deep dorsal metatarsal veins empty into the anterior tibial veins. The superficial veins run in the subcutaneous tissue and have many valves. They are anastomotically linked to the deep veins via their many valves.

The venosum plantar network (*f*) is a very fine network closely adherent to the deep aspect of the skin in the sole of the foot that empties partly into the deep veins and partly into the medial (*g*) and lateral (*h*) marginal veins that run backwards behind the malleolus to the leg, while anteriorly they are tributaries of the plantar venous arch (*i*) that runs between the fat pads of the toe at the level of the transverse bundles of the plantar aponeurosis. The arch receives superficial branches of the plantar digitals and is connected to the dorsal digital veins (*m*) via the intercapitular veins (*l*).

The dorsal digitals join dorsally to form common digital veins (*n*) that empty into the dorsal venous arch, composed of an irregular chain of anastomoses between the common digitals and the medial and lateral marginal that corresponds to the distal portion of the metatarsus. Proximal to this arch is the irregular venosum dorsal network (*o*), which receives many tributaries from the deep venous vessels and continues proximal into the venosum anterius network of the leg (*p*). The network empties at the sides into the lateral and medial marginal veins that give rise to the small and the great saphenous veins, respectively.

The start of the great saphenous vein is medial premalleolar. It receives small vessels from the venosum plantar network and deep vessels from the medial plantar veins. It then runs superficial to the medial aspect of the tibia as far as the thigh, where it empties into

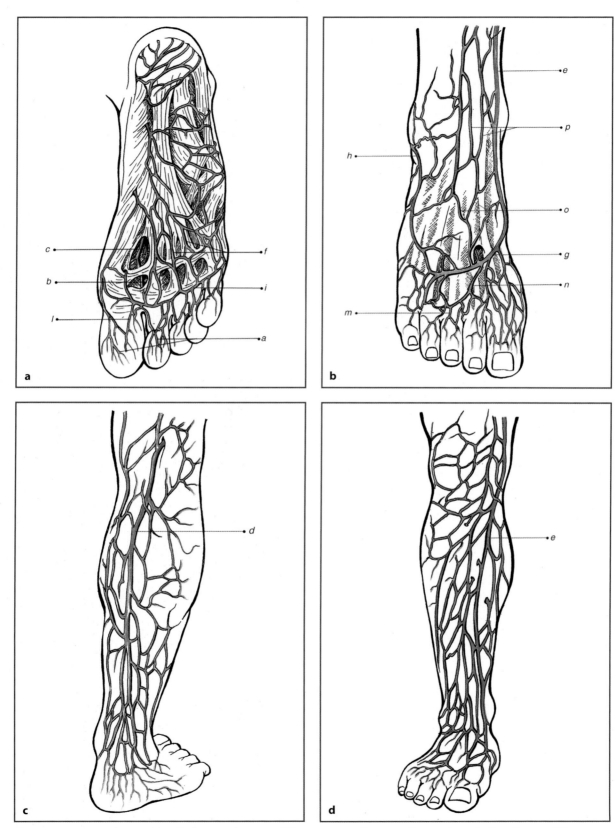

Fig. 36.2. Veins. **a** Plantar veins; **b** dorsal veins; **c** small (posterior) saphenous; **d** great (anterior) saphenous. The names of the individual veins are set out in the text [1]

the femoral vein. It anastomoses several times with the lesser saphenous on its way through the leg.

The small saphenous vein is the continuation behind the lateral malleolus of the lateral marginal vein, though some superficial branches of the venosum plantar network and a branch anastomotic with the deep lateral plantar veins also contribute to its constitution. It proceeds proximal to the leg wrapped in a doubling of the fascia cruris before emptying into the popliteal vein.

Lymphatic Vessels

The superficial and deep lymphatic vessels of the sole and back of the foot pass to the medial and the lateral collector that then proceed to the leg to reach the superficial and deep lymph nodes.

The superficial lymphatics (Fig. 36.3) run from the cutaneous lymphatic network to the subcutaneous panniculus adiposus and alongside the superficial fascia. They are tributaries of the two saphenous veins and form a network over the whole of the upper surface of the foot. Most follow the course of the great saphenous vein and debouch into the superficial inguinal nodes. The others accompany the small saphenous vein and empty into the popliteal nodes.

The sole is also completely covered with a network of superficial lymphatics. Most proceed to the back of the foot, pass round its medial and lateral margin and empty into the superficial inguinal nodes. A few follow the course of the small saphenous vein.

The deep lymphatics are fewer in number. They proceed from the periosteum, joints, muscles and aponeuroses, and are satellites of the blood vessels (Figs. 36.1, 36.2).

Compartments of the Foot

The vessels of the foot are comprised of compartments bounded by neighboring structures (Fig. 36.4) [2–4].

The plantar fascia is inserted proximal to the tuber calcanei. It is composed of three parts divided by lengthwise grooves.

The narrower intermediate component diverges anterially with five bundles that lead to the toes with two terminal bandlets that run on the medial and lateral surfaces of the metatarsophalangeal joints dorsal to the joint and fuse with the fibrous sheath of the extensors. The lateral component dwindles and passes to the lateral margin of the fifth toe. The me-

dial component is thinner proximally, passes to the first toe and coalesces with the corresponding terminal bandlet of the intermediate component.

Two sagittal septa descend to the calcaneus navicular, first cuneiform and first metatarsal from the medial margin of the intermediate component, and to the fifth metatarsal and the sheath of the long peroneal muscle from the lateral margin. They form the boundaries of the medial, lateral and intermediate compartments.

The intermediate compartment is deep in the metatarsal region. It is divided into superficial plantar compartments: lateral (*a*), medial (*b*), superficial intermediate (*c*) and deep intermediate (*d*).

The lateral compartment is bounded by the lateral component of the plantar fascia, which continues laterally with the superficial dorsal fascia, by the lateral intermuscular septum and by the fifth metatarsal. It is comprised of (from plantar to dorsal): the abductor, flexor brevis and little toe opposing muscles. There are no vessels or nerves of any importance.

The medial compartment is bounded by the medial component of the plantar fascia, which continues proximal with the ligamentum laciniatum and medial with the superficial dorsal fascia, by the medial intermuscular septum, and dorsal by the navicular, first cuneiform and first metatarsal. It comprises the bellies of the oblique head of the abductor, the adductor and flexor hallucis brevis. The tendon of the flexor longus enters via the medial septum after a short passage through the intermediate compartment, while the distal insertions of the posterior tibial and the peroneus longus are also present. The vessels and nerves consist of the medial plantar artery, veins and nerve.

The superficial intermediate compartment is bounded by the intermediate component of the plantar fascia, the medial and lateral intermuscular septa, and the deep component of the plantar fascia. It comprises (from plantar to dorsal): the flexor brevis digitorum, the quadratus plantae, the tendon of the flexor longus digitorum with its digitations to the four lateral toes, the lumbricals originating from the tendons of the common flexor and, below these, the transverse head of the adductor hallucis and the tendon of the peroneus longus. The vessels and nerves consist of the lateral plantar artery, veins and nerve.

The deep intermediate compartment is bounded by the deep component of the plantar fascia and (dorsally) by the interossei with their fascia. Four sagittal septa stem from the dorsal aspect of the deep component of the plantar fascia to their insertions on the second, third and fourth metatarsals and divide this compart-

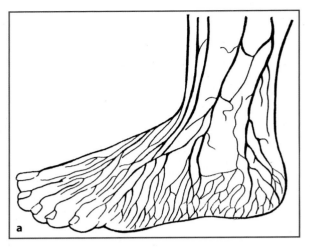

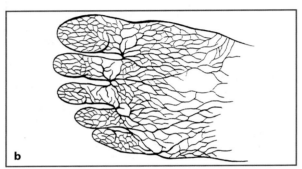

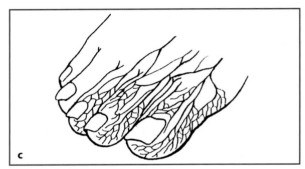

Fig. 36.3. Lymphatics. **a** Lateral lymphatics; **b** plantar lymphatics of the toes; **c** dorsal lymphatics of the toes; **d** posterior and plantar lymphatic system; **e** anterior and dorsal lymphatic system [1]

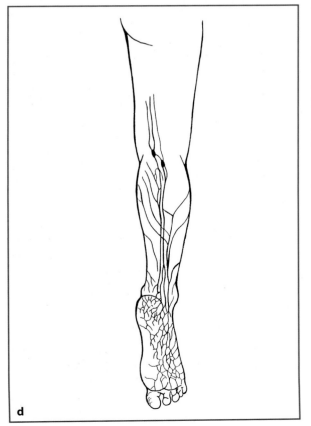

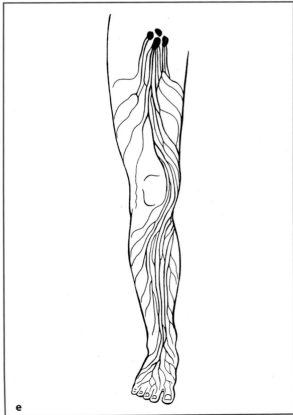

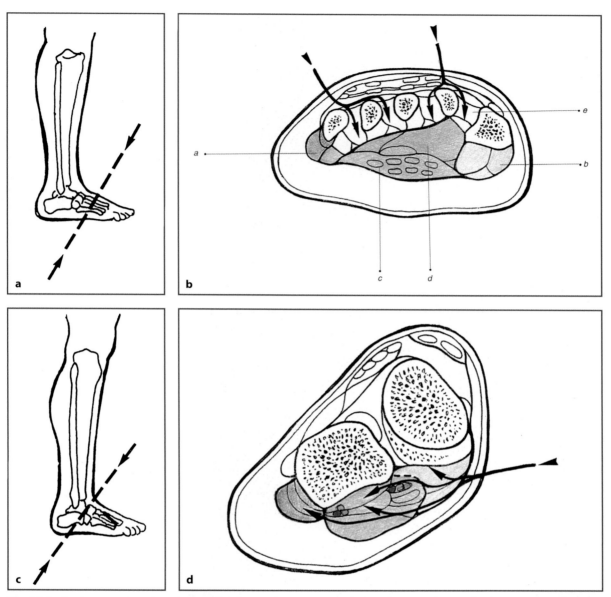

Fig. 36.4. Foot compartment anatomy. **a** Section at the metatarsus; **b** dorsal approaches to the intermetatarsal spaces; **c** section at the tarsus; **d** approaches to the plantar compartments [1]

ment into four metatarsal chambers (*e*) containing the respective plantar and dorsal interossei muscles. The vessels and nerves consist of the lateral plantar artery, the metatarsal arteries and veins, and the deep branch of the lateral plantar nerve with its branches.

Only the lateral compartment can be regarded as independent, apart from small orifices for the passage of small nerves and vessels. The medial and intermediate compartments communicate via the orifices of the tendons of the longus hallucis and digitorum flexors. They communicate with each other and with the posterior compartment of the leg via the orifices of the sulcus calcanei.

Observations

Vessels, of course, are not the surgeon's only concern. His attention must equally be directed to the nerves, muscles, tendons, aponeuroses, etc., encountered during any approach to the foot. A proper understanding of their distribution and correlations, however, is the first line of defense against apprehension and the causing of damage.

Vascular malformations are often defined as compartmental. Correct definition of vascular areas and knowledge of the approaches to each compartment are thus essential (Fig. 36.4) [2–5].

Each disorder must be addressed via a specific approach [4, 6]. Classic skin incisions have been elaborated to secure access to the area concerned, without impairing the deep structures. The extended surgical routes are illustrated schematically in Figures 36.5 and 36.6. The protean nature of vascular malformations often requires a resort to alternative and atypical approaches.

Figure 36.7 shows the clinical and phlebographical appearance of widespread subcutaneous infiltrating vascular malformations in the medial malleolar and plantar region of a 25-year-old woman. The wide cutaneous approach (represented schematically) is indispensable for exposure of the lesion, which probably extends to the medial and superficial intermediate compartments.

Figure 36.8 shows the clinical and radiographic appearance after direct injection of a cavernous lymphangioma in the great toe in a 6-year-old girl. The wide "S" incision (represented schematically) ensures medial dorsal and lateral exposure of the lesion and its environment.

Figure 36.9 shows the clinical and phlebographic appearance of widespread subcutaneous sole-infiltrating arteriovenous malformation in the medial malleolar and calcaneal regions. Here, too, a wide "S" incision is essential for total exposure.

Figure 36.10 shows intra- and subcutaneous venous malformation in the left foot of a 26-year-old woman. Arteriography revealed arteriovenous fistulae along the anterior tibial artery and in the lateral malleolar region. In this case two incisions were needed to secure complete exposure in the right foot.

Since blood in the foot, by contrast with the leg, is drained from the deep to the superficial veins, these must be preserved during surgery. The lymphatics, too, are not always referred to in the expositions of the access routes, whereas they are often the origin of postoperative edema.

Its many arterial and venous anastomoses endow the foot with an abundant circulation that can be well compensated even if a major trunk is damaged. This also means that the skin can be incised lengthwise, obliquely, transversely and S-wise, and to any extent. The so-called "boomerang" incision for lateral exposure of the calcaneus, for example, provides a flap that is excellently vascularised from the peroneal, while conservation of the small saphenous safeguards the venous return and the lymphatic branches that run with this vein. The lateral-dorsal-plantar "S" flap used to approach the first metatarsophalangeal is also well vascularised, prior to its division into the digitals, by branches from the first metatarsal artery. The dorsolateral digital must ob-

viously be preserved by stripping the flap adhering to the capsule. Dissection of the extensor digitorum brevis to gain access to the sinus tarsi and the subtalar joint preserves the artery of the sinus which, together with the motor branch for the muscle, penetrates at its superomedial corner.

Full-field dorsal or plantar transverse incisions as a distal approach to the metatarsus are also harmless if made distal to the venous arches near the base of the toes, with subsequent prosecution of the longitudinal approach to preserve the numerous communications between the dorsal and plantar retia: obviously a transverse incision only as far as the subcutaneous layer, through which the dissection is taken longitudinally along the axis of the necks of the metatarsals to preserve the subcutaneous arteries, veins and lymphatic ducts that can then be shifted as required during the operation. The wide proximal flaps are supplied by the metatarsal arteries from the plantar and dorsal arches, the distal flaps by the perforating digital branches of the opposite plantar arches. Venous drainage is similar via the many connections of the dorsal and plantar retia, both digital and deep. Attention must be directed to the lateral marginal vein, which continues as the small saphenous. It runs at the border of the dorsal and medial region of the foot and must be carefully preserved during medial approaches to the tarsus.

The lymphatics are more responsible for postoperative edema than the veins, especially in the elderly, due to structural alterations, particularly of the precollectors.

The network of the lymphatic vessels, in addition to their distribution in the subcutaneous tissue, makes them vulnerable in blunt dissections, which cause more damage than an open approach incision. Wide approaches are preferable with the skin loaded on wires, and in the absence of distractive maneuvers that often dissect the subcutaneous tissue. Knurled, atraumatic forceps must be used instead of the conventional traumatic surgical kinds [7, 8].

As always in foot surgery and when handling vascular malformations, the surgeon must employ approaches that allow easy, elective management of the lesion, especially when dealing with vessel alterations which are localized intracutaneously and that may impair the integrity of the skin. A clinical and instrumental vascular assessment of the trophic risks is also necessary, through evaluation of the vascular axes so as to avoid the risk of cutaneous necrosis. Nerves must be spared, especially their more exposed sensitive branches, not only for the residual hypoanesthetic damage, but also to conserve the proprioceptive function controlling vasomotoricity and skin

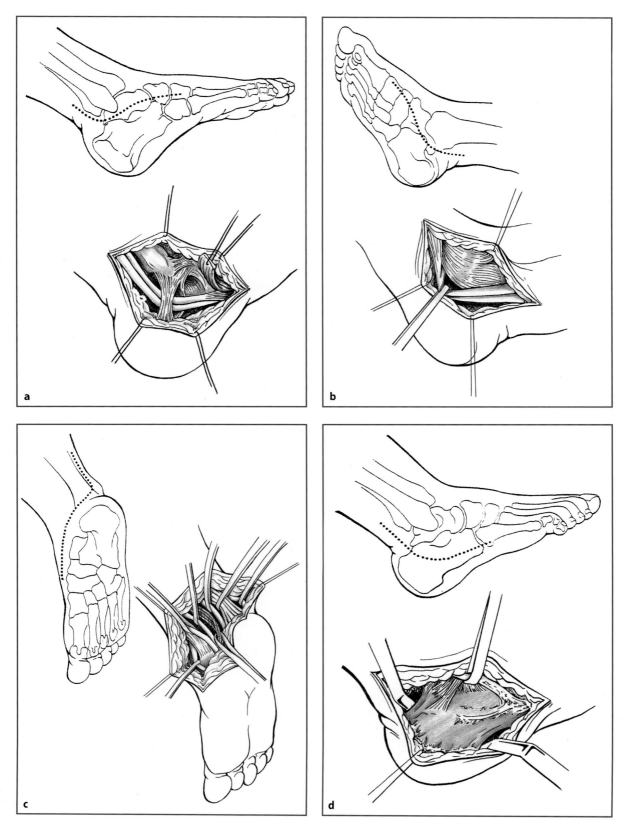

Fig. 36.5. Approaches to the foot. **a** Approach to the peroneals; **b** medial approach; **c** latero-postero-medial approach; **d** approach to the calcaneus [1]

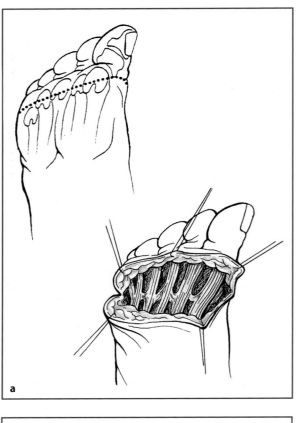
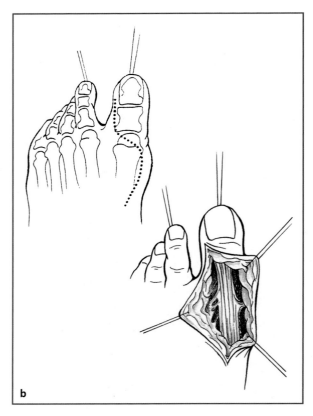
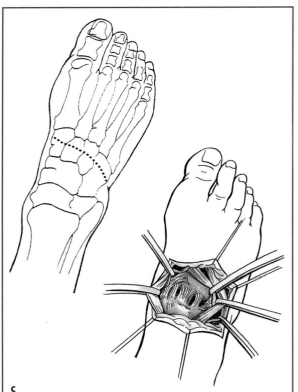
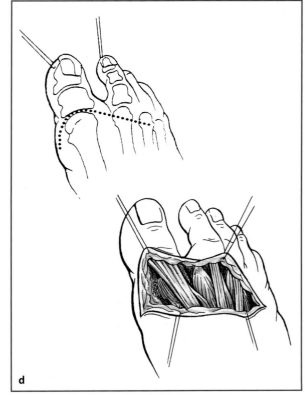

Fig. 36.6. Approaches to the foot. **a** Plantar approach to the metatarsal heads; **b** approach to the first metatarsopha-langeal joint; **c** dorsal approach to the tarsus; **d** dorsal approach to the forefoot [1]

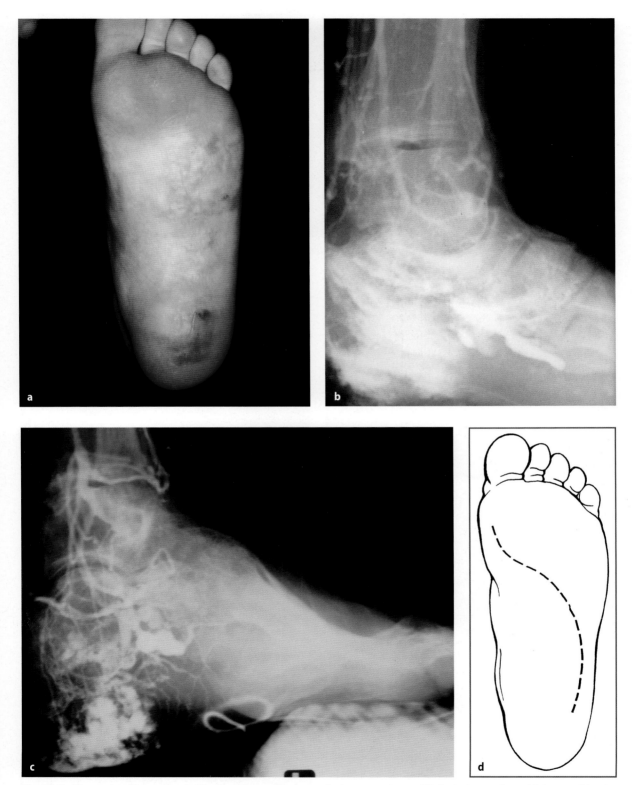

Fig. 36.7. Venous malformation infiltrating the malleolar and plantar region. **a** Clinical picture; **b, c** phlebographic picture; **d** completed incision [1]

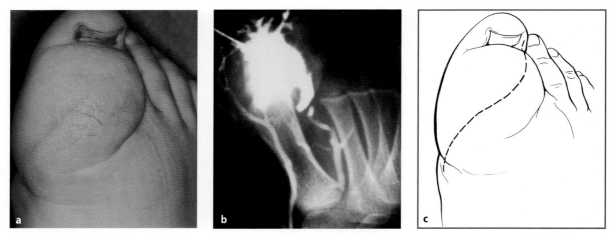

Fig. 36.8. Cavernous lymphangioma of the great toe. **a** Clinical picture; **b** radiographic picture; **c** completed incision [1]

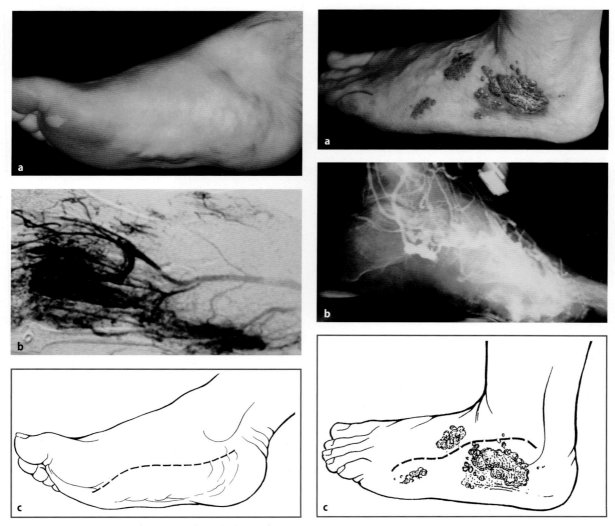

Fig. 36.9. Arteriovenous fistulae. **a** Clinical picture; **b** arteriographic picture; **c** completed incision [1]

Fig. 36.10. Venous malformation. **a** Clinical picture; **b** phlebographic picture; **c** completed incision [1]

tropism. In the event of multiple approaches, the incisions must be sufficiently spaced to avoid distress of over-reduced interposed skin flaps.

Incisions should be traced out to suit the loading zones of the foot wherever possible. Preference should be accorded to zones not subjected to axial traction to prevent the development of pathological scars. Lastly, thought should be directed to the relationship between the site of a scar and the use of footwear.

References

1. Pisani G, Loose DA (2002) Il piede. In: Malformazioni vascolari ed emangiomi. Testo-atlante di diagnostica e terapia. Springer-Verlag Milano, pp 180–193
2. Pisani G (1998) Fusschirurgie. Thieme, Stuttgart, New York
3. Brunner U (1982) Der Fuss. Diagnostische und therapeutische Aspekte der Arteriologie, Phlebologie und Lymphologie. Hans Huber, Bern, Stuttgart, Wien
4. Loose DA (2001) Modern tactics and techniques in the treatment of angiodysplasias of the foot. Chir del Piede 25:1–17
5. Loose DA (1998) Diagnostik und Therapie von Wundheilungsstorungen im Fussbereich bei Angiodysplasien. Vortrag auf dem 2. Hamburger Wundheilungsforum, Hamburg
6. Tasnádi G (1991) Clinical investigations in epidemiology of congenital vascular defects. In: Balas P (ed) Progression in angiology. Edizioni Minerva Medica, Turin, pp 391-394
7. Belov S (1967) Chirurgische Behandlung der kongenitalen Angiodysplasien. Zbl Chir 26a:1959–1602
8. Belov S (1992) Treatment of vascular defects in the lower extremities. Communication at the 9th International Workshop for the Study of Vascular Anomalies, Denver, Colorado

Diagnosis and Management of Vascular Malformations of Bone

37

Wayne F. Yakes

Abstract

Vascular malformations of bone are extremely complex lesions that can present with a myriad of symptomologies. Ethanol endovascular and direct puncture embolization can cure or significantly obliterate these lesions at long-term follow-up. Further, ethanol sclerotherapy in conjunction with coil embolization can treat massive lesions and cure them at long-term follow-up. In low-flow lesions, direct puncture injection of the vein malformation can be curative, lead to new bone formation or obliteration of the vascular cyst, and obviate the need for complex surgeries and their attendant complications.

Vascular malformations, whether of soft tissues or bones, should be managed in centers that routinely treat these lesions. In this fashion, complications can be better managed, minimizing patient morbidity, and practitioners can gain greater experience. Significant experience leads to improved judgment and the refinement of techniques for the management of these challenging lesions.

Introduction

Vascular malformations of bone are an uncommon entity. Both high-flow lesions (arteriovascular malformations [AVM] and arteriovenous fistulae [AVF]) and low-flow lesions (venous malformations) exist in bone. There is much confusion in the literature with regards to the terminology of these vascular lesions of bone. Therapeutic options to manage these vascular lesions of bone have involved surgery as well as embolization.

High-flow AVMs can be extremely striking on arteriography. Significant therapeutic dilemmas are presented by the extent to which the bones and periosteum are involved. Low-flow lesions of bone may be difficult to diagnose due to the fact that the arteriograms are normal. Magnetic resonance imaging (MRI) is the diagnostic imaging procedure of choice to evaluate these lesions; however, this is not always thought of as a diagnostic option prior to attempted therapy, either surgical or interventional.

A complicated array of terms further confuses the picture. The so-called vertebral body hemangioma is actually a venous malformation of bone and not a pediatric hemangioma. Pediatric hemangiomas are tumors of infancy that appear within the first month of life, go through a rapid proliferative phase, then slowly involute. Usually by 5–7 years of age the vast majority of these lesions have totally involuted [1]. Another area of confusion is the so-called hepatic hemangioma. Again, this is a venous malformation of the liver and not a pediatric hemangioma. Confusion also exists in the true classification of lesions of unicameral bone cysts and aneurysmal bone cysts. Once again these are vascular malformations, largely of the venous and capillary-venous type in bone.

If vascular malformations can exist in soft tissues, there is no reason to believe they cannot exist in bone. Even in highly developed tissues such as the brain, high-flow vascular malformations and low-flow vascular malformations exist. The high-flow lesions are consistent with AVMs as well as AVF of the congenital type. The misnomers "cavernous angioma" and "cavernoma" are confusing and should be replaced with the term "venous malformation".

Etiology

Vascular malformations, regardless of the tissues they involve, are congenital lesions related to primitive

R. Mattassi, D.A. Loose, M. Vaghi (eds.), *Hemangiomas and Vascular Malformations*.
© Springer-Verlag Italia 2009

vascular elements that were incompletely resorbed in an early stage of fetal development. These immature blood vessels of whatever type (arterial, capillary, venous, lymphatic) are functional in the early stages of fetal development; however, as organogenesis progresses these abnormal vascular elements are resorbed and replaced with a more mature vascular system appropriate to the level of development. When a failure occurs with this resorptive mechanism, the lesions are incorporated into the more mature vascular system that should have completely replaced them. This explains the congenital nature of these lesions [2–4].

These lesions may be symptomatic or asymptomatic. The age of presentation in these patients is usually dependent upon when symptoms develop and when the patient is worked-up. Vascular malformations of bone can present with pathologic fractures through a cystic cavity of the long bone, skin ulcerations that are non-healing in extremities affected by high-flow lesions, pain syndromes, skin hemorrhages, and if lesions are extensive and large enough, high-output failure. The so-called vertebral body hemangioma, a venous malformation of a vertebral body in the spine, can extend into the epidural space and cause spinal cord and/or nerve recompression with long track signs in the lower extremities as well as bowel and bladder dysfunction. A myriad of clinical presentations can occur depending on the anatomy affected by vascular malformations of bone.

The vascular origins of unicameral bone cysts are already appreciated by several authors [5–10]. The etiology of the unicameral bone cyst is unclear and several mechanisms have been advocated for its development: a traumatic hematoma which undergoes cystic resorption [5] or a vascular obstruction of an intramedullary venous drainage system of the bone [6]. A cystic degeneration of a pre-existing benign tumor is a possible etiology [7]. Invagination of the synovial membrane of a large joint through the epiphyseal plate during osseous growth and its later separation has also been suggested as an etiology, based on the observation that unicameral bone cysts are located exclusively in the metaphyseal areas of long bones [9, 10].

Histologically, the unicameral bone cyst's wall is composed of endothelial-like cells and some authors believe that this cell is entirely separated from the circulation. However, other authors, including myself, have noted that direct injection of contrast shows that there is communication with the normal venous system [11, 12]. The intracystic fluid of the unicameral bone cyst has components similar to

serum, rather than to synovial fluid. Within bone, a unicameral bone cyst is similar to a stagnant venous lake that communicates with a normal outflow venous system, a characteristic shared by soft tissue vein malformations. The intracystic pressure of the serum-like fluid in a unicameral bone cyst is slightly higher than the intramedullary bone marrow pressure of a normal contralateral bone [7]. Some authors have felt that this slightly increased pressure leads to slow bone resorption and enlargement of the cystic cavity, thus causing the cortical bone to thin until a fracture occurs [7]. The expansion of bone due to vascular malformation is also present in aneurysmal bone cysts. In vertebral body hemangiomas, thickened trabeculae are identified on plain film radiography without enlargement of the vertebra itself. If long track signs are present in a patient, imaging with MRI will demonstrate the epidural expansion of vein malformation compressing the cord and/or nerve roots that accounts for the patient's symptoms.

The theories on the etiology of the unicameral bone cyst described by previous authors are extremely interesting. However, the most plausible theory is that these are merely congenital vascular malformations of bone, rather than being related to a mechanism causing an acquired vascular malformation of bone as theorized by other authors. It is proven that vascular malformations of the soft tissues are congenital lesions. Therefore, it would seem logical that vascular malformations, when they occur in bone, could also be congenital in origin. Endovascular approaches using ethanol as an embolic agent are known to routinely cure soft tissue malformations at long-term follow-up. As can be logically inferred, the same endovascular techniques can be applied to bone vascular malformations and are equally effective.

High-Flow Lesions of Bone

Congenital AVMs and AVF are both high-flow lesions of bone. AVMs that involve the intramedullary cavity can also involve the periosteum and extend into the soft tissues. While any bone can be affected, in our experience the bones of the extremities are the most often affected. The lesion can be in the metaphyseal region and involve the epiphyseal plate, as well as the mid-shaft of the long bones. An interesting observation in our patient series is that approximately 40% of patients thus far have exhibited multiple AVMs often affecting multiple bones of the involved extremity. For this reason, it is mandatory to perform exhaustive arteriography of the affected extremity to determine the presence or absence of multiple AVMs.

Patients with an AVM of bone can present with a variety of symptoms, including pain, non-healing skin ulcerations, hemorrhages from these ulcerations, repeated soft tissue infections of the extremity's affected area, neuropathy and pathologic fractures. In patients with extensive AVMs, involvement of bone leads to elevated cardiac outputs and lowered systemic vascular resistance that can cause a hyperdynamic cardiac state with exercise intolerance and resultant myocardial chronic injury.

Surgery was the first form of therapy used to manage these lesions. However, complete removal of an AVM requires a total resection of the affected bone, leading to significant deformity and functional loss. Thus, post-surgical recurrences are routine and often the symptoms worsen at the time of recurrence. With the advent of transvascular and direct puncture approaches to these lesions, significant ablation or cure is possible, as seen in soft tissue AVM. Embolization of these lesions with agents other than ethanol has led to temporary palliation [13]. In our patient series, in the larger lesions that demonstrate single outflow vein physiology, coil embolization coupled with ethanol embolization can be curative at long-term follow-up (Fig. 37.1) [14–22]. In smaller lesions that demonstrate multiple venous outflow channels, ethanol has been extremely effective as the sole embolic agent (Fig. 37.2).

Proximal arterial ligation by surgery has no role in the management of these lesions. This is never cu-rative and the patient will be worse symptomatically at follow-up as new collaterals are formed to reach the intraosseous AVM. Similarly, transarterial coil embolization of the arterial supply proximal to the AVM has no role. This is physiologically identical to proximal surgical arterial ligation procedures and must be avoided. Not only is this endeavor fruitless, it will make endovascular procedures more difficult because arterial access to the lesion has been interrupted.

Venous Malformations of Bone

As has been stated, venous malformations of bone have not been described in the literature. Previously, these malformations have been given many names, including unicameral bone cyst (Fig. 37.3), aneurysmal bone cyst and vertebral body hemangioma. Patients with unicameral bone cysts and vertebral body hemangiomas often have normal arteriograms with only mild late venous phase pooling of contrast. This is similar to arteriography of venous malformations of the soft tissues. In aneurysmal bone cysts, the arteriogram can show increased vascularity with more prominent contrast puddling in the venous phase. This arteriographic picture is similar to the intramuscular venous malformation subtype (known in the literature as "intramuscular hemangioma") [23]. These lesions of soft tissue and bone suggest that the malformation may be capillary-venous due to the increased vascularity and lack of AV shunting.

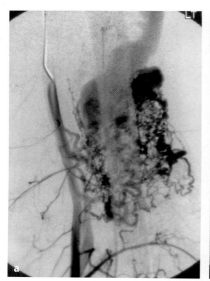
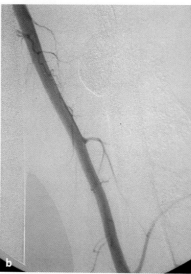

Fig. 37.1. Thirty-two year-old male with pain and swelling in the left lower extremity and exercise intolerance. **a** Massive arteriovenous malformation involving the midshaft of the femur. This is a superficial femoral artery injection demonstrating the multiple AV fistulae within the AVM and single outflow venous drainage. **b** Arteriogram 5 years post-therapy demonstrating normal vascularity and absence of AVM. Cures are possible in these significantly large lesions. Reproduced from [14]

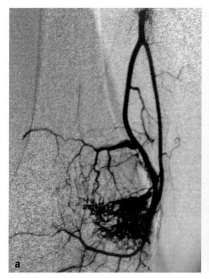
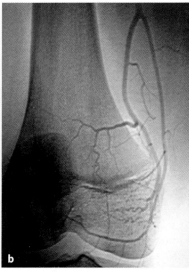

Fig. 37.2. Eighteen year-old male with left knee pain related to arteriovenous malformation. **a** Branch of the superficial femoral artery injection. High-flow arteriovenous malformation is identified in the medial femoral condyle involving the epiphyseal plate. **b** Arteriogram demonstrating cure of AVM at 6 month follow-up. Reproduced from [14]

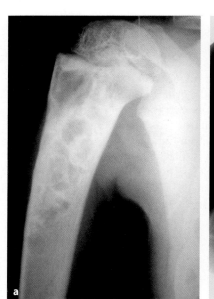
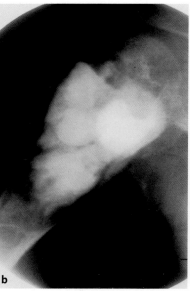
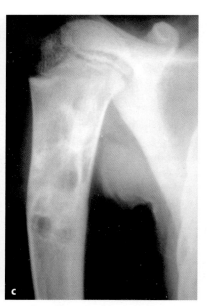

Fig. 37.3. Six year-old male with pain and weakness in the right upper extremity. **a** Plain films demonstrated multiple cystic lesions in the proximal right humerus accounting for the patient's symptoms. **b** Direct puncture injection into multiple channel venous malformation of the proximal humerus. Note the contrast is within these multiple septated segments. **c** Plain film radiograph 2.5 years post-embolization demonstrates osseous infiltration in the cystic cavities that were treated. The pain symptoms no longer exist and the right upper extremity is totally functional. The patient continues to be evaluated by his physicians. Reproduced from [14]

MRI is the modality of choice to image these lesions of bone, especially when there are extensions into the soft tissue from the bone. Venous malformations of bone can occur concurrently with venous malformations of the soft tissues and may be multifocal. The optimal MRI sequence is the T2 weighted fast spin echo, with fat suppression. The suppression of fat (that has a bright signal on T2 weighted sequences) can distinguish fat from the malformation in the soft tissues as well as in the intramedullary cavity, in which a significant amount of fat can exist. Fat suppression is therefore mandatory in order to prevent any confusion between the fat and the coexisting vein malformation. One must also be aware that synovial joint fluid has increased signal on T2 and should be distinguished from venous malformation of bone. MRI is an excellent tool, not only for the diagnosis of these lesions and determination of the extent of involvement, but also as a follow-up imaging modality to determine the efficacy of therapy and the amount of malformation that has been ablated. This is evidenced by decreased signal in the T2 weighted sequences and can be compared with the MRI carried out prior to therapy.

The primary approach for the management of these low-flow lesions of bone is direct puncture into the venous malformation. Direct puncture angiograms can then be performed showing the extent of the lesion and its venous outflow into normal tissues. Further, these lesions of bone may be compartmentalized, requiring multiple direct punctures to determine the full extent because of the septae separating the various compartments. This is an important issue for treatment, in that all cavities must be accessed and ethanol injected into each individual cavity for the malformation to be ablated. Once this is successfully accomplished, then serial x-rays may show bone healing, despite the presence of pathologic fractures, and the cystic cavities become filled with newly formed bone (Fig. 37.3).

Venous malformations of vertebral bodies (vertebral body hemangioma) also respond to transpedicular ethanol injection. A needle is advanced through the pedicle of the affected vertebral body, often using a bilateral transpedicle approach, allowing a direct puncture angiogram to be performed. The amount of ethanol can be calculated based on the volume of contrast injection before epidural veins appear. After successful transpedicular direct puncture ethanol injection of these venous malformations of the vertebral body, shrinkage of the epidural masses occurs and improvement of the patient's symptoms or a reversion to complete normalcy of the long track signs can occur [24].

Thus, unicameral bone cysts, aneurysmal bone cysts, and vertebral body venous malformations can all be effectively managed with the use of ethanol by direct injection. Long-term follow-up demonstrates a high success rate and permanence using this technique. This obviates the need for difficult surgeries such as vertebral body resections (corpectomy) with the use of stabilization metal devices for the spine. The resection of unicameral bone cysts with the placement of prostheses in the affected extremity of a pediatric patient can also be obviated through the use of this simple technique.

References

1. Mulliken JB, Golawacki J (1982) Hemangiomas and vascular malformations in infants and children: a classification based on endothelial characteristics. Plast Reconstr Surg 69:412–422
2. DeTakats G (1932) Vascular anomalies of the extremities. Surg Gynecol Obstet 55:227–237
3. Wollard HH (1922) The development of the principal arterial stems in the forelimb of the pig. Contrb Embryol 14:139–154
4. Reid MR (1925) Studies on abnormal arteriovenous communications acquired and congenital. I Report of a Series of Cases. Arch Surg 10:601–638
5. Boseker EH, Bickel WH, Dahlin DC (1968) A clinical pathologic study of simple unicameral bone cysts. Surg Gynecol Obstet 127:550–560
6. Broder HM (1968) Possible precursor of unicameral bone cysts. J Bone Joint Surg 50A:503–507
7. Chigira M et al (1983) The etiology and treatment of simple bone cysts. J Bone Joint Surg 65B:633–637
8. Cohen J (1960) Simple bone cysts; studies of the cyst fluids and six cases with a theory of pathogenesis. J Bone Joint Surg 42A:609–616
9. Mirra JM (1980) Bone tumors: diagnosis and treatments. Lippincott, Philadelphia, pp 462–477
10. Gebhart M, Blaimont P (1996) Contribution to the vascular origin of the unicameral bone cyst. Acta Orthopaedica Belgica 62:137–142
11. Yakes WF (1992-2008) Personal observation in Budapest (Hungary), Garbagnate (Italy), and Denver (Colorado, USA) during direct injection of multiple unicameral bone cysts of the humerus, vertebral body hemangioma, tibial and aneurysmal bone cysts.
12. Spence KF, Sell KW, Brown RH (1969) Solitary bone cysts: treatment with freeze-dried cancellous bone allegraft. J Bone Joint Surg 51A:87–96
13. Widlus DM, Murray RR, White RI Jr et al (1988) Congenital arteriovenous malformations: tailored embolotherapy. Radiology 169:511–516
14. Yakes WF (2002) Diagnosi e terapia delle malformazioni vascolari ossee. In: Mattassi R, Belov S, Loose DA, Vaghi M (eds) Malformazioni vascolari ed emangiomi. Testo-atlante di diagnostica e terapia. Springer-Verlag Milano, pp 60–65
15. Yakes WF, Rossi P, Odink H (1996) How I do it: arteriovenous malformation management. Cardiovasc Intervent Radiol 19:65–71
16. Yakes WF, Luethke JM, Merland JJ et al (1990) Ethanol embolization of arteriovenous fistulas: a

primary mode of therapy. J Vasc Intervent Radiol 1:89–96

17. Yakes WF (1996) Diagnosis and management of vascular anomalies. In: Castaneda-Zuniga WR, Tadavarthy SM (eds) Interventional radiology. Williams and Wilkins, Baltimore, pp 103–138

18. Yakes WF, Pevsner PH, Reed MD et al (1986) Serial embolizations of an extremity AVM with alcohol via direct percutaneous puncture. AJR 146:1038–1040

19. Yakes WF, Luethke JM, Parker SH et al (1990) Ethanol embolization of vascular malformations. Radio Graphics 10:787–796

20. Yakes WF, Luethke JM, Merland JJ et al (1990) Ethanol embolization of AVF: a primary mode of therapy. JVIR 1:89–96

21. Keljo DJ, Yakes WF, Andersen JM, Timmons CF (1996) Recognition and treatment of venous malformations of the rectum. J Pediatr Gastroenterol Nutr 23:442–446

22. Yakes WF, Krauth L, Ecklund J et al (1997) Ethanol endovascular management of brain AVMs: initial results. Neurosurgery 40:1145–1154

23. Connors JJ, Khan G (1977) Hemangioma of striated muscle. South Med J 70:423–1424

24. Heiss JD, Doppman JL, Oldfield EH (1994) Brief report: relief of spinal cord compression from vertebral hemangioma by intralesional injection of absolute ethanol. N Engl J Med 331:508–511

The Role of Syndromes

38

Massimo Vaghi

Abstract

Vascular malformation syndromes with particular involvement of anatomical areas, genetic peculiarities and specific therapies are given eponyms. There are capillary, arterial, venous, lymphatic and arteriovenous syndromes.

Introduction

Eponyms are widely used in medical literature and in medical search engines to define some types of vascular malformations (VMs). Although the extensive use of eponyms for the description of VMs should be discouraged because they are often the cause of confusion, their use can be admitted in case of a linkage to particular anatomical involvement or anatomopathological, genetic or therapeutic peculiarities. Eponyms thus define only a specific clinical picture and should be used specifically. Unfortunately, very often, due to a lack of knowledge or incomplete diagnostics, syndrome eponyms are used to define other VMs that are not characteristic of the syndrome. The most common incorrect diagnosis is "Klippel-Trenaunay syndrome", followed by "Parkes-Weber syndrome". A list of the main syndromes follows.

Capillary Malformations

Sturge Weber syndrome is characterized by the presence of a cutaneous port wine stain in the area of the first trigeminal branch (sometimes including also the second and the third trigeminal root), associated with vascular anomalies of the leptomeninges and ipsilateral ocular anomalies. Epilepsy episodes begin in the first year of life and decrease after puberty. Cognitive deficit and mental retardation and motor deficit controlateral to the meningeal involvement follows the onset of seizures [1, 2].

Klippel-Trenaunay syndrome is characterized by the presence of a cutaneous nevus (capillary malformation), associated with VMs (venous insufficiency) and sometimes with lymphatic malformations. The limbs present an overgrowth and visceral involvement is possible. Many different types of VMs are often erroneously described as Klippel-Trenaunay syndrome [3, 4].

Proteus syndrome is characterized by overgrowth of bones in the extremities (fingers, toes) and with spinal cord and skull-associated subcutaneous benign tumors such as fibroma, lipoma and epidermal nevus which can assume a cerebriform aspect in the extremities [5].

Cutis marmorata teleangiectasica congenita is characterized by the presence of teleangiectasia in the limbs presenting a purplish reticular network. This nevus is linked to hypotrophy of the affected limb. VMs may be present and there is some association with glaucoma and neurological anomalies [6].

Rendu Osler disease is an autosomal dominant disorder which is characterized by skin and mucosal teleangiectasias. The predominant symptomatology is epistaxis. The teleangiectasia may also involve the gastro intestinal tract and can be the cause of visceral hemorrhage. In some patients, the opening of arteriovenous (AV) shunts in the lungs, brain and liver are possible [7, 8].

Ataxia teleangiectasia is an autosomal recessive disease which is characterized by ocular and cutaneous teleangiectasia, progressive cerebellar ataxia and immune deficiency. Heterozygous carriers of the syndrome are at high risk of malignancy, especially breast cancer [9].

R. Mattassi, D.A. Loose, M. Vaghi (eds.), *Hemangiomas and Vascular Malformations*.
© Springer-Verlag Italia 2009

Anderson-Fabry disease is a lysosomal storage disorder linked to the X chromosome and is characterized by the absence or a deficit of alfa galactosidase A. In men the symptomatology is evident in childhood and is characterized by the presence of a diffuse angiokeratoma, acroparestesia, hypo- or anhidrosis [10].

Visceral involvement such as stroke, renal insufficiency, heart and pulmonary impairment is significant. Diagnosis is based on the detection of the deficit of alfa galactosidase A in leucocytes and plasma. It is possible to give these patients replacement therapy; this is more efficient before the onset of visceral impairment.

Lymphatic Malformations

Gorham Stout syndrome (vanishing bone syndrome) consists of bone invasion and destruction caused by lymphatic and sometimes venous vessels. In case of vertebral involvement it is possible to observe complications such as chyloascites and chylothorax [11].

Venous Malformations

Bean syndrome or blue rubber bleb nevus syndrome consists of multiple venous lesions of the skin presenting as hyperkeratotic spots, blebs and dilated veins. The involvement of the gastrointestinal tract is usual and bleeding is the natural consequence. In neonates the intestinal lesions may cause intussception and volvulus. The skin involvement is visible at birth and the lesions increase in number and diffusion with age [12, 13].

Maffucci syndrome is characterized by firm blue nodules in the skin. The radiological workup of these lesions is characteristic of VMs with phleboliths and hyperintense signals in T2-weighted magnetic resonance images. The other feature of the syndrome is the presence of bone enchondromas localized in the diaphysis and metaphysis [14].

Arterio-Vascular Malformations (AVMs)

Parkes-Weber syndrome is characterized by the presence of skin nevi, limb hypertrophy, venous dilatation and AV shunting. According to the studies of Tasnadi, it represents the evolution of venous hypertension in childhood which decompensates further with the opening of AV shunts in puberty.

Cobb syndrome is an AV metameric syndrome at the trunk level which links the superficial AVMs with AVM in the spine [15].

Bonnet-Dechaume-Blanc syndrome is a metameric syndrome with diffuse AV shunts which involve the face, the retina and the brain [16].

Arterial Malformations

Arteries are commonly involved in congenital anomalies of the connective tissue such as Marfan syndrome, Ehler-Danlos syndrome and pseudoxanthoma elasticum. In these cases the common response of the arteries is aneurysmatic enlargement. Congenital anomalies are also represented by popliteal artery entrapment and medial dysplasia.

The specific meaning of each VM syndrome should be well known in order to give a correct diagnosis and avoid the incorrect and misleading use of these terms.

References

1. Etchves HC, Vincent C, Le Douarin NM, Couly GF (2001) The cephalic neural crest provides pericytes and smooth muscle cells to all blood vessels of the face and forebrain. Development 128:1059–1068
2. Ville D, Enjorlas O, Chiron C, Dulac O (2002) Prophylactic antiepileptic treatment in Sturge Weber disease. Seizure 11:145–150
3. Berry SA, Pearson C, Mize W et al (1998) Klippel Trenaunay syndrome. Am J Med Gen 79:319–326
4. Maari C, Frieden IJ (2004) Klippel-Trenaunay: the importance of geographic stains in identifying lymphatic disease and the risk of complications. J Am Acad Dermatology 51:391–398
5. Turner JT, Cohen MM, Biesecker LG (2004) Reassessment of the Proteus syndrome literature: application of diagnostic criteria to published cases. Am J Genet 130:111–122
6. Devillers AC, deWaard-van der Speck, Oranj AP (1999) Cutis marmorata teleangiectasica congenita: clinical features in 35 cases. Arch Dermatol 135:34–38
7. Bayrak-Todemir P, Mao R, Lewin S, McDonald J (2004) Hereditary hemorrhagic teleangiectasia: an

overview of diagnosis and management in the molecular era for clinicians. Genet Med 6:175–191

 8. Begbie ME, Wallace GM, Shovlin Cl (2003) Hereditary hemorrhagic teleangiectasia: a view from the 21st century. Postgraduate Med J 79:18–24

 9. Gungor T, Buhring I, Cremer R et al (1997) Pathogenesis, diagnosis, clinical and therapeutical aspects of ataxia teleangiectasia. Klin Padiatr 209:328–335

10. Linthorst GE, De Rie MA, Tjam KH et al (2004) Misdiagnosis of Fabry disease: importance of biochemical confirmation of clinical or pathological suspicion. Br J Dermatol 150:575–577

11. Hirayama T, Sabokbar A, Itonaga I et al (2001) Cellular and humoral mechanism of osteoclast formation and bone resorption in Gorham Stout disease. J Pathol 195:624–630

12 Ertem D Acarv Y, Kotiloglu et al (2001) Blue rubber bleb nevus syndrome. Pediatrics 107:418–420

13. Domini M, Aquino A, Fakhro A et al (2002) Blue rubber web nevus syndrome and gastrointestinal haemorrhage: which treatment? Eur J Pediatr Surg 12:129–133

14. Wassef M, Vanwijck R, Clapuyt P, Boon L, Magalon G (2006) Vascular tumors and malformations, classification, pathology and imaging. Ann Chir Plast Esthet 51(4–5):263–281

15. Bhattacharya JJ, Luo CB, Suh D (2001) Wyburn-Mason or Bonnet-Dechaume-Blanc as cerebro facial artero venous metameric syndromes. Intervent Neuroraradiol 7:5–17

16. Rodesch G, Hurth M, Alvarez H et al (2002) Classification of spinal cord arteriovenous shunts: proposal for a reappraisal. The Bicetre experience with 155 consecutive patients treated between 1981 and 1999. Neurosurgery 51:374–379

Conclusions

Raul Mattassi, Dirk A Loose, Massimo Vaghi

When a curious tourist travels through an unknown country using a guidebook, at the end of his trip he may have a number of different feelings. If the land he visited was interesting and the guidebook brought him to the most remarkable places and clearly explained to him the meaning of what he was seeing and how to move through the country, he probably would have remained interested in his trip, loved the new country and would want to return to it in order to explore it more in detail. If the guidebook was unclear, did not to give him the correct explanations or guide him to remarkable places, he may leave without an interest in the land, lay down his guidebook and not come back.

The goal of this atlas is to guide the reader through the difficult field of hemangiomas and vascular malformations, to help him to understand them and give him answers to questions, mainly concerning the practical approach to these diseases. All the authors involved have attempted to explain their topics in the simplest way with pictures and text.

If we succeed in our effort and this small atlas is appreciated by readers, we will be happy to have accomplished the goal given to us by our teacher and friend, Professor Stefan Belov. He dedicated his life to study these diseases and strongly wished to publish an atlas to help colleagues to understand hemangiomas and vascular malformations in order to extend knowledge and treatment possibilities. He passed away before he could see his idea become reality, but we hope that our efforts will have fulfilled his wishes.

R. Mattassi, D.A. Loose, M. Vaghi (eds.), *Hemangiomas and Vascular Malformations*.
© Springer-Verlag Italia 2009

Subject Index

A

Activin receptor-like kinase 1 (ALK1) 100, 105
Aneurysm of arteries
- aberrant left subclavian 211
- aorta 209, 253
- brachial 210, 254
- carotid 209
- intracranial 209, 210
- persistent sciatic 210, 211
- pulmonary 209
- subclavian 210
- vertebral 209
- visceral 210
Aneurysm of veins
- banding technique 226
- popliteal 114
- tangential resection 145, 149, 210, 226, 227, 229
Angiogenesis 3-7, 54
Aplasia and hypoplasia 24, 112, 113, 123, 226
- of arteries 145, 209, 211
  • abdominal aortic 210
  • carotid 210
  • pulmonary 210
  • vertebral 210
- of veins
  • deep 141, 146, 227, 252, 255, 271
  • iliac 257
Arteriovenous fistulae 9-11, 53, 94, 101, 105, 112, 129, 140, 150, 153-156, 161, 164, 166, 175, 176, 191, 192, 195-204, 206, 216, 218-220, 225, 227, 228, 252, 268, 269, 290, 291, 295, 312, 316, 319, 321
Arteriovenous malformations (AVM) 7, 29, 100, 101, 105, 123, 140, 159, 163, 165, 184, 185, 195-204, 215-220, 231, 268, 278, 282, 288, 290, 291, 295, 296, 312, 321, 322
Arthroscopy 303
Anti-angiogenic therapy 7
Autosomal-dominant hereditary 18, 100-105

C

Capillary-lymphatic malformations 99, 112, 183, 184, 231, 271, 272, 325
Capillary malformation 24, 36, 85, 99-101, 105, 109, 110, 112, 113, 129, 167, 181-185, 192, 195, 206, 236, 255, 278, 280, 283, 284, 319-321, 325
- hyperkeratotic 101, 103, 182-184, 188, 269, 326
Cardiac failure 24, 31, 35, 43, 44, 54, 185, 277, 283, 295
Cartilage 3, 32, 65, 68, 72, 79, 80, 206, 256, 299
Caucasian infant 17, 18
Cerebral cavernous malformation (CCM) 100-103
Cystic hygromas 187, 265, 294

D

Destructive angiodysplastic arthritis 299-303

E

Endoglin (ENG) 100, 105
Endothelial cells 3-5, 37, 62, 101, 102, 171
- activated 4, 6
- sprouting 4, 5, 102, 103
Erysipelas 29, 72, 183

F

Facial nerve 40, 207, 275
Foot compartment 305-317
FOXC2 100, 104, 107

G

Genetic bases 7, 99-106, 325
Glomangioma 23, 26-28, 30, 191, 259, 261
Glomulin (GLMN) 103, 104
Glomuvenous malformations (GVM) 30, 99, 100, 102, 103, 106, 191, 259, 260

H

Hand function 287
Hemangioma
– anogenital 24, 30, 32, 33, 49, 50, 66, 93-95
– dangerous 49
– diagnosis 32, 35-37, 85
– differential diagnosis 23, 25-28, 30, 37, 42, 45, 46, 76
– duplex sonography 24, 25, 27, 29, 50, 52, 71, 93, 94, 115, 116, 120, 129, 135, 140, 173, 175, 179, 184, 224, 226, 228, 234, 241, 243, 256
– eye 87
– extracutaneous 39
– facial 19, 32, 40, 60, 76, 82, 85-90
– Glut-1 23, 26, 28, 37, 42, 43, 46, 89
– immunohistochemical analysis 37, 42, 43, 61
– indeterminate 18, 19
– intra-articular 24, 30, 31, 206, 299-301
– intra-osseous 24, 30, 31, 156, 164, 205, 206, 240, 287, 289, 290, 321
– liver 26, 30-32, 39, 42-45, 54, 60, 61
– localized 18, 27, 85, 86
– mesenchymal origin 50, 53, 54
– MRI 35-37
– multifocal 18, 19
– nasal tip 87
– NICH 24, 27-29, 31, 35-37, 50, 52, 55, 69, 75, 79, 80, 86, 89, 278
– non-involuting congenital hemangioma (NICH) 24, 27-29, 31, 35-37, 50, 52, 55, 69, 75, 79, 80, 86, 89, 278
– parotis 59, 88
– PELVIS 33, 94
– PHACE 17, 19, 20, 33, 60, 86, 88
– physical examination 37, 39, 46, 60, 85
– problem zones 50
– proliferative phase 26, 36, 42, 46, 79, 80, 82, 86
– psycho-social impact 40, 82, 86, 87, 89
– rapidly involuting congenital hemangioma (RICH) 24, 27-29, 31, 35-37, 43, 50, 52, 55, 86, 89, 278
– regression 23-32, 35, 40, 42, 44, 49-55, 60, 61, 65, 69, 71, 72, 77, 88, 181, 190, 265, 293-296
– RICH 24, 27-29, 31, 35-37, 43, 50, 52, 55, 86, 89, 278
– segmental 17-19, 39, 86, 88
– spontaneous course 50, 52
– subglottal and tracheal 55, 58, 76, 78, 88, 279
– strawberry 23, 35
– subcutaneous growth 25-27, 67
– ulceration 17-19, 24-27, 31-33, 50, 53, 54, 57, 66, 85-87, 93-95, 142, 166, 184, 196, 199, 203, 269, 296, 320, 321

Hemangiomatosis
– "benign" neonatal (BNH) 26, 31
– "disseminated neonatal" (DNH) 31, 32
– systemic 23, 30, 31, 33
Hereditary hemorrhagic telangiectasia (HHT) 100, 105, 186
Hypertrophy 9, 10, 32, 101, 104, 109, 112, 128, 183, 184, 186, 252, 255, 256, 268-271, 280, 326
– limb 326
– somatic 9
Hypotrophy 9, 109, 127, 184, 240, 252, 255, 257, 325

I

Infection 10, 24, 29, 31-33, 51, 57, 60, 66, 72, 82, 93, 94, 104, 109, 188, 210, 235, 236, 239, 253, 265, 277, 280, 321
Integrin 5, 6, 101, 102, 106
Intraosseous AV fistulae 24, 31, 156, 164, 206, 290, 321
Intussusceptive angiogenesis 5

J

Joint pathologies 299-303
Joint replacement 299, 301, 303

K

Kaposiform hemangioendothelioma 24, 27, 29, 30, 32, 33, 89, 278
KRIT1 100-102

L

Larynx 24, 76, 88, 188, 191, 207, 279-281
Laser
– bare fiber contact vaporization 182, 185, 188, 190
– Chimney effect 70
– CO_2-laser 52, 68, 184
– continuous ice cube cooling 71-76
– continuous wave (cw-Nd:YAG) 66, 68-70, 183, 185, 187, 188, 191
– endoscopy 42, 76, 182, 185, 88, 191
– exposure time 65, 68, 69, 185, 190
– flash lamp pumped pulsed dye laser (FLPDL) 65-67, 182-184
– fluid cooling cuvette 66, 68-70, 183
– igloo effect 70
– impression technique 69, 73, 74, 76, 182, 188, 190, 192
– interstitial coagulation 185, 187-190, 192
– interstitial puncture technique 69, 72, 74, 75
– intraluminal procedure 182, 187-191
– intravascular absorption 53, 65

– frequency doubled Nd:YAG ("KTP") 65-67, 69, 70, 182-185, 191
– optimal total dose 72
– photobiological reactions 181
– photon density 68
– pulsed Nd:YAG 65, 66, 68, 73, 182-186, 191
– side effects 66, 72, 186, 189
– skin temperature 73, 74, 185, 269
– specific absorption 52, 65, 68, 70
– superselective systems 65
– transcutaneous direct application 69, 76
– tracheotomy 55, 76, 282
– wavelength 52, 65
– Werner procedure 188, 191
Limb length discrepancy 10, 109, 145, 220
Lymphangioma 10, 23, 26, 28, 29, 187, 191, 231, 232, 245, 248, 265-267, 312, 316
– circumscriptum 26, 183
Lymphedema 100, 104, 109, 151, 228, 231-240, 245, 247, 248
Lymphovenous shunt 124, 126, 129, 131

M

Macrocystic 104, 187, 189, 240-245, 248, 281
Malcavernin 100, 101
Marginal vein 115, 123, 135, 137, 139-141, 146, 174, 177, 189, 223, 226-228, 237, 246, 247, 255-257, 271, 307, 309, 312
Meningitis 277, 279
MGC4607 101
Microcystic 104, 187, 188, 191, 240-243, 245, 248, 282, 282
MMP 5-7

N

Nevus 9, 10, 42, 94, 102, 109, 111, 136, 184, 190, 191, 229, 254, 256, 257, 269-271, 325, 326
Nidus 105, 125, 141, 146, 149, 150, 154-156, 161, 163, 165, 166, 191, 192, 196, 198, 215-218, 282, 283, 295, 296

P

Paradominant inheritance 103, 106
PDCD10 100-102
Pelvis 125, 126, 138, 154, 205, 208
Pharynx 31, 32, 51, 185, 188, 191, 279-281
p120RasGAP (RASA1) 100, 101
Phakomatoses 184
Port wine stains 23, 25, 36, 135, 182-185, 226, 254, 283
Premature birth 18

S

Second somatic hit model 106
SOX18 100, 104
Sporadic venous malformation (VM) 99-106, 261
Staples 220, 256
Syndrome of
– Anderson-Fabry 326
– Ataxia teleangiectasia 25, 27, 28, 184, 325
– Bean (blue rubber bleb nevus) 42, 102, 190, 229, 326
– Bonnet-Dechaume-Blanc 254, 326
– Budd-Chiari 227, 258
– Cobb 254, 326
– Cutis marmorata telangiectasia congenita 25, 27, 28, 184, 325
– Ehler-Danlos 253, 326
– Gorham Stout 188, 326
– Kasabach-Merritt 29, 30, 33, 50, 60, 73, 75, 76, 89
– Klippel-Trenaunay 101, 111-113, 183, 184, 231, 233, 254-257, 271, 325
– Mafucci 102, 111, 326
– Parkes-Weber 113, 251, 234, 268, 269, 271, 325, 326
– Proteus 100, 106, 284, 325
– Pseudoxanthoma elasticum 326
– Rendu-Osler 325
– Rothman-Thompson 186
– Sturge-Weber 19, 101, 111, 112, 182, 184, 254, 255, 283, 325
– Telangiectasia macularis eruptiva persistans 186
– Wyburn-Mason 184

T

TIE2 (TEK) 100-103, 106, 107
Tip cell 5
Tissue heterogeneity 106
Treatment of hemangiomas
– antiangiogenic drugs 7, 52, 54, 55
– antiproliferative drugs 54
– bleeding 19, 31, 42, 45, 46, 52, 54, 55, 57, 75, 79, 80, 82, 89
– bleomycin 62
– compression 52-54, 65-67, 70
– corticosteroids 19, 41, 44, 57-61, 79, 80, 83, 86-88
– cryotherapy 45, 49-53, 57, 60, 95
– cyclophosphamide 57, 61
– "dog ears" 81
– dosage 58, 60
– embolization 11, 36, 44, 45, 49, 50, 52-54, 60
– hemostatic squeezing 80-82
– imiquimod 52, 54
– indications 40, 55, 57, 65, 69, 79, 82, 94

– interferon 6, 40, 44, 45, 52, 54, 57, 60, 61, 86
– interstitial corticoid crystals 52, 54
– interstitial magnesium seeds 54
– laser therapy 33, 45, 49-55, 58-60, 65-77, 79, 80, 83, 94, 106, 149, 153
– ligation 52, 53
– neurotoxicity 60, 61
– prednisone 50, 58, 76
– purse string closure 80-82
– round-block technique 80-82
– scarification techniques 51, 52, 54
– sclerotherapy 42, 49, 50, 52, 54
– side effects 50, 54, 55, 57, 58, 60, 61, 66, 72, 93, 94
– special clamp 80, 81
– surgical excision 41, 44-46, 49, 50, 79-82
– tyrosine kinase inhibitors 62
– vincristine 57, 60, 86-89
– wound management 93-95
– X-ray therapy 49, 52, 53
Treatment of vascular malformation
– complex decongestive therapy (CDT) 237-239, 245, 248
– direct puncture 11, 124, 143, 146, 149, 156, 160, 166, 167, 187, 188, 215, 216, 223, 224, 232, 247, 266, 289, 291, 294, 296, 312, 319-323
– embolization 129, 140, 141, 143, 146, 149, 151, 153-156, 159, 161, 163-168, 182, 184, 185, 191, 192, 195-202, 210, 215, 216, 219, 220, 225, 283, 287, 294-296, 319, 321, 322
   • catheter devices 153, 154
      balloon-tipped 154, 166, 296
      coaxial combinations 153, 154
      tracker catheters 153, 154
   • coils 153, 154, 160, 161, 165, 166, 176, 296
   • Ethibloc 153-157, 159, 172
   • glue 216, 282, 283, 287, 289, 296
   • lipiodol 155, 156, 224
   • post embolization syndrome (PES) 156, 216
– laser 181-192, 195, 215, 216, 223, 226, 255, 260, 265, 282-284, 287, 291
– multidisciplinary team 168, 198, 238
– non surgical 195, 196, 198, 207, 238
– sclerotherapy 103, 117, 124, 143, 149, 153, 156, 171-179, 182, 187-190, 195, 198, 215, 216, 223-226, 229, 231, 235-248, 259, 260, 265, 275, 281, 282, 287, 291, 292, 294-296, 319
   • ethanol 153, 154, 160-168, 171-173, 195, 198, 216, 224, 225, 235, 237, 240-245, 247, 248, 259, 260, 265, 289, 294-296, 319-323
   • microfoam 171-179
   • OK432 171, 172, 179, 235, 240-245, 247, 248, 265, 266
   • polidocanol 171-174, 224, 245

   • sclerosing agents 117, 124, 149, 156, 171, 172, 240, 241, 242, 259, 265, 294, 295
   • sodium tetradecyl sulphate 171-174, 224, 294-296
– strategy 145, 153, 215, 223, 240, 293, 295, 296
– surgery
   • arthroscopy 301
   • Belov IV technique 200, 302
   • Blalock suture 150, 200
   • combined therapy 141, 153, 160
   • combined treatment 195-204
   • devascularization 145, 146, 165
   • Doppler, intraoperative 206
   • hemodynamic procedures 146, 149, 196
   • Loose II technique 197, 220
   • microsurgical techniques 206, 288, 289
   • multidisciplinary 205-208
   • neurolysis 287, 290, 292
   • resection 103, 124, 136-138, 145, 146, 150, 157, 160, 187, 188, 205, 207, 210, 216, 220, 226, 228, 229, 243, 246, 265, 282
   • revascularization 145, 146
   • skin sparing 288, 289
   • synovectomy 291, 292
   • tourniquet 224, 287, 288, 291
Tufted angioma 24, 27-29, 31, 33, 37, 60, 89, 278
Tumor suppressor gene PTEN 100, 105, 106

V
Vascular bone syndromes 319-323
Vascular malformations
– avalvulia 141
– classification 140, 141
   • complex combined 112
   • congenital vascular malformation (CVM) 9-11, 109, 111-113, 121, 129, 135-143, 145-149, 151, 153, 161, 205-208, 215, 231, 235, 236, 245, 287, 289-292, 305-317
   • embryological development 111-113
   • extratruncular 24, 28, 29, 53, 109, 110, 112, 113, 114, 115, 117, 120-122, 125, 145, 149, 150, 174-178, 181, 185, 187, 189, 192, 198, 199, 215, 216, 218, 223, 225, 226, 228, 231, 232, 235-237, 239, 240, 243-248
   • Hamburg classification 135
   • hemolymphatic 112, 231, 234, 237, 244, 246
   • high flow 36, 112, 115, 116, 121, 123, 124, 140-142, 153, 154, 164, 166, 175, 280, 296, 319, 320, 322
   • infiltrating 145, 149, 150, 167, 174-176, 178, 179, 198-201, 205-207, 218, 219, 223, 229
   • limited 259, 261, 265, 269

- Mulliken and Glowacky 17, 111-114
- slow flow 99, 100, 102, 112
- truncular 24, 28, 53, 110, 112, 113,114, 120, 121, 135, 145-147, 176, 181, 187, 189, 191, 192, 198, 199, 209, 215, 216, 226, 231-240, 245-248
- complications and side effects 153, 159, 160, 189
  - cutaneous necrosis 159, 171-173, 195-198, 242, 294, 312
  - neural damage 159
- diagnostic
  - activity-time curves 121, 124
  - albumin radio-labelled with 99m-technetium 129
  - angioscintigraphy 130
  - arteriography 10, 135, 139-143, 153, 155-157, 159, 160, 164, 166, 167, 181, 196, 199, 200, 202, 203, 217, 218, 225, 233, 234, 312, 316, 319, 321
    sub-selected series 141
  - clinical examination 135
  - cold (lesion) 123
  - CT scan 117, 120
  - dermal diffusion ("backflow") 128-130, 146, 238
    microspheres 129, 131
  - duplex scan 115, 116, 129, 140, 224, 226, 228
  - dynamic sequence 124
  - functional tests 115
  - invasive diagnostics 129, 131, 135-143, 232, 300, 303
  - isometric exercise (hand grip) 128
  - iterative rebuilding algorithms 124
  - lymphography 140, 141, 263
  - lymphoscintigraphy 121, 125, 127, 128, 130, 228, 234, 237, 238, 245, 246, 262, 263
  - micelles of purified human albumin 126
  - morphofunctional tests 115
  - MRI 101, 117-120, 135, 140, 143, 157, 161, 164, 166, 167, 178, 181, 207, 208, 219, 233-235, 241-247, 259, 260, 270, 280, 300, 303, 319, 320, 322, 323
  - multihead gamma camera 124
  - nuclear medicine imaging (NMI) 124
    radiolabelled cells 123, 124, 126
  - phlebodynamometry 137, 141
  - phlebography 10, 135-141, 143, 160, 174, 181, 202, 225, 227, 247, 256, 257, 259, 272, 294, 302, 312, 315, 316
  - phleboliths 116, 117, 135, 139, 259, 277, 326
  - plain film 135, 137-140, 142, 320, 322
  - pressure measurements 115, 140, 141
  - pulsatility index 115
  - radiotracer 123-131
  - resistance index 115
  - spot scan 131
  - three-dimensional rebuilding 131
  - transarterial lung perfusion scintigraphy (TLPS) 121, 129, 131, 233, 234, 245
  - ultrasound 99, 115-117, 135, 140, 143, 173, 175, 179, 183, 201, 234, 241-243, 260, 265, 295
  - varicography 136, 138, 140, 141
  - volume measurements 115
  - volumetric asymmetry 106, 130
  - whole body blood pool scintigraphy (WBBPS) 121-123, 233, 234, 244-246
- epidemiology 109, 110
- incidence 99-102, 105, 106, 109
Vascular tumors 10, 17, 18, 23-33, 41-46, 49-55, 60, 65-77, 85, 89, 99, 157, 181, 189, 190, 278
Vasculogenesis 3-5, 99
VEGF 5-7, 62, 101, 106
VEGFR-3 (or FLT-4) 100, 104, 248

W
"Wait and see" 49, 50, 86, 87, 93, 94
Wasp sting symptom 29

Printed in February 2009